DENTAL ANATOMY

Its Relevance to Dentistry

SIXTH EDITION

DENTAL ANATOMY

Its Relevance to Dentistry

Julian B. Woelfel, D.D.S.
Professor Emeritus
Sections of Prosthodontics, Dental Materials, and Dental Hygiene
The Ohio State University College of Dentistry
Columbus, Ohio

Rickne C. Scheid, D.D.S., M.A.
Associate Professor
Section of Primary Care, Dental Hygiene; and Restorative Dentistry, Prosthodontics, and Endodontics
The Ohio State University College of Dentistry
Columbus, Ohio

LIPPINCOTT WILLIAMS & WILKINS
A **Wolters Kluwer** Company
Philadelphia · Baltimore · New York · London
Buenos Aires · Hong Kong · Sydney · Tokyo

Publisher: Susan Katz
Managing Editor: Jacquelyn Merrell
Marketing Manager: Anne Smith
Production Editor: Paula C. Williams
Compositor: Maryland Composition, Inc.
Printer: Quebecor World

351 West Camden Street
Baltimore, Maryland 21201-2436 USA

530 Walnut Street
Philadelphia, Pennsylvania 19106 USA

Printed in the United States of America.

Library of Congress Cataloging-in-Publication Data
Scheid, Rickne C.
     Dental anatomy : its relevance to dentistry.–6th ed. / Rickne C. Scheid, Julian B. Woefel.
          p. cm.
     On 5th ed. Woelfel appears first.
     Includes bibliographical references and index.
     ISBN 0-7817-2797-9
     1. Teeth–Anatomy. 2. Mouth–Anatomy. I. Woelfel, Julian B. II. Title.

   QM311 .W64 2001
   611′.314–dc21   2001038187

The publishers have made every effort to trace the copyright holders for borrowed material. If they have inadvertently overlooked any, they will be pleased to make the necessary arrangements at the first opportunity.

To purchase additional copies of this book call our customer service department at **(800) 638-3030** or fax orders to **(301) 824-7390**. International customers should call **(301) 714-2324**.

00 01 02 03 04
1 2 3 4 5 6 7 8 9 10

Julian B. Woelfel, D.D.S.

Professor Emeritus Woelfel, known primarily for his expertise on complete dentures, research and occlusion, taught clinical dentistry for 40 years in the College of Dentistry, The Ohio State University, Columbus, Ohio. He served as an Army prosthodontist for two years, conducted clinical research for the American Dental Association at the National Bureau of Standards in Washington, D.C. for two years, and was a visiting professor in Japan, Taiwan, England, and Brazil. Dr. Woelfel has lectured in eighteen foreign countries. He has published seventy-five scientific articles, four editions of Dental Anatomy and chapters in five books. He holds patents on two inventions which are used in Europe and the United States for accurately recording jaw relations. In addition to his love for students and teaching, he conducted a part-time private practice limited to partial and complete dentures for 33 years. One of his proudest accomplishments is this textbook. In 1967, he was the first recipient of the International Association of Dental Research Award for Research in Prosthodontics, and became a Life Member of the Nihon University Dental Alumni Association. In 1972, the New York Prosthodontic Society selected him for the Jerome and Dorothy Schweitzer Award for Outstanding and Continuing Research in Prosthodontics. In 1992, the Ohio Dental Association chose Dr. Woelfel for the prestigious Callahan Award. He is a Life Member of several professional societies including Sigma Xi, the International Association for Dental Research, the American Prosthodontic Society, and the A.D.A., F.D.I., F.I.C.D., and F.A.C.D.

Rickne C. Scheid, D.D.S., M.Ed.

Dr. Rickne Scheid received his D.D.S. in 1972 at The Ohio State University and was inducted into the dental honorary fraternity, Omicron Kappa Upsilon. After serving in the U.S. Navy Dental Corps, he went into part-time practice and has taught at his alma mater since 1974. His appointments at the College of Dentistry have been in the Department of Operative Dentistry, the Division of Dental Hygiene and, currently, he holds a dual appointment in the Section of Restorative Dentistry, Prosthodontics and Endodontics, and the Section of Primary Care in Dental Hygiene. While teaching, he received his Masters in Education with honors in 1980. He has authored or co-authored nearly fifty scientific papers and abstracts. Throughout his teaching career, he has developed and directed twelve different courses, and most recently, has taken on the responsibility of directing the dental anatomy course, which is presented each year to 130 dental and dental hygiene students. Further, he helped develop and annually co-directs over 184 hours of continuing education, including a dental hygiene review course and an expanded functions course for dental auxiliaries. He was inducted into the dental hygiene honorary, Sigma Phi Alpha, in 1989, and has received numerous dental and dental hygiene student teaching awards, as well as the peer-evaluated Postle Teaching Award in 1996.

Preface to the 6th Edition

Dental Anatomy: Its Relevance to Dentistry is primarily intended as a study guide for dental students, dental hygiene students, dental assistants, and dental laboratory technicians in the study of tooth morphology and related structures. The text is designed to help the reader appreciate the relationship of teeth to one another, and to the bones, muscles, nerves, and vessels closely associated with the teeth and face. This edition also includes considerable emphasis on the application of dental morphology to the practice of dentistry. The book is organized to be used by instructors of dental anatomy courses as a teaching manual during lectures, discussion periods, laboratory sessions, and in early clinical experiences. It is also useful as a reference in a dental office.

How the book is organized:

Chapter 1 begins with a very brief overview of the teeth: just enough to help the reader appreciate the relationship of the teeth to the head and neck anatomy presented in the remaining sections of this chapter. Topics include the bones of the skull and associated bony landmarks, the temporomandibular joints, chewing muscles, and the nerves, blood supply, and lymph drainage associated with the oral cavity. **Chapter 2** includes the location and description of *normal* oral structures observed during a head and neck cancer screening examination in the dental office, followed in **Chapter 3** by a more detailed description of general terminology of normal tooth morphology, and ideal tooth and occlusal relationships. **Chapters 4 through** 7 include detailed descriptions of each type of adult tooth, with drawings, photographs, and charts designed to illustrate the normal characteristics of each tooth type. These chapters also help the reader appreciate the variation which can occur between the same type of teeth in different mouths. The roots of the adult teeth are discussed in more detail in **Chapter 8**, where the importance of root morphology is presented relative to both periodontal and endodontic treatment. **Chapter 9** includes the discussion of deciduous or primary teeth, along with eruption patterns occurring throughout the time when mixed dentition is present. **Chapter 10** provides a contemporary overview of occlusion. Here, the authors describe the relationship of the jaws and teeth during various normal and abnormal relationships, including a discussion of treatment modalities used to correct malocclusion or temporomandibular joint dysfunction. Next, in **Chapter 11**, there is an extensive discussion of many commonly encountered dental anomalies. The importance of dental anatomy and terminology related to operative and restorative dentistry is presented in **Chapter 12**. **Chapter 13** includes helpful techniques for learners to draw, sketch, and carve teeth, and **Chapter 14** provides an introduction of the importance of tooth morphology within the field of forensic dentistry.

Each chapter includes methods designed to help you, the reader, master the content and put it to practice immediately.

- **Topic List:** Each *chapter* begins with a list of topics which are presented within that chapter. The topics are presented in the same order as the section outline headings within that chapter.
- **Learning Objectives:** In each section, the authors have included important learning objectives developed to help you appreciate what you can expect to learn as you read. You can refer to the objectives to ensure that you are mastering the appropriate knowledge and skills.
- **New terms:** As each new term is encountered for the first time, it is highlighted in bold print, and is defined within the text at that time, often with references to figures or diagrams to improve understanding. The bold print is helpful when using the text as a reference for understanding terms that can be found within the text's index.
- **Index (instead of a glossary):** The extensive index has been used instead of a glossary since the authors feel that many terms in dentistry required reference to illustrations or photographs for complete understanding. In most cases, the first page where a term is referenced in the index is the page where you can find the term (in bold) and can refer to the suggested illustrations for the best learning.

- **Pronunciations**: New terms which the author's feel are difficult to pronounce have phonetic suggestions placed within brackets [like this] immediately after the word is first encountered.
- **Learning questions with answers**: Each chapter or section ends with a series of learning questions to test the learner's mastery of the objectives. These questions, in many cases, cover topics similar to those included on past dental and dental hygiene national examinations. For the convenience of quick and convenient feedback, the answers are presented immediately following the questions (but upside down).
- **Learning exercises**: Practically every chapter provides the reader with a series of learning exercises. These exercises are presented with the body of each chapter at intervals where the authors feel an active learning experience would be helpful for you to understand and/or apply the topic. These exercises may suggest that you examine extracted teeth or tooth models, or skulls (or skull models), or perform specific self or partner examinations. More advanced exercises (as in Chapter 13) provide methods for drawing, sketching, and carving them teeth from wax, helping you to become intimately familiar with tooth shape and terminology.
- **Tables**: Throughout the text, the author's have placed numerous tables to help summarize the many facts presented within the text. These tables are helpful when reviewing the highlights of content found within each section.
- **Illustrations and drawings**: For complete understanding and clinical application of each topic, the authors have included a variety of photographs, illustrations, and original drawings selected and designed to illustrate key points and improve learning. Since a picture is worth a thousand words, it is critical that you refer to figures whenever they are referenced within the text in order to maximize your learning. Many figures are designed so you can cover up the names of structures and test yourself. In some instances, important additional information is presented or clarified in the legends.
- **Appendix of Comparative Dental Anatomy**: The text's unique appendix is designed to help you visualize the many tooth similarities and differences that are often difficult to understand with words alone. Each adult tooth type is referenced on two appendix pages. The first page includes characteristics (each labeled with a different letter) that are *common* to all other teeth within that class. The second page is devoted to the *differences* (each identified with a letter) between teeth within each class and arch. Two additional appendix pages are included that illustrate the unique characteristics of anterior and posterior primary teeth. The layout on these pages make it easy to compare the differences between teeth because various views of each tooth type are lined up on the same page next to other teeth in that class. As each tooth characteristic is described within the chapters on tooth morphology (Chapters 4-7 and 9), reference is frequently made to the illustrated representation of that characteristic on an appendix page as follows: the word "Appendix" is followed by the page number and letter denoting items being discussed (for example, "Appendix 1a" refers you to the appendix, page 1, item "a"). Appendix pages are printed on heavier, perforated paper to permit removal and placement in a separate loose-leaf notebook. When used in this fashion, these pages provide you with increased *convenience* (since fewer page turns are required when referencing tooth characteristics within each chapter), *easier learning* (since the complex terminology used to describe each characteristic is best learned by visualizing that characteristic and comparing it to other similar teeth), and as a separate *study guide* (since all labeled characteristics for each type of tooth are described on the back of each appendix page).
- For learning the form of individual teeth, the best learning resource is a collection of as many intact **extracted teeth** as you are able to acquire. A dentist, if presented with a quart jar of bleach, will remember his or her own student days and will probably be glad to put extracted teeth in the jar. Do not expect these teeth to be clean or sorted out; sorting is your job. While handling these teeth, it *is critical that the guidelines for infection control be followed*:

Using protective gloves, tooth specimens should be scraped clean with a knife. Soaking for several hours in hydrogen peroxide before scraping is helpful. After scraping to remove hard deposits and soft tissue, tooth specimens should be further cleansed by soaking for 20 minutes in 4 ounces of household bleach containing 2 tablespoons of Calgon (a water softener). Teeth can then be placed in water (in a beaker covered with tin foil) to be autoclaved for 40 minutes at 121°C and 15 psi [Pantera E and Schuster G, J Dent Ed, vol. 54, No. 5, 1990, p. 284]. Once prepared, teeth should be kept moist, either by soaking in water, or, as suggested by Dr. Kim Loos, DDS, soaked in 25% glycerin and 75% water [parentsplace.com on Feb. 28, 2001].

As you begin learning the characteristics which differentiate each type of tooth as described in Chapters 4 through 7, you need to be aware of the considerable variation in tooth morphology which can occur from one patient to the next. You must keep in mind that relative tooth sizes and characteristics cited within the text do *not* apply to *all* patients' teeth, but are based on average sizes, or particular morphology occurring with the greatest frequency. This text is unique in providing you with both original and reviewed research findings based on the study of thousands of teeth, casts, and mouths. The data from these studies are presented throughout the text in *brackets* [like this] and provide a scientific basis for understanding the frequency and extent to which differences from the norm occur. For example, the text states that "a mesial marginal groove is a distinguishing characteristic of the maxillary first premolar [but this occurred in only 97% of the 600 premolars checked, which means that, on the average, 3% may not have this groove], whereas the maxillary second premolar is not nearly as likely to have this groove [but 37% do have it]."

As you read the description of tooth morphology, identify each structure not only visually, but also use a dental explorer on an actual tooth or model to feel the contours being described, since you will eventually be required to evaluate, reproduce and/or clean the surfaces of these tooth contours with specific dental instruments. As you become familiar with the many similarities and differences of tooth morphology, you can later apply this information during patient treatment, evaluation, and education.

Hopefully, you will spend some time thinking about and comprehending the concepts as you read. After all, you are learning the "foreign" language of dental anatomy that you will be using for the rest of your professional lives. Have fun looking at teeth as though you were a tooth detective. Take notes, sketch different views of each tooth, and take advantage of all learning exercises, references to figures, and the appendix. Ask questions until your curiosity is satisfied. Most importantly, the authors hope this book will stimulate your interest and involvement in the wonderful and fascinating field of dentistry, and that you will consider it to be a worthwhile addition to your library even after your formal education is complete.

Rickne C. Scheid
Julian B. Woelfel

Comments may be submitted to Dr. Scheid on e-mail [scheid.2@osu.edu].

Contents

Introduction to the 6th Edition

During my first year teaching at the Ohio State University College of Dentistry in 1974, I was fortunate to be assigned to teach in a laboratory for dental anatomy where I worked with, and was mentored by, Dr. Julian Woelfel. Little did I realize that in 1994, I would be selected by him to co-author the fifth edition of a text on the very topic I began teaching in 1974: dental anatomy. During the preparation for the fifth, and now the sixth edition, Julian has permitted me great latitude in reorganizing the text to reflect my teaching style since I use this text as I teach over 130 dental and dental hygiene students each year. During this major reorganization, I was careful to maintain the unique aspects that he had incorporated into previous editions. This includes the results of his personal, science-based research which formed the basis for many of the conclusions presented within this text: on everything from the average mandibular hinge opening, to the frequency of Carabelli cusp formation, and the comparative sizes of deciduous and permanent (or secondary) teeth.

I would like to express my appreciation to all of the contributors to this and previous editions of this book. Obviously, my thanks goes to Dr. Woelfel for selecting me as his co-author and teaching me to be meticulous and for his many contributions to this sixth edition; to his wife, Marcile, who has helped tremendously in typing and editing previous editions; and to Drs. Lewis Claman, Robert Rashid, Al Reader, and Theodore Berg, Jr. for their chapters. I would also like to recognize Miss Dorothy Permar, who conceived and wrote the first edition in 1974.

Rickne C. Scheid, D.D.S. M.Ed.

Structures That Form the Foundation for Tooth Function

Topics covered within the six sections of this chapter include the following:

I. Naming teeth based on location within the normal, complete human dentition
   A. Complete primary dentition
   B. Complete permanent dentition
II. Bones of the human skull (with emphasis on the sphenoid, temporal, maxillae, and mandible bones)
   A. Bones of the neurocranium
   B. Bones of the face (visceral apparatus)
III. The temporomandibular joint (TMJ)
   A. Anatomy of the temporomandibular joint
   B. Ligaments that support the joint and limit joint movement
   C. Development of the temporomandibular joint
IV. Muscles of chewing (mastication)
   A. Muscles involved in mastication (chewing)
   B. Other muscles affecting mandibular movement
   C. Other factors affecting tooth position or movement
   D. Summary of muscles that move and control the mandible
V. Nerves of the oral cavity (with emphasis on cranial nerves V, VII, IX, and XII)
   A. Trigeminal nerve (fifth cranial nerve)
   B. Facial nerve (seventh cranial nerve)
   C. Glossopharyngeal nerve (ninth cranial nerve)
   D. Hypoglossal nerve (twelfth cranial nerve)
   E. Summary of nerve supply to the tongue
VI. Vessels associated with the oral cavity (arteries, veins, and lymphatic system)
   A. Arteries
   B. Veins
   C. Lymph

This chapter introduces the readers to the structures that form the foundation for tooth function: gross anatomy of the bones, muscles, nerves, blood supply, and lymph drainage of the head and neck. Emphasis is placed on the importance of these structures as they relate to the functioning of the jaws and teeth.

SECTION I. Naming Teeth Based on Location Within the Normal, Complete Human Dentition

OBJECTIVES

This section is designed to prepare the learner to perform the following:
- Based on location in the normal, complete *primary* dentition, name all 20 teeth by dentition, arch, quadrant, class, and type.

- Based on location in the normal, complete *permanent* dentition, name all 32 teeth by dentition, arch, quadrant, class, and type.

Prior to a discussion of the structures that support the teeth, it is necessary to familiarize yourself with a brief description of the names of teeth based on their location in the human skull and mouth. This overview is necessary to appreciate and understand the full description of the bones, nerves, and blood vessels presented in this chapter, as well as the description of oral landmarks described in Chapter 2. A more in-depth description of all teeth begins in Chapter 3.

In general, each human tooth has a **crown**, the portion of the tooth projecting beyond the gum line, and a **root**, the portion hidden below the gum line. All of the teeth in the mouth together are referred to as the **dentition** [den TISH un]. Humans have two dentitions throughout life: one during childhood, called the **primary dentition**, and one that will hopefully last throughout adulthood, called the **permanent dentition**. The teeth in the upper jawbones (called the maxillae) collectively form an arch shape known as the **maxillary** [MAK sei lair ee] **arch**, and those teeth in the lower jawbone (called the mandible) collectively form the **mandibular** [man DIB yoo ler] **arch**. Each arch can further be divided into the left and right halves (also known as left and right **quadrants**, since each quadrant contains one-fourth of all teeth in that dentition).

A.   COMPLETE PRIMARY DENTITION

The *complete* primary dentition is normally present in a child from the ages of about two to six years old. There are 20 teeth in the entire primary dentition (shown in Fig. 1-1): ten in the maxillary arch and ten in

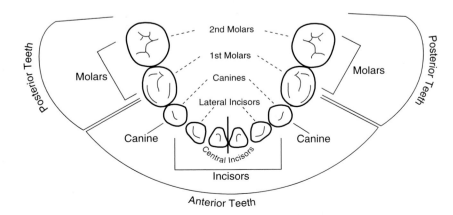

FIGURE 1-1. Maxillary and mandibular primary dentition (chewing surfaces).

the mandibular arch. This dentition is also called the **deciduous** [de SIDJ oo us] **dentition**, referring to the fact that all of these teeth are eventually shed by age 12 or 13, being replaced sequentially by teeth of the permanent dentition. The complete primary dentition has five teeth in each quadrant. The primary teeth in each quadrant are further divided into three *classes*: incisors, canines, and molars. Based on location, the two front teeth in each quadrant of the primary dentition are **incisors** (I), followed by one **canine** (C), then two **molars** (M). Using these abbreviations for the classes of teeth, followed by a ratio comprised of a top number representing the number of teeth in each upper quadrant and the bottom number representing the number of teeth in each lower quadrant, a formula can be used to represent the teeth in the human primary dentition as follows:

$$ I\frac{2}{2}\,C\frac{1}{1}\,M\frac{2}{2} = 10 \text{ teeth on either side; 20 teeth in all} $$

The classes of primary teeth containing more than one tooth per quadrant (incisors and molars) are subdivided into *types* within each class. Each type can also be identified by its location within the complete quadrant. The primary incisor closest to the midline separating the right and left quadrants is called a **central incisor**; the incisor next to or lateral to the central incisor is called a **lateral incisor**. Next in each quadrant is a canine, followed by two molars: a **first molar** behind the canine and then a **second molar**.

LEARNING EXERCISE

Using either models of the complete primary dentition, or Figure 1-1 while covering up the labels, identify each primary tooth based on its location in the arch. To identify each tooth accurately, include the dentition (primary), arch (maxillary or mandibular), quadrant (right or left), class (incisor, canine, or molar) and type of incisor (central or lateral), and type of molar (first or second).

B. COMPLETE PERMANENT DENTITION

The complete permanent (or secondary) dentition is present in the adult. It is composed of 32 teeth: 16 in the maxillary arch and 16 in the mandibular arch (shown in Fig. 1-2). The permanent dentition has eight teeth in each quadrant, which are divided into four *classes*: incisors, canines, **premolars** (PM; a new class for permanent teeth) and molars. Based on location, the two permanent front teeth in each quadrant are *incisors* (I), followed by one *canine* (C), then two *premolars* (PM), and finally three *molars* (M). The dental formula for the human permanent dentition is:

$$ I\frac{2}{2}\,C\frac{1}{1}\,PM\frac{2}{2}\,M\frac{3}{3} = 16 \text{ teeth on either side, 32 teeth in all} $$

The classes of permanent teeth containing more than one tooth per quadrant (namely, incisors, premolars, and molars) are subdivided into *types* within each class. Each type can also be identified by location within the quadrant. As in the primary dentition, the permanent incisor closest to the midline between the right and left quadrants is called a **central incisor**; the incisor next to or lateral to the central incisor is called a **lateral incisor**. Next in the arch is a **canine**, followed by a **first premolar**, then a **second premolar**. Continuing around toward the back in each quadrant are three molars: a **first molar**, **second molar** and, finally, a **third molar** (sometimes referred to as a wisdom tooth).

As noted by comparing the formulas for deciduous and permanent teeth, differences exist. Although central and lateral incisors and canines are similarly positioned in both dentitions, permanent dentitions have a new category of teeth called premolars, which are located between canines and molars. Premolars are positioned in the spaces left where the primary molars had been located earlier in life. Behind the premolars, there are three instead of two molars.

Two other terms are used to categorize or distinguish groups of teeth by their location: anterior and posterior teeth. **Anterior teeth** are those teeth in the front of the mouth, specifically, the incisors and the canines. **Posterior teeth** are those in the back of the mouth, specifically, the premolars and the molars.

It is interesting to note that animal dentition can be represented by the same type of formula as described above. Look at the formulas for animals in Table 1-1 and note that cows have no upper incisors or upper canines. They have three upper and three lower premolars on each side. Did you know that dogs

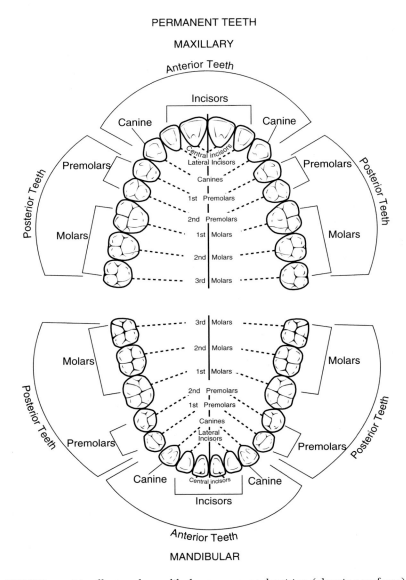

FIGURE 1-2. Maxillary and mandibular permanent dentition (chewing surfaces).

have twice as many premolars as humans if you include uppers and lowers, as well as the right and left sides?

LEARNING EXERCISE

Using either models of the complete permanent dentition, or Figure 1-2 while covering up the labels, identify each permanent tooth based on its location in the arch. To identify each tooth accurately, include the dentition (permanent), arch (maxillary or mandibular), quadrant (right or left), class (incisor, canine, premolar or molar) and type of incisor (central or lateral), type of premolar (first or second), and type of molar (first, second, or third).

Table 1-1

SOME DENTAL FORMULAE (ORDER OF TEETH PER QUADRANT) AND INTERESTING FACTS ABOUT TEETH IN ANIMALS[33-35]

Animal	Formula		Animal	Formula
Humans, Old World monkeys, and apes	$I\frac{2}{2}\,C\frac{1}{1}\,P\frac{2}{2}$	$M\frac{3}{3}$	Porcupines and beavers	$I\frac{1}{1}\,C\frac{0}{0}\,P\frac{1}{1}$ $M\frac{3}{3}$
New World monkeys	$I\frac{2}{2}\,C\frac{1}{1}\,P\frac{3}{3}$	$M\frac{3}{3}$	Bears and pandas	$I\frac{3}{3}\,C\frac{1}{1}\,P\frac{4}{4}$ $M\frac{2}{3}$
Dogs, wolves, and foxes	$I\frac{3}{3}\,C\frac{1}{1}\,P\frac{4}{4}$	$M\frac{2}{3}$	Squirrels	$I\frac{1}{1}\,C\frac{0}{0}\,P\frac{2}{1}$ $M\frac{3}{3}$
Cats	$I\frac{3}{3}\,C\frac{1}{1}\,P\frac{3}{2}$	$M\frac{1}{1}$	Rabbit‡	$I\frac{2}{1}\,C\frac{0}{0}\,P\frac{3}{2}$ $M\frac{3}{3}$
Cows	$I\frac{0}{3}\,C\frac{0}{1}\,P\frac{3}{3}$	$M\frac{3}{3}$	Mice and rats	$I\frac{1}{1}\,C\frac{0}{0}\,P\frac{0}{0}$ $M\frac{3}{3}$
Horses and zebra*	$I\frac{3}{3}\,C\frac{1}{1}\,P\frac{4}{4}$	$M\frac{3}{3}$	Moles	$I\frac{3}{3}\,C\frac{1}{1}\,P\frac{4}{4}$ $M\frac{3}{3}$
Walruses	$I\frac{1}{0}\,C\frac{1}{1}\,P\frac{3}{2}$	$M\frac{0}{0}$	Vampire bats	$I\frac{1}{2}\,C\frac{1}{1}\,P\frac{2}{3}$ $M\frac{0}{0}$
Elephants	$I\frac{1}{0}\,C\frac{0}{0}\,Dm†\frac{3}{3}$	$M\frac{3}{3}$	Shrews	$I\frac{3}{1}\,C\frac{1}{1}\,P\frac{3}{1}$ $M\frac{3}{3}$

* Pigs and hippopotami have the same formula, except that they have two or three upper and two or three lower incisors.
† Elephants have deciduous molars but no premolars. An elephant's skull is larger than necessary to house his brain. The size is needed to provided mechanical support for the tusks (one-third of their length is embedded in the skull) and the enormous molars. Each molar weighs about 9 pounds and is nearly a foot long mesiodistally on the occlusal surface. Tusks (the central incisors) can be as long as 11 ½ feet and weigh 440 pounds (42).
‡ Guinea pigs have the same formula, except that they have only one maxillary incisor.

The beaver has four strong curved incisors. They have very hard, bright orange enamel on the labial surface and much softer exposed dentin on the lingual surface. As the dentin wears off, this leaves very sharp cutting edges of enamel. The incisors continue to grow throughout life. The posterior teeth have flat, rough edges on the occlusal surface, and they stop growing at 2 years of age. There is a large diastema immediately posterior to the incisors, and flaps of skin fold inward and meet behind the incisors to seal off the back part of the mouth during gnawing. Therefore, splinters are kept out. The flaps of skin relax for eating and drinking. Most of the wood beavers gnaw is nonedible.

The shrew has two hooked cusps on the upper first incisor. Its deciduous dentition is shed in utero. The shrew's 1–1½-year life span is limited by the wear on their molars. Death occurs by starvation once the molars wear out. Also, their small body can store only enough food for 1–2 hours, so they must feed almost continually. Their diet consists of small invertebrates, woodlice, and fruit.

The vampire bat has large canines, but its highly specialized upper incisors, which are V-shaped and razor-edged, are what remove a piece of the victim's skin. The bat's saliva contains an anticoagulant, and its tongue rolls up in a tube to suck or lap the exuding blood.

Some vertebrates do not have any teeth (complete anodontia) but have descended from ancestors that possessed teeth. Birds have beaks but depend on a gizzard to do the grinding that molars would usually perform. Turtles have heavy jaw coverings, which are thin edged in the incisor region and wide posteriorly for crushing. The duck-billed platypus has its early-life teeth replaced by keratinous plates, which it uses to crush aquatic insects, crustaceans, and molluscs. The whalebone whale and anteaters also have no teeth, but their diets do not require mastication.

LEARNING QUESTIONS

Select the one best answer.

1. How many teeth are present in one quadrant of a complete adult (permanent) dentition?
   a. 5
   b. 8
   c. 10
   d. 20
   e. 32

2. What class of teeth is present in the permanent dentition that is NOT present in the primary dentition?
   a. incisors
   b. canines
   c. premolars
   d. molars

3. In a permanent dentition, the fifth tooth from the midline is a:
   a. canine
   b. premolar
   c. molar
   d. incisor

4. Posterior teeth in the permanent dentition include which of the following?
   a. premolars only
   b. molars only
   c. premolars and molars only
   d. canines, premolars, and molars
5. What permanent tooth erupts into the space previously held by the primary second molar?
   a. first molar
   b. second molar
   c. first premolar
   d. second premolar

Answers: 1-b, 2-c, 3-b, 4-c, 5-d.

SECTION II. Bones of the Human Skull

OBJECTIVES

This section is designed to prepare the learner to perform the following:
- Describe and identify each bone seen on an intact human skull.
- Describe and identify each bony structure highlighted in bold in this chapter. Emphasis is placed on structures of the mandible, maxillae, temporal, and sphenoid bones.
- Describe and identify the location of the attachment of chewing muscles and ligaments attached to the mandible.
- Describe and identify the foramen of the nerves and arteries that supply the teeth and oral cavity.

LEARNING EXERCISE

To obtain a clear understanding of the bones of the skull and their relationship to one another and to the teeth, it is best to have a skull at hand to examine while reading this chapter. If you touch and trace each bone with your fingers as you read, you are not apt to forget its characteristics.

There are 206 distinct bones in our skeleton, 28 of which are in the skull if we count the malleus, stapes, and incus bones of each ear. The skull bones can be divided into two parts: the **neurocranium** [NOOR o CRAY ne um] surrounding the brain and the **facial** (or visceral) **apparatus** (making up the face).

When studying bones (and teeth), there are many descriptive terms that must be learned. Terms with similar definitions are grouped here to facilitate learning. Since anatomy terms are often similar to common familiar words, the new terms are compared to familiar words whenever possible.

BUMPS — (CONVEXITIES) ON BONES AND/OR TEETH
crest: a projecting ridge along a bone
eminence: a prominence or projection of bone
process: a projection or outgrowth from a larger bone structure
protuberance [pro TU ber ahns]: a prominence or swelling (of bone)
ridge: linear narrow, elevated portion of bone or tooth
tubercle [TOO ber k'l]: a small rounded projection on a bone or tooth

DEPRESSIONS — (CONCAVITIES) IN BONES AND/OR TEETH

alveolus [al VEE o lus] (plural: **alveoli** [al VEE o lie]): small hollow space or socket where the tooth root fits within the jaw bones

cavity: a hollow place within the body of bone (or within a tooth)

fissure [FISH er]: a cleft or groove (crack) between parts

fossa [FOS ah] (plural: **fossae** [FOS ee]): a small hollow or depressed area

fovea [FO ve ah]: small pit or depression

groove: linear depression or furrow

sinus: hollow, air-filled cavity or space within skull bones, or a channel for venous blood

OPENINGS — (HOLES) IN BONES AND/OR TEETH

aperture: an opening; compare a camera lens aperture

foramen [fo RA men] (plural: **foramina** [fo RAM i nah]): a small hole through bone or tooth for passage of nerves and vessels

foramen ovale [o VAL ee]: an oval or egg-shaped foramen (which is bigger than the round [rotundum] foramen)

foramen rotundum: a round foramen; recall a building's rotunda or dome that is relatively round

meatus [me A tus]: a natural passage or opening in the body

RELATIVE LOCATION — FIGURE 1-3 WILL BE HELPFUL IN UNDERSTANDING MOST OF THESE TERMS.

anterior: toward the front of the body

buccal [BUCK al]: related to or near the cheek; the buccal nerve innervates the cheek; the buccinator muscle is within the cheek; the buccal surface of a tooth is the side toward the cheek (also called facial side because it is toward the face that we see)

cervix: of the neck or neck-like; compare a cervical vertebrae in the neck

external: toward the outside of the body; seen from the outside

facial: toward the face; seen when viewing the face side

inferior or the prefix **infra:** located below or beneath; lower than

medial: the surface toward, or closest to, the midline (medial) plane of the body

median plane: a longitudinal plane that divides the body into relatively equal right and left halves

mid-sagittal plane [SAJ i t'l]: same as medial plane

posterior: toward the rear of the mouth or body

retro (prefix): back or behind

sub (prefix): under or beneath

superficial: closer to the surface

superior or the preface **supra:** located above or over; higher or upper

GENERAL TERMS RELATED TO BONES

acoustic [ah KOOS tik]: referring to sounds or hearing

cervical [SER vi kal]: related to the neck; like cervical vertebrae

condyle [KON dile]: an articular prominence of bones resembling a knuckle

coronoid: (compare coronation; where the crown fits or the shape of a crown); for example, the coronoid process of mandible is shaped like the point of a crown

dura: hard , not soft (compare durable)

glenoid [GLE noyd]: socket-like

lacrimal [LAK ri mal] (also spelled lachrymal): referring to the tears (compare lacrimosa)

lamina: a thin layer (compare laminated wood)

lingula [LING gyoo la]: tongue-shaped structure (compare lingual)

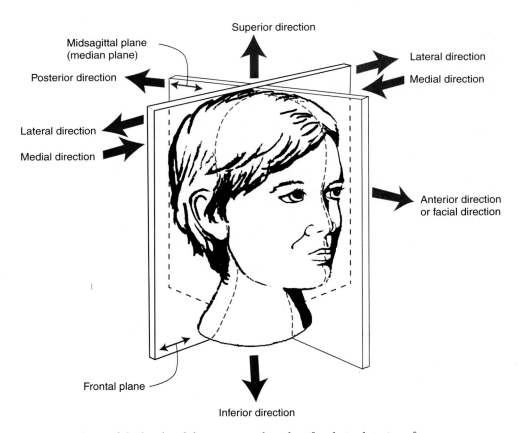

FIGURE 1-3. Planes of the head and directions used to identify relative location of structures or surfaces in the head.

LEARNING EXERCISES, cont.

malar [MAY lar]: referring to the cheek or cheek bone (not to be confused with molar)

meatus: [mee A tus] a pathway or opening

palpebral [PAL pe bral]: referring to the eyelid

piriform [PEER i form]: pear-shaped

septum: a partition (compare separate)

symphysis [SIM fi sis]: fibrocartilaginous joint where opposed bony surfaces are joined (a suture line may not be evident)

trochlea [TROK lee ah]: pulley-shaped

A. BONES OF THE NEUROCRANIUM

The **neurocranium** is the portion of the skull that supports, surrounds, and protects the brain. It is made up of replacement bone (i.e., there is a cartilaginous precursor or model for these bones). Other names for this type of bone are cartilage bone and endochondral bone. The eight bones of the neurocranium are four single bones (sphenoid, occipital, ethmoid, and frontal) and two paired bones (one on each side): temporal and parietal.

The following description of structures on each bone will focus on the location of key muscle and ligament attachments and the passageway (foramen and spaces) for the major cranial nerve branches to the mouth or oral cavity (especially the trigeminal, facial, glossopharyngeal, and hypoglossal nerves). The learner should become familiar with these bony structures in order to understand fully how the muscles move the jaw in each direction and where to apply local anesthetic along the path of a nerve, as described in subsequent sections of this chapter.

1. SPHENOID BONE

This single, irregularly shaped, midline bone cradles the base of the brain and pituitary gland and forms the posterior part of the orbit (eye socket). Its complex shape can only be appreciated by looking at it from several different views (best seen in Figs. 1-4 and 1-5 where it is shaded). The **sphenoid** [SFE noid] **bone** is important to dental professionals because it has processes that serve as part of the attachment for three of the four pairs of major chewing muscles. The sphenoid bone also has foramina (holes) that are the passageway for the nerve branches that supply all teeth and many surrounding structures.

The sphenoid bone has processes or wings projecting laterally. The **lesser wings** can only be seen internally in Figure 1-4. The **greater wings** are also seen internally in Figure 1-4 but are best viewed externally in Figure 1-7. The external surface of the greater wing is part of the **temporal fossa** where the temporalis muscle attaches to the neurocranium. The fissure internally between the greater and lesser wing is called the **superior orbital fissure** (Fig. 1-4), which is the passageway of the ophthalmic nerve (one branch of the trigeminal nerve).

The sphenoid bone also has two processes that project downward from the base of the skull just adjacent to the posterior surface of the maxillae (upper jaw bones). These are called **pterygoid** [TER i goid] **processes** and are best seen in the lateral view of Figure 1-6. (*Hint:* To remember the name of this process, note that it has a scalloped border somewhat like the wings of a *pter*odactyl flying dinosaur.) One pterygoid process contains a fossa about the size of the end of your little finger called the **pterygoid fossa** (Fig. 1-5). This fossa is where one end of a major chewing muscle, the medial pterygoid muscle, attaches. The pterygoid fossa is bounded by a lateral plate of bone known as the **lateral pterygoid plate** (or lamina) and a medial plate of bone (**medial pterygoid plate**). The lateral surface of the lateral pterygoid plate (also called lamina) visible in Figure 1-6 is where one end of the lateral pterygoid muscle attaches.

Two pairs of foramina in this bone are important to dental professionals. Individually these are known as the foramen rotundum and the foramen ovale. The oval, more posterior **foramen ovale** is the skull opening for the passage of the mandibular nerve (part of the trigeminal nerve), a major nerve to the mandibular teeth and jaw, and the chewing muscles. The foramen ovale is best seen internally in Figure 1-4 and externally in Figure 1-5. Pass a pipe cleaner through this foramen and appreciate that it drops inferiorly toward the mandible. It can be identified easily by its proximity to the much smaller foramen known as the **foramen spinosum** [spy NO sum]. The rounder, more medial and anterior **foramen rotundum** [ro TUN dum] (seen only internally in Fig. 1-4) is the opening for the passage of another part of the trigeminal nerve called the maxillary nerve. If you are able to pass a pipe cleaner from the brain through this foramen, it will be somewhat hidden in a space between the pterygoid process and upper jaw (maxilla). This space between the pterygoid process and the posterior wall of the maxillae (which is covered in part by vertical projections of the palatine bones) is known as the **pterygopalatine** [TER i go PAL eh tine] **space** labeled in Figure 1-6. The maxillary nerve that exits the skull through the foramen rotundum proceeds through this space as it gives off branches to the upper jaw (maxillae) and teeth.

The **sphenoidal** [SFE noid al] **(angular) spine** is a sharp, small process on the inferior surface of the sphenoid bone just posterior to the foramen ovale and foramen spinosum, as seen inferiorly in Figure 1-5. This spine is the superior attachment of the *spheno*mandibular ligament, which extends inferiorly to the medial surface of the lower jaw (mandible).

2. TEMPORAL BONES

The **temporal bones** are a pair of complex bones that form part of the sides and base of the skull (best seen laterally in Fig. 1-7 where it is shaded). The **temporal fossa** is a large, very shallow depression in the temple region formed by the lateral part of the temporal bone, along with a portion of the sphenoid (greater wing), and the adjacent portions of the parietal and frontal bones described later. The temporal fossa is where one end of another major chewing muscle (the temporalis) attaches.

The paired temporal bones are important to dental professionals since each has a **mandibular fossa**

FIGURE 1-4. Human skull: bones of neurocranium, superior view. The **sphenoid bone** is shaded in this figure.

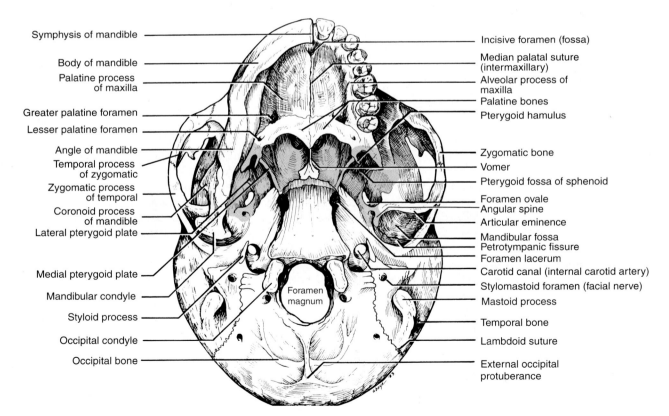

FIGURE 1-5. Human skull: inferior surface with half of the mandible removed on the right side of the drawing to permit easier viewing of the **sphenoid bone**, which is shaded.

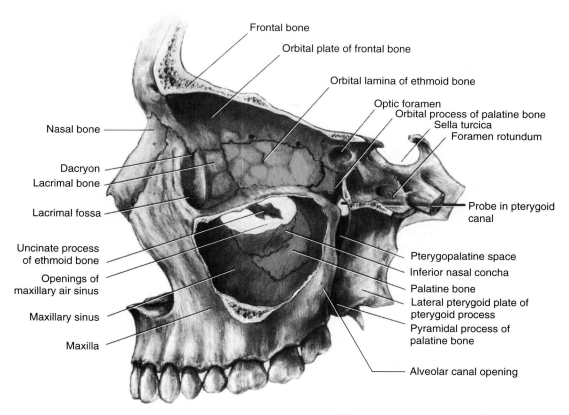

Frontal bone

Orbital plate of frontal bone

Orbital lamina of ethmoid bone

Optic foramen
Orbital process of palatine bone
Sella turcica
Foramen rotundum

Nasal bone

Dacryon
Lacrimal bone

Lacrimal fossa

Probe in pterygoid canal

Uncinate process of ethmoid bone

Openings of maxillary air sinus

Pterygopalatine space
Inferior nasal concha
Palatine bone
Lateral pterygoid plate of pterygoid process
Pyramidal process of palatine bone

Maxillary sinus

Maxilla

Alveolar canal opening

FIGURE 1-6. Part of human skull, lateral view, with the lateral wall of the left maxilla removed exposing the large **maxillary sinus**. Note the lateral surface of the **lateral pterygoid plate** just behind the maxilla. Also, note that the floor of this sinus is in proximity to the maxillary posterior teeth, but that it does not extend as far forward as the maxillary anterior teeth. The opening of this sinus (into the nasal chamber) is located superiorly on the medial wall of the sinus. Finally, the process of the palatine bone indicated in the illustration is the vertical part of the **palatine bone** located on the posterior surface of each maxilla. (Reproduced by permission from Clemente CD, ed. Gray's anatomy of the human body. 30th ed. Philadelphia: Lea & Febiger, 1985:166.)

(one is labeled on the right side of Fig. 1-5). The mandibular fossae (right and left) are located on the inferior aspect of the temporal bones. It is within these fossae that the lower jaw (or mandible) articulates with and moves against the temporal bones on the base of the neurocranium. This jaw joint (actually a joint on each side) is called the temporomandibular joint (TMJ). Each mandibular fossa can be divided into two parts by the **petrotympanic fissure**. The anterior two-thirds is the important functional part called the **articular** (or glenoid) **fossa**. Each articular fossa has a ridge of bone forming its anterior border, which is called the **articular eminence**.

Each temporal bone has several processes. The **zygomatic** [zy go MAT ik] **process** (Fig. 1-7) is the finger of bone anterior to the mandibular fossa that joins with another bone, the zygomatic, to form an arch called the **zygomatic arch** (sometimes referred to as the cheekbone). This is the attachment of one end of the large muscle of mastication, the masseter. The **mastoid process** (Fig. 1-7), seen inferiorly and posteriorly to the mandibular fossa, is the attachment for one end of a major neck muscle, the sternocleido*mastoid* muscle. You can feel the bump of the mastoid process behind the ear lobe. The **styloid process** (Fig. 1-5), shaped like a small skinny pencil (or stylus), is the attachment for one end of a ligament (*stylo*mandibular ligament) that extends to the lower jaw.

Several paired foramina are of importance on this bone. Laterally, the **external acoustic meatus** [a KOO stik me A tus] is the opening into the ear canal (Fig. 1-7). On the inferior surface, the **stylomastoid foramen** (Fig. 1-5), located between the styloid and mastoid processes, is where the facial

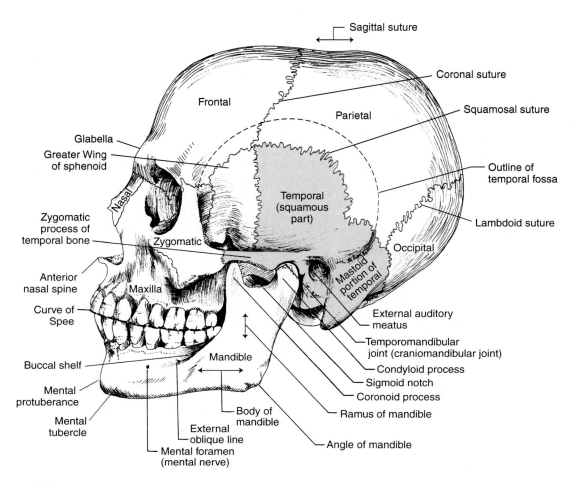

FIGURE 1-7. Human skull, left side. Note the outline of the shallow **temporal fossa**, which includes part of the temporal and sphenoid bones, as well as the adjacent portions of the frontal and parietal bones.

nerve exits the temporal bone. Internally, this nerve enters the temporal bone through the **internal acoustic meatus** (Fig. 1-4).

3. FRONTAL BONE

This single, large midline bone forms the "forehead" and eyebrow region (Fig. 1-7). A small portion of this bone in the temporal fossa region serves as part of the attachment for one end of the temporalis muscle.

4. PARIETAL BONES

These large, paired bones protect the brain laterally and posteriorly (Fig. 1-7). Like the frontal bone, part of this bone is located within the temporal fossa, which is where one end of the temporalis muscle attaches.

5. OCCIPITAL BONE

This bone provides the articulating surface between the skull and vertebral column at the **occipital condyle** [ahk SIP eh tal KON dile] (seen on the inferior surface in Figure 1-5). The large **foramen magnum** serves as the passageway for the spinal cord. Lateral to the foramen magnum (between the occipital and temporal bones) is the large **jugular** [JUG you lar] **foramen** (Fig.1-4), the passageway of the glossopharyngeal nerve.

6. ETHMOID BONE

This single, hollow, sinus-filled bone is located on the midline beneath the anterior part of the brain and extends between the eye sockets and helps separate the halves of the nasal cavities. The most superior aspect of this bone is visible within the brain case at the midline as the sieve-like **cribriform** [KRIB ri form] **plate** (Fig 1-4) surrounding the triangular projection called the **crista galli** [KRIS ta GAL li]. The cribriform plate is full of holes providing the passage from the nasal cavity for the fibers of the olfactory nerve (the nerve for smell). Inferior to the cribriform plate, this bone spreads out to form part of the medial aspect of each orbit (orbital lamina of the ethmoid bone is visible in Fig. 1-6). It also has scrolled processes extending into the nasal cavity similar in appearance to the inferior nasal concha described later in this section. Finally, a vertical midline plate of the ethmoid bone extends downward into the nasal cavity to form (along with the separate vomer bone) the **nasal septum** (Fig. 1-8), which separates the right and left nasal cavities.

7. SUTURE LINES BETWEEN BONES

Suture lines of the neurocranium are lines of fibrous connective tissue that join two bones of the skull immovably together best seen in Figure 1-7. **Coronal sutures** are located between the frontal and two parietal bones [*Hint:* This location is where a crown might fit during a *corona*tion]. **Squamosal** [skwa MO sal] **sutures** are located between the temporal and parietal bones (squamous refers to the fish-scale shape that this portion of the temporal bone resembles). The **sagittal suture** (best seen on the

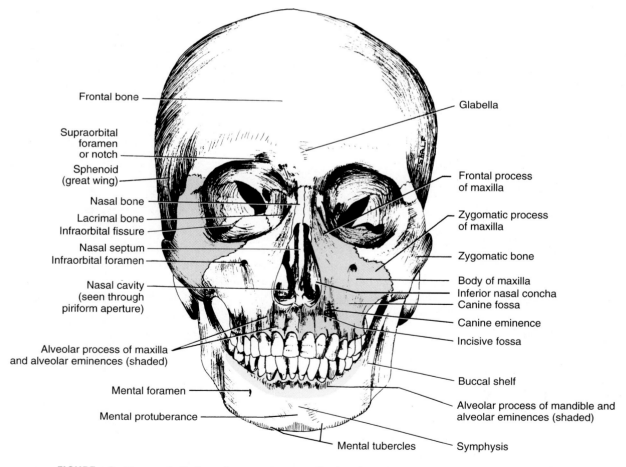

FIGURE 1-8. Human skull, frontal aspect. One **maxilla** (on the right side of the drawing), one **zygomatic bone** (on the left side of the drawing), and the facial surface of the arch-shaped **alveolar process of the mandible** and the left **maxilla** have been shaded.

top of the skull) joins the right and left parietal bones on the top midline of the skull, parallel to the sagittal plane of the skull. The **lambdoid** [LAM doid] **suture** joins the occipital bone with the parietal bones. Its shape from the posterior view resembles an upside-down "V" and can be compared to the shape of the Greek letter lambda (λ).

B. BONES OF THE FACE (VISCERAL APPARATUS)

The form of facial bones gives us our appearance. They function in both respiration and digestion and are made up of dermal or intramembranous bone, the type that is not preceded by cartilage. The facial bones are located anterior and inferior to the forehead and make up the major anterior part of the skull. There are fourteen facial bones. Two single bones are the mandible (lower jaw) and the vomer. Six paired bones are the palatine, zygomatic, nasal, and lacrimal bones, as well as the maxillae (upper jaw) and inferior nasal concha (turbinates). The mandible and maxillae are most important when considering the foundation for teeth and tooth function, so they will be discussed in more detail. The mandible is the largest bone in the face. Each maxilla (right and left) is the second largest bone in the face.

1. MAXILLAE (RIGHT AND LEFT MAXILLA)

Each maxilla (right or left) consists of one large, hollow central mass called the *body* and four projecting *processes* or extensions of bone. It is best seen shaded in Figure 1-8.

a. Body of the Maxilla

The *body* of the maxilla is shaped like a four-sided, hollow pyramid with the base oriented vertically next to the nasal cavity and the apex or peak extending laterally into part of the cheekbone (or zygomatic bone). Part of the maxilla forms the floor of the orbit of the eye (Fig. 1-8) where an **infraorbital fissure** is located. It disappears anteriorly to become the **infraorbital canal** (not visible in Fig. 1-8). Important nerves and vessels enter this fissure and canal, give off branches within the canal which supply some of the maxillary teeth and surrounding tissue. The nerves and vessels exit the maxilla on to the face through the **infraorbital foramen** (Fig. 1-8). This foramen is on the anterior surface of the body, inferior to the eye and just superior to the canine fossa.

The entrance to the **alveolar** [al VEE o lar] **canals** (Fig. 1-6) where the nerves to the maxillary teeth (posterior superior alveolar nerves) enter the maxilla are very small **foramina** located posterior and superior to the third molar.

b. Bony Processes on Each Maxilla

There are four processes extending out from the body of the maxillae: The first three described below are best viewed in Figure 1-8.

(1) Frontal (or Nasofrontal) Process
The **frontal (nasofrontal) process** derives its name from the fact that its medial edge joins with the nasal bone, extending superiorly to also articulate with the frontal bone. The medial or nasal surface forms part of the lateral wall of the nasal cavity and half of the opening of the nasal cavity (called the piriform aperture because of its pear shape).

(2) Zygomatic Process
The zygomatic process forms part of the anterior or facial surface of each maxilla. It extends laterally to join with the maxillary process of the zygomatic bone.

(3) Alveolar Process
The **alveolar processes** of the right and left maxillae (and also of the mandible described later) extend to form an arch shape of bone that surrounds the roots of the maxillary dental arch of teeth (seen shaded on one maxilla in Fig. 1-8). The roots of the teeth are embedded in individual **alveoli** (tooth sockets). The shape of each alveolus or thin bony socket naturally corresponds closely with the shape of the roots of the tooth it surrounds. **Alveolar** [al VEE o lar] **eminences** are raised ridges of bone overlying tooth root convexities. The alveo-

lar eminence over the canine tooth on each side is called the **canine eminence** (Fig. 1-8). Anterior to the canine eminence is a shallow fossa over the root of the maxillary lateral incisor called the **incisive** [in SI siv] **fossa**. Posterior to the canine eminence is a fossa over the roots of maxillary premolars named the **canine fossa**.

The alveolar process is made up of several bony layers (Fig. 1-9). Supporting bone is made up of the thickened inner (lingual) and outer (facial) dense **cortical plate** with less dense **trabecular** [trah BEK u lar] **bone** sandwiched in between. Trabecular bone is composed of many plate-like bone partitions that separate the irregularly shaped marrow spaces located within this bone. Synonyms for trabecular bone include cancellous or spongy bone.

The **lamina dura** (Fig. 1-9) is the much thinner, compact bony layer that lines the wall of each tooth socket (or alveolus). The only space between the outer layer of tooth root (which is covered with cementum) and this alveolar bone is occupied by a periodontal ligament that suspends each tooth within its alveolus by attaching the circumference of each tooth root to the surrounding lamina dura. The **periodontal ligament** is very thin [between 0.12 and 0.33 mm thick] and is composed of thousands of fibers. Synonyms for lamina dura include alveolar bony socket, alveolar bone, true alveolar bone, alveolar bone proper, and cribriform plate of the alveolar process.

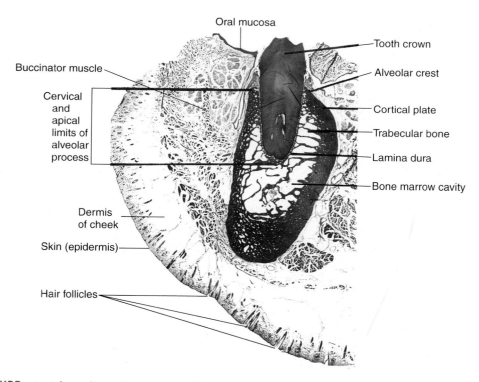

FIGURE 1-9. A buccolingual cross-section [about 30 μm thick] of a human mandible and a molar. To the left of the mandible is the soft facial tissue of the cheek. Note the extent of the **alveolar process**: only the part of the mandible that surrounds the tooth root. The thick **cortical plate** surrounds the entire facial (left) and medial (right) surfaces of the mandible, while the thin **lamina dura** layer of bone lines the socket that surrounds the tooth root. A **periodontal ligament** (averaging only twice as thick as this page [0.2 mm]) extends between the lamina dura and outer layer of tooth root, and supports the tooth within its socket. [Tooth enamel was destroyed by the decalcification of the specimen with nitric acid preparatory to embedding and sectioning.] For further information on the histology of these structures, refer to references 10, 23, and 37–41.

(4) Palatine Process of the Maxilla

Refer to Figure 1-10 while reading about the palatine process. Each **palatine** [PAL a tine] **process** is a thin, bony shelf of bone that projects horizontally from the inner surface of each maxilla to form most of the anterior hard palate and floor of the nasal passage. The antero-posterior line of fusion between the right and left palatine processes of the maxillae and the horizontal plates of the palatine bones is the **intermaxillary** (or midpalatine) **suture**. It is located on the midline running posteriorly from the incisive foramen. The **incisive foramen** is a centrally located hole at the most anterior part of this suture, just posterior to the central incisors. It transmits branches of the artery and nasopalatine nerve that supply adjacent palatal soft tissue.

An embryonic **premaxilla** cannot normally be distinguished in the adult skull. It is the anterior part of the maxillary bone, which contains the incisors. When visible, a suture line separates the premaxilla from the palatine processes of the two maxillae.

c. Maxillary Sinus or Antrum

Sinuses are hollow spaces within bones and are found within the sphenoid, frontal, and ethmoid bones, as well as within each maxilla. The **maxillary sinus**, located within the body of each maxilla, functions to (a) lighten the skull, (b) give resonance to the voice, (c) warm the air we breathe,

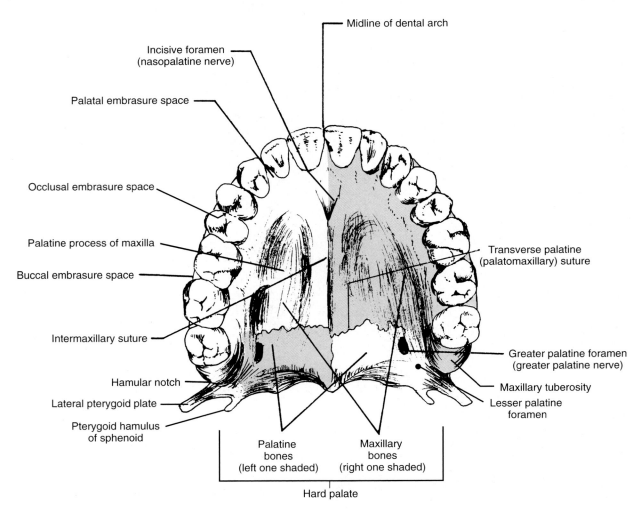

FIGURE 1-10. Inferior view of the hard palate with maxillary teeth. The **palatine process of one maxilla** (on the right side of the drawing) and the **horizontal process of one palatine bone** (on the left side of the drawing) are shaded.

and (d) moisten the nasal cavity. [The average size of each maxillary sinus in an adult is about 25 mm from side to side, 30 mm from front to back, and 30 mm high, with an average capacity of 15 ml (range: 9.5–20 ml),[1] or about 1 tablespoon.]

Refer to Figure 1-6 while reading about the maxillary sinus. This large four-sided, pyramid-shaped cavity is located within the body of each maxilla. One wall forms the sinus cavity floor. It extends inferiorly onto the superior portion of the maxillary alveolar process, where many projections of the ends (apices) of the molar roots, and sometimes premolar roots, are found. The most intimate relationship between the teeth and maxillary sinus is seen in Figure 1-11. Only very thin bone lies between the floor of the sinus and the apices of the roots of the maxillary molars. In rare cases, no bone separates the root apices from the sinus. There is always soft tissue, made up of the periodontal ligament on the tooth root and the mucous membrane lining the sinus cavity, between the root and the space of the cavity. Sometimes when a dentist extracts a molar and the root breaks off, he is unjustly accused of pushing the root into the sinus. It may have been located in the maxillary sinus prior to the extraction. The other three walls of the pyramid-shaped sinus are toward the orbit of the eye, toward the face, and posteriorly and laterally, next to the infratemporal space.

The maxillary sinus is a significant structure because of the close relationship it has to the teeth. The nerve and blood supply to the upper teeth travels just beneath the membrane lining of the sinus or through bony canals within the walls of the sinus. An infection in either place can spread to the other. Pain caused by a maxillary sinus infection can be mistaken for pain originating in any one or all of the molars or premolars on that side. Unfortunately, healthy teeth are sometimes extracted in a futile attempt to alleviate pain that was caused by a chronic maxillary sinus infection.

A

B

FIGURE 1-11. A. Three views of part of the left **alveolar process** of the maxilla surrounding maxillary first and second molar, and second premolar, roots. Note the root tips (apices) shown by arrows extending out of the maxilla into what would have been the floor of the **maxillary sinus** space in an intact skull. **B.** Radiograph of the maxillary molar region showing the roots of the first molar several millimeters deep into the maxillary sinus (dark area). Part of the roots of the second molar are also within the sinus cavity. The root tip of the second premolar root is in the sinus as well. This is a common relationship.

The maxillary sinus is lined with specialized cells (ciliated columnar epithelium) similar to those found in the respiratory tract. The mucous film it secretes moves spirally and upward (against gravity) across the membrane to the *opening* of the sinus located on the anterosuperior wall (Fig. 1-6), where it drains into the nasal cavity. If humans walked on all fours with the head forward like many animals, this opening for drainage would be on the floor of the sinus, not near the roof, and humans would have fewer sinus problems. Many people can get pain relief by placing their head in a prone position for several minutes to permit more rapid drainage of the maxillary sinuses.

2. MANDIBLE

The single horseshoe-shaped **mandible** [MAN de b'l], seen anteriorly in Figure 1-8, is the largest and strongest bone of the skull. Generally speaking, it is bilaterally symmetrical. It bears the mandibular teeth and is attached only by ligaments and muscles to the relatively immovable bones of the neurocranium. The temporomandibular joints between the mandible and the temporal bones are movable articulations, the only visible movable articulations in the head. The mandible is the only bone of the skull that can move. The other bones of the skull move only when the whole head is moved, and then they move in unison.

The mandible has three parts: one horizontal *body* and two vertical **rami** [RAY mee] (singular, **ramus** [RAY mus]) (see Fig. 1-12). The landmarks of the mandible will be discussed according to their location: external surface of the body, then ramus, then the internal surface.

a. Body: External Surface

As with the maxillae, an **alveolar** [al VEE o lar] **process** surrounds the tooth roots (shaded in Fig. 1-8), and **alveolar eminences** are visible as vertical elevations over tooth roots on the facial surface. The prominent elevations overlying the roots of the canines are called the **canine eminences**.

The bulky, curved horizontal body and the flattened vertical ramus join at the angle of the mandible on either side. The **angle** of the mandible is located where the inferior border of the body joins the posterior border of the ramus (Fig. 1-7). The roughened portion of the lateral surface near the angle of the mandible is where one end of the powerful masseter muscle attaches. The posterior border of the ramus is also the location of the attachment of the stylo*mandibular* ligament (whose other end attached to the styloid process of the temporal bone).

The **symphysis** [SIM fi sis] is the line of fusion of the right and left sides at the midline where the two halves of the mandible fuse (join together) during the first year after birth. It is therefore usually not visible. Near the symphysis, two mental tubercles and one mental protuberance make up the human chin (Fig. 1-8). No other mammal has a chin. Two **mental tubercles** lie on either side of the midline near the inferior border of the mandible. The **mental protuberance** is centered on the

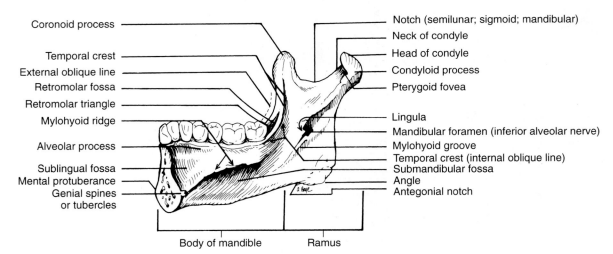

Coronoid process —
Temporal crest —
External oblique line —
Retromolar fossa —
Retromolar triangle —
Mylohyoid ridge —
Alveolar process —
Sublingual fossa —
Mental protuberance —
Genial spines or tubercles —

— Notch (semilunar; sigmoid; mandibular)
— Neck of condyle
— Head of condyle
— Condyloid process
— Pterygoid fovea

— Lingula
— Mandibular foramen (inferior alveolar nerve)
— Mylohyoid groove
— Temporal crest (internal oblique line)
— Submandibular fossa
— Angle
— Antegonial notch

Body of mandible   Ramus

FIGURE 1-12. Mandible, medial surface. Notice the major parts of a mandible called the **body** (horizontal part) and the **ramus** (vertical part). The mylohyoid ridge beneath the mucosa can be felt by gently pressing laterally with a finger beneath your tongue.

midline between the two mental tubercles but is about 10 mm superior. The protuberance and the tubercles are more prominent on men than on women.

An **external oblique** [ob LEEK] **ridge** (Fig. 1-7) extends from the canine region to the anterior border of the ramus. The nearly horizontal ledge of bone in the molar region between the external oblique ridge and alveolar process is named the **buccal shelf**. This is the proximity of the buccal nerve in the cheek.

The **mental foramen** is located near the root end (apex) of the second premolar (Fig. 1-7). On dental radiographs (x-rays) this foramen appears as a small dark circle next to the premolar root and must be distinguished from a periapical abscess (infection destroying bone near the root apex), which may appear very similar to the normal mental foramen. The nerves and vessels (inferior alveolar) that traverse the mandibular canal within the mandible divide while within the mandible, and a branch (mental branch) exits through this mental foramen in an outward, upward, and posterior direction. Place a flexible probe carefully into this canal of your skull model to confirm this direction. The mental foramen is located at practically the same level on most humans: 13–15 mm superior to the inferior border of the mandible. [In a study of 40 skulls,[2] the mental foramen was found most often to be directly under the second premolar (42.5% of the time) or between the apices of the first and second premolars (40%). Infrequently, it was located distal to the apex of the second premolar (17.5%), and was never found under the apex of the first premolar.]

b. Ramus: External Surface

Refer to Figure 1-7 while reading about this surface. There are two processes on the superior end of each ramus. The **coronoid** [KOR o noyd] **process** is the more pointed, anterior process on the upper border. The second more rounded and posterior process of the ramus is the **condyloid** [KON di loyd] **process** (also called the **mandibular condyle**). This process is composed of a bulky condyle head and a narrow neck that attaches the head to the ramus. A portion of one of the important chewing muscles, the lateral pterygoid, attaches to the front of the neck of the condyloid process. As stated earlier when discussing the temporal bone, the head of the mandibular condyle fits into and functions beneath the articular (glenoid) fossa of the temporal bone. The **sigmoid notch** (also called the mandibular or semilunar notch) is located between the coronoid process and the condyloid process.

c. Internal or Medial Surface of Mandible

Refer to Figure 1-12 while reading about this surface. The **mandibular foramen** is a prominent opening located on the medial surface of the ramus inferior to the sigmoid notch near the center of the ramus. It is the entrance into the mandibular canal where the inferior alveolar vessels and nerves pass into the mandible. The mandibular **lingula** [LING gu lah] is a sharp ridge or projection of bone just anterior and slightly superior to the mandibular foramen. This is where one end of the sphe-no*mandibular* ligament attaches to the mandible. The other end attaches to the angular (sphenoidal) spine on the sphenoid bone. The **mylohyoid groove** is a small groove running inferior and anterior from the mandibular foramen. The mylohyoid nerve rests in this groove.

The **temporal crest** is a ridge extending from the tip of the coronoid process onto the medial surface of the ramus and terminating near the third molar. The tendon from the fibers of the wide, flat, fan-shaped temporalis muscle attaches here. The inferior one-fourth of the temporal crest is called the **internal oblique line**. It is most important as a radiographic, rather than an anatomic, landmark. It appears on radiographs as a short, curved line somewhat inferior to the image of the external oblique line. The internal oblique line *is not synonymous with the mylohyoid ridge,* as incorrectly stated in some radiographic textbooks.

The **retromolar fossa** is a roughened shallow fossa distal to the last molar and bounded medially by the lowest portion of the temporal crest and laterally by the external oblique ridge. The **retromolar triangle** is in the lowest most anterior, and only horizontal, portion of the retromolar fossa. A **buccinator** [BUCK sin a tor] **crest** is a barely discernible ridge of bone that divides the smaller retromolar triangle from the rest of the larger retromolar fossa. The most posterior fibers of the buccinator (a pouch-shaped cheek muscle) muscle attach here.

Genial [JEE ne al] **spines** or tubercles are located on either side of the midline on the internal surface of the mandible. Two large muscles (the genioglossus and the geniohyoid) attach to the genial spines and the elevated and roughened bone near them.

The **mylohyoid ridge** extends downward and forward from the molar region to the genial tubercles. The mylohyoid muscle, which forms part of the floor of the mouth, attaches from the mylohyoid ridge on the right internal side of the mandible to the ridge on the left internal side (somewhat like a hammock). A shallow **sublingual** [sub LING gwal] **fossa** is found just superior to the mylohyoid ridge and lateral to the genial tubercles on each side. The sublingual salivary gland rests in this fossa. A shallow **submandibular fossa** is found just inferior to the mylohyoid ridge in the premolar and molar regions. This is where the large submandibular gland rests.

3. ZYGOMATIC BONE

The **zygomatic bone** (one on each side of the face, shaded on the left side in Fig. 1-8) forms the prominence of each cheek. The temporal process of the zygomatic bone forms an arch along with the zygomatic process of the temporal bone. This **zygomatic arch** is where the superior end of the masseter muscle attaches to the skull. As stated previously, its lower end is connected to the lateral angle of the mandible.

4. PALATINE BONE

Refer to Figure 1-10 while reading about the **palatine bone**. The horizontal processes of the paired palatine bones form the posterior one-fourth of the bony shelf called the **hard palate**. The entire hard palate (bony roof of the mouth) is made up of the inferior surfaces of these palatine bones, along with the right and left palatine processes of the maxillae. A **palatomaxillary** [PAL ah toe MAK si ler ee] (**transverse palatine**) **suture**, at right angles to the intermaxillary suture, is the junction between the palatine processes of the maxillae and the horizontal processes of the palatine bones.

The superior surfaces of the hard palate form the floor of the nasal cavity. The shape of the palate and the shape of the maxillary arch vary in length, breadth, and height. The hard palate blends smoothly with the palatal portion of the maxillary alveolar process. Part or all of the palatine processes are absent in a person who was born with a cleft palate.

The palatine bones also have vertical processes that are practically hidden from view on the intact skull. These vertical processes lie against the posterior wall of each maxilla (barely visible on Fig. 1-6). These vertical processes are separated from the pterygoid process of the sphenoid bone by a space called the **pterygopalatine** [TER i go PAL ah tine] **space**, mentioned earlier when discussing the maxillae. Recall that this space is an important passageway of the major nerves from the brain to the maxillary teeth and surrounding structures.

The **greater palatine** [PAL ah tine] **foramina** (Fig. 1-10) are located posteriorly on each side near the angle where the right and left palatine bones meet the alveolar processes of the hard palate. They transmit the descending palatine vessels and greater (anterior) palatine nerves to the palate. The **lesser palatine foramina** are located on the palatine bone just behind and lateral to the greater palatine foramen. They transmit the middle and posterior palatine nerves.

5. VOMER BONE

The **vomer bone** (Fig. 1-5) is a midline bone which, along with the vertical projection of the ethmoid bone, forms the **nasal septum**. This septum separates the right and left halves of the nasal cavity. A deviated septum may limit breathing and require surgery.

6. NASAL BONES

The two **nasal bones** form the bony bridge of the nose (Fig. 1-8).

7. LACRIMAL BONES

The **lacrimal** [LAK ri mal] **bones**, small rectangular bones at the medial corner of each orbit, contain a depression for tear glands (Fig. 1-6).

8. INFERIOR TURBINATES

The **inferior nasal conchae** [CONG kee]; singular concha [KONG kah] (or **turbinates**), are scrolled bones in the nasal cavity forming part of the maxillary sinus wall. These are best seen through the opening to the nasal cavity (piriform aperture) (Fig. 1-8). Along with other scrolled processes of the ethmoid bone, they increase the area of mucous membrane inside the nasal cavity to warm and moisten air that we breathe.

9. HYOID BONE

The **hyoid** [HI oid] **bone** (see Fig. 1-23) is not really a bone of the skull but floats alone above the laryngeal prominence of the thyroid cartilage (known to many as the Adam's apple or voice box). All of the bones of the skull, except the mandible and hyoid, are firmly attached to one another by irregular sutures. The hyoid bone is not connected to the bones of the skull except via soft tissue. Muscles extend in a superior direction (suprahyoid muscles) from the hyoid bone to the mandible (e.g., the geniohyoid) and in an inferior direction (infrahyoid muscles) from the hyoid to the sternum (breastbone) and clavicle. Like the bones of the neurocranium, the hyoid bone has a cartilaginous model precursor.

LEARNING QUESTIONS

Select the one best answer.

1. Which of the following bones does not form part of the temporal fossa?
   a. parietal
   b. frontal
   c. sphenoid
   d. temporal
   e. occipital

2. The mental foramen is located where?
   a. on the external surface of the mandible
   b. on the internal surface of the mandible
   c. on the palatal surface of the maxilla
   d. on the external surface of the maxillae
   e. on the sphenoid bone

3. What space does the maxillary nerve pass through immediately after exiting the foramen rotundum?
   a. nasopalatine canal
   b. mandibular canal
   c. maxillary sinus
   d. infraorbital canal
   e. pterygopalatine space

4. What bony process of the maxilla surrounds tooth roots?
   a. nasofrontal process
   b. frontal process
   c. alveolar process
   d. zygomatic process
   e. palatine process

5. Which structures are NOT located on the sphenoid bone?
   a. foramen ovale
   b. foramen rotundum
   c. greater wing
   d. pterygoid process
   e. articular fossa

ANSWERS: 1–e, 2–a, 3–e, 4–c, 5–e

LEARNING EXERCISES

Each of the following bony landmarks can be seen or felt underneath the soft tissue on the face or in the mouth and could be used to describe the location of abnormalities during a clinical examination. First, describe the location, then identify each of the following landmarks on an actual skull (or figures within this text). Use the referenced figures to confirm that you have correctly located each landmark.

- canine eminence of the mandible and maxillae — Figure 1-8
- mental protuberance—Figure 1-8
- maxillary tuberosity—Figure 1-10
- external auditory meatus—Figure 1-7

Each of the following landmarks is the attachment of a major muscle or ligament of importance to the dental professional. First, describe the location, then identify each of the following landmarks on an actual skull (or figures within this text). Use the referenced figures to confirm that you have correctly described the location of the attachment on the skull. When possible, also feel or point to the landmark's location on your own head.

- Angle of the mandible, lateral surface (masseter muscle)—Figure 1-7
- Zygomatic arch (masseter muscle)—Figure 1-7
- Angle of the mandible, medial surface (medial pterygoid muscle)—Figure 1-12
- Medial surface of the lateral pterygoid plate and adjacent pterygoid fossa (medial pterygoid muscle)—Figure 1-5
- Temporal fossa (temporalis muscle)—Figure 1-7
- Coronoid process and temporal crest of mandible (temporalis muscle)—Figure 1-12
- Lateral surface of the lateral pterygoid plate of the sphenoid bone (lateral pterygoid muscle)—Figure 1-6
- Anterior neck of mandibular condyle (lateral pterygoid muscle)—Figure 1-12
- Spine of the sphenoid (sphenomandibular ligament)—Figure 1-5
- Lingula of the mandible (sphenomandibular ligament)—Figure 1-12
- Styloid process (stylomandibular ligament)—Figure 1-5
- Mastoid process (sternocleidomastoid muscle)—Figure 1-7
- Mylohyoid ridge (mylohyoid muscle)—Figure 1-12
- Genial spines (some suprahyoid muscles)—Figure 1-12

Each of the following foramen or spaces is the passageway for nerves and blood vessels of importance to the dental professional. First, describe the location, then identify each of the following foramina or spaces on an actual skull (or figures within this text). Use the referenced figures to confirm that you have correctly located the foramen, canal, or space on the skull.

- foramina rotundum (for the maxillary division of trigeminal nerve)—Figure 1-4
- foramina ovale (for the mandibular division of trigeminal nerve)—Figures 1-4 and 1.5
- mandibular foramina (for the inferior alveolar nerve)—Figure 1-12
- mental foramina (for the mental nerve)—Figure 1-8
- greater palatine foramina (for the greater palatine nerve)—Figure 1-10
- incisive foramen (for the nasopalatine nerve)—Figure 1-10
- pterygopalatine space (for the maxillary division of trigeminal nerve)—Figure 1-6
- infraorbital foramina (for the infraorbital foramen)—Figure 1-8

SECTION III. The Temporomandibular Joint (TMJ)

OBJECTIVES

The objectives for this section are to prepare the reader to perform the following:
- Describe and locate (on a skull) the articulating parts of the temporomandibular joint (TMJ).
- Describe the location and functions of the articular disc.
- Palpate the lateral and posterior surfaces of the condyle of the mandible during movement of the jaws.
- On a skull, describe and locate the attachments of the ligaments of the temporomandibular joint.

A joint, or articulation, is a connection between two separate parts of the skeleton. The **temporomandibular joint** is the articulation between the mandible and the two temporal bones. The mandibular articulation with the skull on each side may also correctly be termed the **craniomandibular articulation**, since it is the articulation between the movable mandible and the stationary cranium or skull.[3] It is a bilateral articulation: the right and left sides work as a unit. It is the only visible free-moving articulation in the head; all others are sutures and are immovable.[4] The coordinated movements of the right and left joints are complex and usually controlled by reflexes. Within some limit or range, the great adaptability of the joints permits the freedom of movement of the mandible required during speech and mastication (chewing). One can learn, however, to move the mandible voluntarily into specific, well-defined positions or pathways.[5-9] Both the maxillae and mandible support teeth whose shape and position greatly influence the most closed portions of mandibular movements.[3] Proper functioning of the temporomandibular joints has a profound effect on the occlusal contacts of teeth which involve nearly all phases of dentistry.

A. ANATOMY OF THE TEMPOROMANDIBULAR JOINT

There are three articulating parts to each temporomandibular joint: the mandibular condyle, the articular fossa with its adjacent eminence (or tubercle) of the temporal bone, and the articular disc interposed between the bony parts (Figs. 1-13 and 1-14). These parts are enclosed by a fibrous connective tissue capsule.[1,4,7]

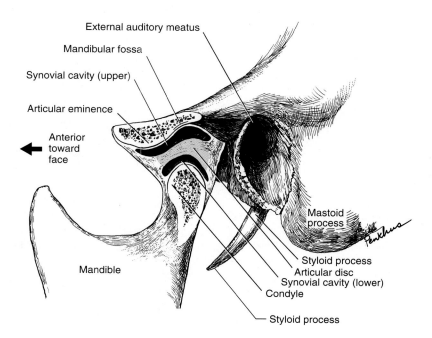

External auditory meatus
Mandibular fossa
Synovial cavity (upper)
Articular eminence
Anterior toward face
Mastoid process
Styloid process
Articular disc
Synovial cavity (lower)
Condyle
Styloid process
Mandible

FIGURE 1-13. Temporomandibular joint, sagittal section. The facial surface is to the left. The sectioned temporal bone (with mandibular fossa and articular eminence) forms the superior part of the joint, and the sectioned head of the condyle forms the inferior part. The articular disc is shaded. The upper and lower synovial cavity surround the disc. (Reproduced by permission from Clemente CD, ed. Gray's anatomy of the human body. 30th ed. Philadelphia: Lea & Febiger, 1985:340.)

Upper space   Disc

Temporal bone   Lower space   Articular fossa   Articular eminence

Loose bilaminar   Condyle   Fibrous covering   Direction of face ➡ (Anterior)

FIGURE 1-14. Temporomandibular joint, photomicrograph of the lateral aspect. Anterior is toward the right of the picture. The white area across the top is the space of the brain case. Notice the thicker **fibrous covering** and underlying compact bone on the **functional** part of the posterior inferior articular eminence and superior, anterior part of the mandibular condyle. [This specimen was removed in a block of tissue, fixed in formalin, demineralized, embedded in celloidin, sectioned at a thickness of about 25 mm, and stained with hematoxylin and eosin.] (Courtesy of Professor Rudy Melfi.)

1. MANDIBULAR CONDYLE

The **mandibular condyle** [KON dile] is about the size and shape of a large date pit with the greater dimension mediolaterally (Fig. 1-15). From the side, it looks like a round knob (Fig. 1-12). From the posterior aspect, it is wide and narrow mediolaterally with a narrow neck. The upper surface of the mandibular condyle is strongly convex anteroposteriorly, and mildly convex mediolaterally. [Note the width of the condyle and its depth beneath the skin in Figure 1-15. It is a large solid structure, about 10 mm thick anteroposteriorly and 20.4 mm wide mediolaterally. Although the average depth of the outer surface of the condyle is 15 mm beneath the skin, it is readily palpated, and its movements are visible (seemingly just beneath the skin) when eating. Research by Drs. Woelfel and Igarashi on 25

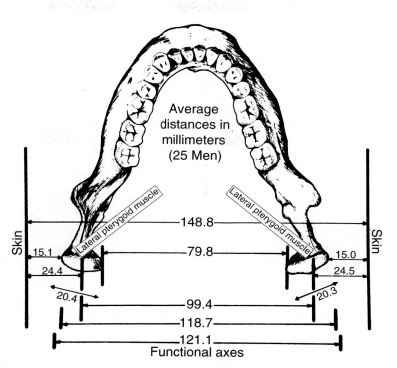

FIGURE 1-15. Depth (beneath the skin) of the landmarks of the head of the mandibular condyle and relative **direction of the lateral pterygoid muscle** fibers from their insertion on the neck of the condyle toward their origin (not seen, but on the pterygoid fossa of the sphenoid bone). [To obtain these measurements, metal markers were placed on the skin and some teeth on 25 men prior to taking submental vertex cephalometric radiographs for analysis, tracing, and measuring. The location of the center of rotational opening of the mandible (the hinge axis) was found to pass through or near the center of the heads of the condyles. The functional axes were determined from pantographic recordings. Resultant articular settings were found to be wider than the outer poles of the condyles. This means that lateral and protrusive excursions are controlled by ligaments and muscles, rather than by bone, as previously reported. This research was conducted by Drs. Woelfel and Igarashi and supported by the Ohio State University College of Dentistry and Nihon University School of Dentistry in Tokyo.]

men found the average depth of the outer surface of the mandibular condyle on each side to be 15.0 mm; the range was 10.3–21.4 mm beneath skin.]

Carefully examine the photomicrograph of a human temporomandibular joint seen in Figure 1-14. The condyle is in the position it would occupy when the teeth come together as tightly and as comfortably as possible (maximum intercuspation), about 1 mm anterior to its most retruded position. The functioning regions are covered with fibrous connective tissue. The fibrous layers of the joint and the disc are avascular (devoid of blood vessels and nerves),[10] indicating that considerable force occurs on these surfaces of the joint. This fibrous, avascular type of connective tissue is adapted to resist pressure. It is particularly thick on top of the condyle over the region where most function occurs when the condyle is forward from its resting position, as when we bite our front teeth or incisors together. Notice on the photomicrograph that this same type of fibrous covering lines the head of the condyle (superior and anterior surfaces), the posterior articulating surfaces of the articular eminence and adjacent fossa, as well as the center portion of the disc.

2. ARTICULAR FOSSA (NONFUNCTIONING PORTION) AND ARTICULAR EMINENCE (FUNCTIONING PORTION)

Study the right side of Figure 1-5 where half of the mandible has been removed, exposing the maxillary teeth, tuberosity, and articular fossa and eminence. The **articular** (glenoid) **fossa** (the anterior three-fourths of the larger **mandibular fossa**) is considered to be a nonfunctioning portion of the joint because, when the teeth are in tight occlusion, there is no tight contact among the head of the condyle, the disc, and the concave part of the articular fossa. [The fossa is about 23 mm mediolaterally and extends 15 mm posteriorly from the eminence. The intracapsular surface area is two to three times greater than on the very mobile mandibular condyle. The anterior part of the capsule attaches 10 mm in front of the crest of the articulating eminence.[11]]

The **articular eminence** or transverse bony ridge is located just anterior and inferior to the articular fossa (Fig. 1-13). As stated earlier, its surface is padded or lined by a thickened layer of fibrous connective tissue, more than the rest of the articular fossa, indicating that this is the functional portion of the joint when we are chewing food with the mandible in a protruded and/or lateral position. The thickest functional part of this lining is on the posterior inferior portion of the articular eminence. This is where the anterior-superior portion of the mandibular condyle rubs against it, but only indirectly since the articular disc is normally interposed between the two functioning bony elements.

3. ARTICULAR DISC

Examine a skull with the posterior teeth fitting together (in occlusion) and study how the mandibular condyle fits loosely into the articular fossa. The disc is not present in a prepared dry skull because the disc is not bone. There should be a visible space between the mandibular condyle and the articular fossa that in life was occupied by the disc.

The disc (Figs. 1-13 and 1-14) is a tough oval pad of dense fibrous connective tissue acting as a shock absorber between the mandibular condyle and the articular fossa and articular eminence. The disc surfaces are very smooth. It is thinner in the center than around the edges. Its periphery is thinner anteriorly and laterally but thicker medially and posteriorly. Rarely, it may become perforated. The center of the disc has no blood supply[10]; however, it is richly supplied elsewhere.

The *upper* contour of the disc is concave-convex anteroposteriorly to conform to the shape of the articular eminence and fossa. In other words, it is concave anteriorly to fit under the articular eminence, and convex posteriorly, conforming to the shape of the articular fossa that it loosely rests against. The *lower* surface of the disc is concave in both directions, thus adapting to the upper surface of the convex mandibular condyle.

The disc forms one natural wedge anterior to the condyle head and a second wedge posterior to the condyle. Because of the extremely slippery surfaces, these two wedge portions help the disc move harmoniously with the condyle. When the wedge portions become flattened or the center of the disc thickens, the disc fails to move synchronously with the condyle, resulting in popping or grating noise (**crepitus**), which is quite annoying yet a fairly common occurrence (Table 1-2). With an elastic posterior attachment, the disc moves with the head of the condyle during function but only about half as far.

The articular disc has many functions.[11,12] It divides the space between the head of the condyle and the articulating fossa into upper and lower spaces (synovial cavities seen in Fig. 1-13), which permits complex functional movements of the mandible.[12] Because the anterior and posterior portions of the disc contain some specialized nerve fibers called **proprioceptive** [PRO pri o SEP tiv] **fibers,** which help unconsciously to determine the position of the mandible, the disc helps regulate

Table 1-2

PREVALENCE OF CREPITUS DURING MAXIMUM OPENING*

	NONE (%)	BOTH SIDES (%)	RIGHT SIDE (%)	LEFT SIDE (%)	ONE SIDE (R OR L) (%)
594 Dental hygiene students	52.0	13.3	18.2	16.8	35.0
505 Dental students	72.0	4.2	15.9	7.9	23.8
Percentage of all 1099 students	61.2	9.1	17.1	12.7	29.8

* Determinations by Dr. Woelfel, 1970–1986. More than 20% of these professional students had or were undergoing orthodontic treatment.

movements of the condyle. It stabilizes the condyle by filling the space between incongruous articulating surfaces of the convex condyle and concave-convex articular fossa and articular eminence.[12] The disc cushions the loading of the joint at the point of contact (like a shock absorber). The cushioning and lubrication reduce physical wear and strain on joint surfaces. The lining of the capsule surrounding the disc produces synovial fluid that lubricates the movement of the joint.

B. LIGAMENTS THAT SUPPORT THE JOINT AND LIMIT JOINT MOVEMENT

Ligaments are slightly elastic bands of tissue. They do *not* move the joint; muscles move the joint. They do support and confine the movement of the mandible to protect muscles from being stretched beyond their capabilities.

1. FIBROUS CAPSULE (CAPSULAR LIGAMENT)

The **fibrous (or articular) capsule** is a fibrous tube of tissue that encloses the joint best seen in Figures 1-16 and 1-17. It is fairly thin, except laterally, where the thicker **lateral** (formerly temporomandibular) **ligament** is located.[13] The upper border of the capsule is attached to the temporal bone around the circumference of the articular fossa and the articular eminence. The lower border is attached around the neck of the condyloid process, thus enclosing the condyle and completing the tube.

The internal surface of the fibrous capsule is lined with a **synovial** [si NO vee al] **membrane** that covers the bones to the borderline of their articulating surfaces and part of the mandibular neck. This thin membrane secretes a fluid, **synovia**, which lubricates the joint. The coefficient of friction of this fluid makes it three times more slippery than ice. The synovial fluid both lubricates and nourishes the fibrous covering of the articulating surfaces and center of the disc, which lack a blood supply. In a normal joint space, there is only a small amount of fluid (1 or 2 drops).

The articular disc is not attached to the skull, but anteriorly it is attached to the fibrous capsule. Posteriorly, the disc and the capsule are connected by a thick pad of loose elastic vascular connective tissue called the bilaminar zone (Fig.1-14). Laterally and medially, the disc is tightly attached to the lateral and medial sides of the mandibular condyle but not to the capsule. Therefore, the disc follows the movement of the condyle when the lateral pterygoid muscles move the mandible and disc forward or sideways. This design of attachments gives the disc freedom to move anteriorly but limits it from excessive forward movement that could result in its displacement anterior to the head of the condyle.[14]

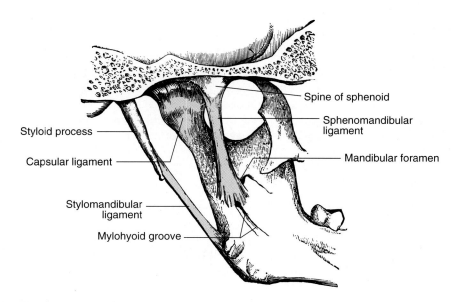

FIGURE 1-16. **Ligaments of the temporomandibular joint** attaching to the medial aspect of the mandible. The fibrous capsule (capsular ligament) surrounds the joint. (Reproduced by permission from Clemente CD, ed. Gray's anatomy of the human body. 30th ed. Philadelphia: Lea & Febiger, 1985:339.)

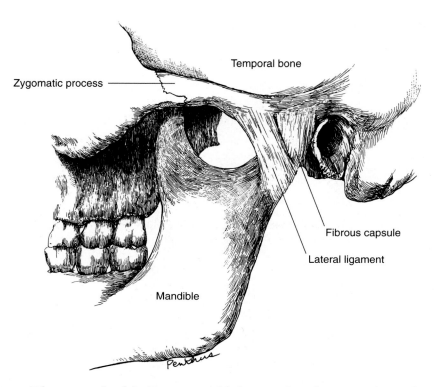

FIGURE 1-17. **Fibrous capsule of the Temporomandibular Joint**, lateral aspect, enclosing the joint, and the thickened, outer **lateral ligament**. (Reproduced by permission from Clemente CD, ed. Gray's anatomy of the human body. 30th ed. Philadelphia: Lea & Febiger, 1985:339.)

The outer layer of the fibrous capsule is a thicker layer of fibrous tissue that is reinforced by accessory ligaments, which strengthen it. The anterior part of this fibrous capsule restricts posterior movement of the condyle of the mandible on wide openings as it becomes taut.

2. LATERAL LIGAMENT (FORMERLY TMJ LIGAMENT)

The **lateral ligament** of the joint is the strong reinforcement of the anterior lateral wall of the capsule (Fig. 1-17). It attaches to the zygomatic arch, then narrows as it drops obliquely down and backward to the lateral and posterior neck of the condyle. It keeps the condyle close to the fossa and helps to prevent lateral and posterior displacement of the mandible. It has no counterpart medially, and seemingly none is needed, since the right and left temporomandibular articulations work together as a unit. The lateral ligament on the opposite side, by failing to stretch, prevents excess medial displacement on the side moving medially.

3. STYLOMANDIBULAR LIGAMENT

The **stylomandibular** [STY lo man DIB yoo lar] **ligament** is posterior to the joint but also gives support to the mandible (Fig. 1-16). It is relaxed when the mouth is closed but becomes tense on extreme protrusion of the mandible.[13] It is attached above to the styloid process of the temporal bone and below to the posterior border and angle of the mandible.

4. SPHENOMANDIBULAR LIGAMENT

The **sphenomandibular** [SFE no man DIB yoo lar] **ligament** is medial to the joint (Fig. 1-16). It gives some support to the mandible and may help limit maximum opening of the jaw. It is attached above to the angular (sphenoidal) spine of the sphenoid bone. Then it spreads out like a fan and attaches on the lingula of the mandible near the mandibular foramen.

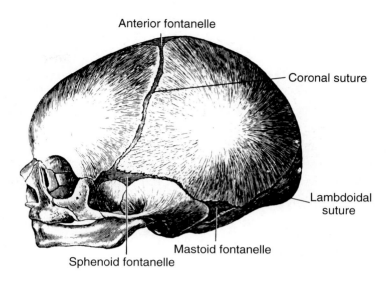

Anterior fontanelle

Coronal suture

Lambdoidal suture

Mastoid fontanelle

Sphenoid fontanelle

FIGURE 1-18. Skull at birth showing fontanelles (membrane-covered openings between bones). Notice that the mandibular condyle is barely higher than the crest of the mandibular ridge.

C. DEVELOPMENT OF THE TEMPOROMANDIBULAR JOINT

In infants, the articular fossa, the articular eminence, and the condyle are rather flat. This flatness allows for a wide range of sliding motions in the temporomandibular joint. Also, this joint is at about the same level as the occlusal plane at birth with relatively no ramus height (Fig. 1-18). During growth, the articular fossa deepens, the articular eminence becomes prominent, the condyle becomes rounded, and the shape of the disc changes to conform to the change in shape of the fossa and condyle. There is also a downward lengthening of the ramus. The condyle contains cartilage beneath its surface, and the condyloid process and ramus lengthen until a person is 20–25 years old. This is one way the mandible grows in depth. As a result of growth in the condyle area, the body of the mandible is lowered from the skull, and the occlusal plane is located about one inch below the level of the condyles in an adult.

LEARNING EXERCISE

Study a skull and see how the mandibular condyle fits into the mandibular fossa. When you examine the fit, notice the space between the mandibular condyles and the articular fossae when the posterior teeth are in tight occlusion. This space is where the disc would have been in life. The condyle, with the disc superimposed and attached to its neck medially and laterally, functions in the anterior part of this fossa. (The anterior part of the mandibular fossa is called the articular fossa.)

On yourself, palpate the temporomandibular joint and feel the movement of the mandibular condyle. First, put your index finger immediately in front of either ear and open and close your mouth. Then move your jaw to the right and left sides. You are feeling the movement of the outer pole (surface) of each mandibular condyle. Next, place your little finger gently inside either ear opening, then open and close your mouth and pull your jaw back or posteriorly. You are feeling the upper and posterior portion of the mandibular condyle, especially when you close or retrude (pull back) your mandible.

LEARNING QUESTIONS

Select the one best answer.

1. What two structures articulate in the temporomandibular joint?
    a. the coronoid process of the mandible with the mandibular fossa of the temporal bone
    b. the condyloid process of the mandible with the mandibular fossa of the temporal bone
    c. the coronoid process of the mandible with the mandibular fossa of the sphenoid bone
    d. the condyloid process of the mandible with the mandibular fossa of the sphenoid bone
    e. the condyloid process of the mandible with the mandibular fossa of the maxillae
2. The ligament that limits the amount of movement of the mandible and attaches from the inferior surface of the neurocranium to the lingula of the mandible is the:
    a. lateral (TMJ) ligament
    b. stylomandibular ligament
    c. sphenomandibular ligament
    d. sternocleidomastoid ligament
3. Where on the temporal bone does the mandible function?
    a. in the anterior third of the mandibular fossa called the articular fossa
    b. in the posterior third of the mandibular fossa called the articular fossa
    c. the posterior inferior portion of the articular eminence
    d. the anterior inferior position of the articular eminence

ANSWERS: 1–b, 2–c, 3–c

SECTION IV. Muscles of Chewing (Mastication)

OBJECTIVES

The objectives for this section are to prepare the reader to perform the following:
*   Identify the four pairs of muscles of mastication.
*   Describe and identify the origin and insertion of each of these muscles of mastication on a skull and be able to palpate each (if possible) on yourself or a partner.
*   Describe and demonstrate the function of each of these muscles.
*   List other factors that contribute to the position of teeth and movement of the mandible.
*   Describe the location and list the functions of the groups of muscles that contribute to facial expression.

The following general terms relate to muscles and will be helpful to know as you read this section:

anguli [ANG gu li]: triangular area or angle of a structure
depressor: acts to depress or make lower
insertion of the muscles of mastication: place of attachment of muscles to the bone that moves, like muscle attachment on the movable mandible
labial [LAY bee al]: related to the lips like the labial surface of a tooth
levator [le VA tor]: acts to raise (cf. elevator)
lingual [LIN gwal]: related to the tongue; for example, the lingual nerve innervates the tongue; the lingual muscle is within the tongue; and the lingual surface of a tooth is the side toward the tongue.

mental: referring to the chin; the mental foramen is the hole in the mandible where the mental nerve passes out of the mandible to the chin; the mentalis muscle inserts into the chin[1]

orbicularis [or BIK u lar is]: round; compare an orbit

origin (of muscles of mastication): are the source, beginning or fixed proximal end attachment of a muscle as compared to its insertion, which is a muscle's more movable attachment or distal end[1]

oris: referring to the edge of the mouth; compare oral

procerus [pro SE rus]: long and slender

The muscles of the body contribute 40–50% of the total body weight.[15] Muscles produce the desired action by pulling or by shortening, never by pushing or by lengthening. **Skeletal** or **voluntary muscles** are made up of specialized cells that contract. Skeletal muscles are very active metabolically and therefore require a rich blood supply.[15] There are two other kinds of muscles, **cardiac and smooth (involuntary) muscles**, which we are unable to control or direct.

Muscle cells are small (10–40 microns [μm] in diameter), elongated contractile fibers, each enclosed in a delicate envelope of loose connective tissue. Many individual parallel muscle fibers make up a bundle, and various numbers of bundles comprise a muscle. The longest muscle fibers are 300 mm (11.4 inches) long. Each contractile bundle of cells can contract about 57% of its fully stretched length.[16] The all-or-none law states that any single muscle *fiber* always contracts to its fullest extent.[11] When a weak effort or contraction is required of the whole muscle, then only a few fibers contract (each to the fullest extent). Many fibers contracting produce greater power as needed. No single muscle acts alone to produce a movement or to maintain posture. Many muscles must work in perfect coordination to produce a steady, well-directed motion of a body part.

When a muscle becomes shorter as it moves a structure, the movement is called an **isotonic contraction**. When a muscle maintains its length as it contracts to stabilize a part, this movement is called **isometric contraction**. As you close your jaw until all teeth contact, the closing muscles work isotonically because they become shorter as the mandible moves superiorly. If you maintain contact of all of your teeth but squeeze them together hard, these same muscles are contracting isometrically because they cannot shorten any more once your teeth are together.

Some portions (a few or more individual muscles fibers) of all of our voluntary muscles are continually or alternately contracting during consciousness. This minimal amount of contraction needed to maintain posture is called muscle **tone** or **tonus**, and the muscles involved are named "antigravity" muscles. As you read this, the muscles of mastication are probably in a state of minimal tonic contraction or balance with each other, with the neck muscles, and with gravity, enabling a comfortable, restful position for your mandible with the teeth apart. This normal resting jaw position varies slightly according to whether you are sitting, lying on your back, or standing up, and depending on how tense or stressed you are. Hopefully, this brief discussion will whet your appetite for seeking further knowledge. The list of references at the end of this chapter offers several choices.

A. MUSCLES INVOLVED IN MASTICATION (CHEWING)

Muscles of mastication move the mandible. They include four pairs of muscles (right and left): masseter, temporalis, medial pterygoid, and lateral pterygoid muscles. These muscles have the major control over the movements of the mandible. Each of these muscles has one end named its origin and the other end named its insertion. The **origin end** of each of the muscles of mastication is the source, beginning or fixed proximal attachment located, in this case, on the bones of the neurocranium, which are relatively immovable. The **insertion end** is the attachment on the movable bone that in this case is attached to, and moves, the mandible.

There are five different ways the mandible moves. We can **elevate** it (closing the mouth), **depress** it (opening the mouth, **retrude** it (retracting or pulling back the mandible), **protrude** it (protracting or moving the mandible anteriorly), and move it into **lateral excursions** (moving the mandible sideways as in chewing).

1. MASSETER MUSCLE

The **masseter** [ma SEE ter] **muscle** (Fig. 1-19) is the largest, most superficial, bulky, and powerful of the muscles of mastication. It is quadrilateral in shape. [Its average volume on 25 males was 30.4 $\pm$ 4.1 cm^3, which was 2.6 times larger than the medial pterygoid muscle (second largest one at 11.5 $\pm$ 2.1 cm^3).[17]]

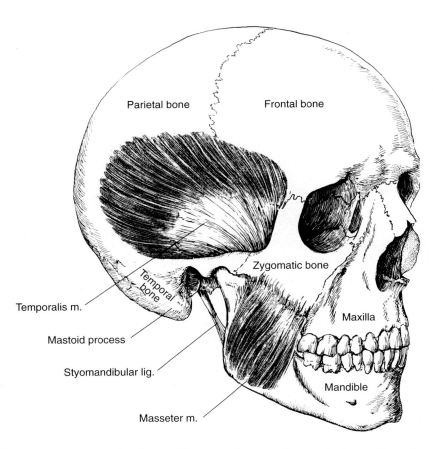

FIGURE 1-19. **Masseter muscle** below and fan-shaped **temporalis muscle** above. (Reproduced by permission from Clemente CD, ed. Gray's anatomy of the human body. 30th ed. Philadelphia: Lea & Febiger, 1985:450.)

Origin: The masseter arises from the inferior and medial surfaces of the zygomatic bone, the zygomatic process of the maxillae, and the temporal process of zygomatic bone (collectively known as the zygomatic arch). From here it extends inferiorly and posteriorly toward its insertion.

Insertion: The masseter inserts on the inferior lateral surface of the ramus and angle of the mandible.

Action: It **elevates** the mandible (closes the mouth) and applies great power in crushing food.[6,8,9]

LEARNING EXERCISE

As you clench your teeth several times, feel the contraction of the masseter by placing a finger on the outside of your cheek posterior to the third molar region. The muscle will produce a noticeable bulge beneath your finger each time.

---

2. TEMPORALIS MUSCLE

The **temporalis** [tem po RA lis] **muscle** is a fan-shaped, large but flat muscle with both vertical anterior (and middle) fibers and more horizontal posterior vertical fibers. Vertical and horizontal fibers are shaded in Figure 1-20.

Origin: The temporalis arises from the entire temporalis fossa (Fig. 1-7) (comprised of the squamous part of temporal bones and the greater wing of the sphenoid bones and the adjacent portions of

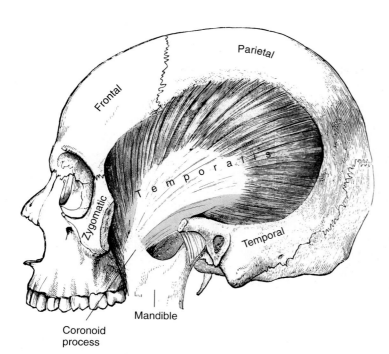

Coronoid
process

Mandible

FIGURE 1-20. Temporalis muscle: vertical (anterior) and horizontal (posterior) fibers. The zygomatic process of the temporal bone and temporal process of the zygomatic bones have been removed. Contraction of the anterior vertically oriented fibers of the temporal muscle act to close the jaw; contraction of the posteriorly placed horizontally oriented fibers act to pull the jaw back or to retract (retrude) the mandible. (Reproduced by permission from Clemente CD, ed. Gray's anatomy of the human body. 30th ed. Philadelphia: Lea & Febiger, 1985:449.)

the frontal and parietal bones). From here, its **anterior** (and middle) fibers are directed vertically downward while its **posterior** fibers are directed more horizontally, mostly anteriorly and somewhat inferiorly, passing medial to the zygomatic arch.

Insertion: The temporalis inserts on the coronoid process of the mandible, medial surface of the anterior border of the ramus, and the temporal crest of the mandible (Fig. 1-12) via one common tendon.

Action: The **anterior** (and middle) vertical fibers contract to act to **elevate** the mandible (close the jaw) especially when great power is not required, and the **posterior** horizontal fibers **retrude** or pull the mandible posteriorly.[6,8,9]

LEARNING EXERCISE

Feel contraction of the temporalis by placing several fingers above and in front of your ear to feel the vertical fibers contract as you gently close your teeth together several times. Then feel the nearly horizontal fibers just above and behind your ears contract as you retrude or pull your mandible posteriorly. This may be more difficult to feel since the bulge is less evident.

3. MEDIAL PTERYGOID MUSCLE

The **medial pterygoid** [TER i goid] **muscle** is located on the medial surface of the ramus (Figs. 1.21 and 1.22). Along with the masseter located on the lateral surface, these two muscles serve as a sling, one on each side of the mandible, and result in similar actions.

Origin: The medial pterygoid muscle arises mainly from the medial surface of the lateral pterygoid plate and the pterygoid fossa between the medial and lateral pterygoid plates (Fig. 1-5) of the sphenoid bone. [Also from the pyramidal process of the palatine bone, with a few fibers to the maxillary tuberosity.[3]] Similar to the masseter, the fibers pass from their origin inferiorly and posteriorly (but laterally) toward their insertion.

Insertion: The medial pterygoid muscle inserts on the medial surface of the mandible in a triangular region at the angle and on the superior adjacent portions of the ramus just above the angle.

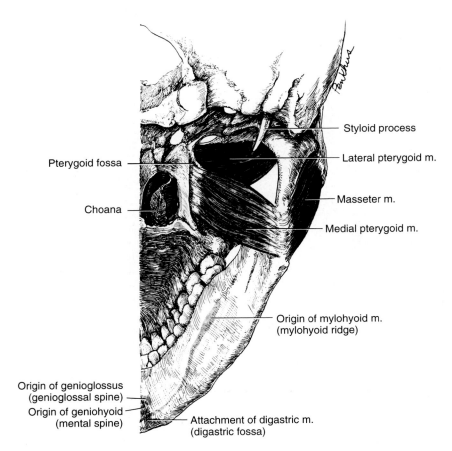

Pterygoid fossa

Choana

Origin of genioglossus
(genioglossal spine)
Origin of geniohyoid
(mental spine)

Styloid process

Lateral pterygoid m.

Masseter m.

Medial pterygoid m.

Origin of mylohyoid m.
(mylohyoid ridge)

Attachment of digastric m.
(digastric fossa)

FIGURE 1-21. The **pterygoid and masseter muscles**, inferior view. Note how the medial pterygoid and masseter muscles form a sling that support the mandible. Also from this view, it is clear that the **lateral pterygoid** muscle has its origin (on the base of the cranium) more medial than its insertion (on the anterior portion of the head of the condyle and articular disc). If this muscle contracts only on the right side, that condyle of the mandible moves toward its origin, thus bodily moving the mandible toward the left or opposite side. (Reproduced by permission from Clemente CD, ed. Gray's anatomy of the human body. 30th ed. Philadelphia: Lea & Febiger, 1985:452.)

Action: It **elevates** the mandible (closes jaw) like the anterior (and middle) fibers of the temporalis and masseter muscles. Although not as large or powerful, it is a synergist of (i.e., works together with) the larger masseter muscle in helping apply the power or great force on closures.

4. **LATERAL PTERYGOID MUSCLE**

The **lateral pterygoid muscle**, unlike the other three pairs of muscles where fibers are oriented primarily vertically, has its fibers aligned mostly horizontally (Fig. 1-22). The lateral pterygoid muscle is a short, thick, somewhat conical muscle located deep in the infratemporal fossa (inferior to the temporal bone and posterior to the maxillae) and is the prime mover of the mandible except for closing the jaw.

Origin: The lateral pterygoid muscle arises from two heads, both located on the sphenoid bone. The smaller superior head is attached to the infratemporal surface of the greater wing of the sphenoid bone; the larger inferior head is attached to the adjacent lateral surface of the lateral pterygoid plate on the sphenoid bone. Fibers pass posteriorly and laterally in a horizontal direction toward their in-

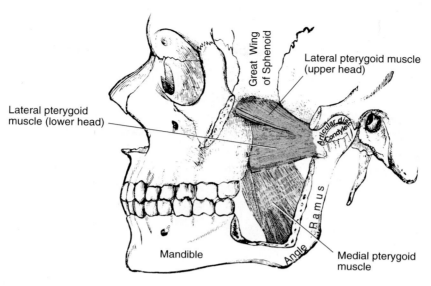

FIGURE 1-22. Medial pterygoid muscle and two heads of lateral pterygoid muscle with zygomatic arch and the anterior part of the ramus removed. Notice the horizontal orientation of the lateral pterygoid fibers (shaded in red) in direct contrast to the vertical direction of the medial pterygoid fibers. Contraction of the medial pterygoid muscle in harmony with the masseter elevates (closes) the mandible. Simultaneous contraction of both lateral pterygoid muscles pulls the condyle (and disc) forward, which causes the mouth to protrude and open. (Reproduced by permission from Clemente CD, ed. Gray's anatomy of the human body. 30th ed. Philadelphia: Lea & Febiger, 1985:451.)

sertion. The direction of these fibers, from their insertion on the anterior surfaces of the heads of the mandibular condyles, is represented by the "lateral pterygoid muscle" labels in Figure 1-15.

Insertion: The lateral pterygoid muscle inserts on the depression on the front of the neck of the condyloid process called the pterygoid fovea (Fig. 1-12) and into the anterior margin of the articular disc. Minor forward contractions of the upper head pulling the disc forward work in concert with the stretching of the elastic band of tissues behind the disc (retrodiscal tissues) permit the disc to accompany the mandible as it moves forward, preventing posterior displacement of the disc.[14]

Actions: When *both lateral pterygoids* contract simultaneously, the action is:

- to **protrude** the mandible. No other muscle or groups of muscles are capable of doing this but can only assist in this action as stabilizers or by controlling the degree of jaw opening during the protrusion.[5,6,8,9,18]

- to **depress** the mandible. They do this by pulling the articular discs and the condyles forward and down onto the articular eminences, which moves the mandible inferiorly and helps rotate it, thereby opening the mouth. The lateral pterygoids are assisted somewhat in this task by other muscles (suprahyoids and infrahyoids).

- When *only one lateral pterygoid* contracts, it pulls the condyle on that side medialward and anteriorly, moving the body of the mandible and its teeth toward the opposite side (since the origin of the lateral pterygoid muscle is medial to its insertion). For example, contraction of the left lateral pterygoid muscle draws the left condyle medially (to the right) and forward, causing the mandible to move toward the right side (into **right lateral excursion**).[8] Conversely, the contraction of the right lateral pterygoid muscle causes the mandible to move to the left side (**left lateral excursion**).[8] No other muscle is capable of moving the mandible sideways, although synergistic (in harmony with) unilateral contraction of the posterior fibers of the temporalis muscle occurs on the side toward which the jaw moves.[8]

LEARNING EXERCISE

Viewing the inferior surface of a skull with movable mandible, imagine elastic bands attached from the location of the origins to the insertions of the lateral pterygoid muscles, right and left side. Since the origin on the base of the skull stays stationary, but the mandible at the insertion can move, confirm that the mandible moves anterior and inferior if both elastic bands were contracted (shortened). Next, see what would happen if only one band was shortened (contracted). If only the right side were shortened, the right condyle would move medially (to the left), closer to its origin on the lateral pterygoid plate, so the body of the mandible and its teeth would also move toward the left side. Practice this until you understand why the jaw moves the way it does when one lateral pterygoid muscle works.

B. OTHER MUSCLES AFFECTING MANDIBULAR MOVEMENT

Other muscles affecting mandibular movement include the suprahyoid and infrahyoid group of muscles. The **suprahyoid** [SOO prah HI oid] **muscle group** extends from the superior surface of the hyoid bone to the mandible, whereas the **infrahyoid muscle group** extends from the inferior surface of the hyoid bone to the clavicle (collarbone) and sternum (breast bone) (Fig. 1-23). The inferior hyoid muscles must stabilize the hyoid bone in order for the suprahyoid muscles to move the mandible. These muscle groups act together with both lateral pterygoid muscles to help depress the mandible (open the mouth), and act with the posterior (horizontal) fibers of the temporalis muscles to retrude (pull back) the mandible.

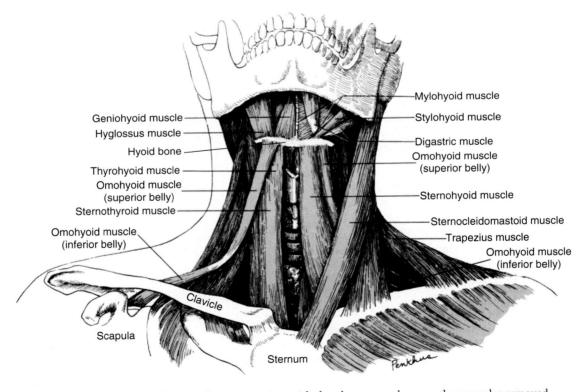

FIGURE 1-23. Muscles of the neck, anterior view, with the platysma and some other muscles removed. Note the **hyoid bone** with some muscles superior to it attaching to the mandible (the **suprahyoid muscle group**) and some muscles attaching inferior to the clavicle and sternum (the **infrahyoid muscle group**). Working together, these muscle groups can help open and retrude the mandible. (Reproduced by permission from Clemente CD, ed. Gray's anatomy of the human body. 30th ed. Philadelphia: Lea & Febiger, 1985:451.)

The suprahyoid muscles include the **stylohyoid** [STY lo HI oid] muscles (which arise on the styloid process), **digastric** [di GAS trik] (the anterior bellies attach near the genial spines or tubercles), **mylohyoid** (arising from the mylohyoid ridges on each half of the medial surface of the mandible and found inferior to the floor of the mouth), and **geniohyoid** [JEE ni o HI oid] (arising from the genial tubercles). The infrahyoid muscles include the **sternohyoid**, **sternothyroid**, **thyrohyoid**, and **omohyoid** muscles that arise from the clavicle (collarbone), sternum (breastbone), and adjacent structures.

C. OTHER FACTORS AFFECTING TOOTH POSITION OR MOVEMENT

Other factors affecting relative tooth positions and movements include the ligaments, fascia, and to a certain extent, the muscles of facial expression. The **ligaments**, including the capsular, temporomandibular, stylomandibular, and sphenomandibular ligaments (Figs. 1-16 and 1-17), provide some limits to protrusive, lateral, and opening movements of the mandible.

Fascia [FASH e ah] is also thought to limit movement of the mandible to some extent. Fascia is connective tissue that forms sheets or bands between anatomic structures. It attaches to bones and surrounds muscles, glands, vessels, nerves, and fat.

Some **muscles of facial expression** (especially in the lips and cheeks) and the tongue muscles are thought to influence development, position, and shape of the dental arches. The muscles of facial expression are shown in Fig. 1-24 and include the following:

FIGURE 1-24. The muscles of facial expression. (Reproduced by permission from Clemente CD, ed. Gray's anatomy of the human body. 30th ed. Philadelphia: Lea & Febiger, 1985:444.)

- **Orbicularis oris** [or BIK u LAR is O ris] is located within the lips around the opening of the mouth and acts to close or purse the lips (as around a straw or around a saliva ejector within the dental office).
- **Buccinator** [BUCK si na tor] attaches on the buccinator crest of the mandible and adjacent soft tissue forming a pouch in the cheeks. When contracting, it pulls the cheek inward to keep food on the chewing surfaces of teeth during chewing.
- *Upper oral group* includes the **zygomaticus** [ZI go MAT i kus] **major and minor, levator labii** [LAB e e] **superioris,** and **levator anguli oris.** All contribute to raising the upper lip and/or angle, as in smiling. The **risorius** [ri SO ri us] retracts (spreads) the angle of the mouth. The **levator anguli oris alaeque** [a LY kwe] **nasi** dilates the nostrils, as in contempt.
- *Lower oral group* (including the **depressor labii inferior** and **depressor anguli oris**) contracts to lower the lower lip or angle, as in a frown. The **mentalis** [men TA lis] is located in the chin and raises or protrudes the chin as in a pout.
- *Nose muscles* include the **nasalis** [na SA lis], which flares the nostrils; the **depressor septi nasi,** which pulls the nares down thereby constricting the opening of the nose (nares); and the **procerus** [pro SE rus] over the bridge of the nose, which lowers the medial eyebrow and wrinkles the nose.
- *Eye muscles* include the **orbicularis oculi** [or BIK u lar is AHK u li], which surrounds the eye and acts to squint the eye, while the **corrugator supercilii** [COR u gay tor su per SIL e e] draws the medial end of the eyebrow down, as in a frown.
- *Ear muscles* include the **posterior, superior,** and **anterior auricular** [aw RIK u lar] muscles, which act to move the ears and/or scalp. Can you wiggle your ears by contracting these muscles? Give it a try.
- The **occipitofrontalis** [ahk SIP i toe fron TAL is] (or epicranial) muscle draws back the scalp, wrinkling the forehead and raising the eyebrows, as in surprise.
- The **platysma** [plah TIZ mah] muscle is a broad muscle that extends from the mouth to the anterior and lateral surfaces of the neck and contacts during a grimace.

The posterior and deep muscles of the neck, as well as the overlying fascia and skin, all have a slight postural influence on the physiologic resting position of the mandible. Other than this, the numerous facial muscles, including the buccinator, do *not* influence any movements of the mandible. However, a person's posture, state of mind, stress, health, and physical and mental fatigue each have a decided effect on the resting posture of the mandible at any given time.[19]

D. SUMMARY OF MUSCLES THAT MOVE AND CONTROL THE MANDIBLE

There are five specifically different ways that we can voluntarily move our mandible. There are limitless combinations of these movements that occur throughout any 24 hours. In review, here are the muscles that contribute to each movement:

1. ELEVATION

Elevation (closing the mouth) results from the bilateral contraction of three pairs of muscles. Right and left temporalis muscles (vertical fibers) bring the mandible upward into position for crushing food. The temporalis muscles are primarily the *positioning* muscles, as they elevate the mandible upward until it is in position to have the real force applied by the other two pairs of closing muscles. Right and left masseter muscles and right and left medial pterygoid muscles act together to apply the power for forceful jaw closures, as in crushing food, such as biting through a carrot.

2. DEPRESSION

Depression (opening of mouth) results primarily from the bilateral contraction of both lateral pterygoid muscles, assisted by suprahyoid and infrahyoid muscles, especially the anterior bellies of the digastric muscles and the omohyoid (infrahyoid) muscles, which help fix or hold the hyoid bone.

3. RETRUSION

Retrusion (retracting the jaw) results from the bilateral contraction of the posterior fibers of the temporalis muscles assisted by the suprahyoids, especially the digastric muscles (anterior and posterior bellies).

4. PROTRUSION

Protrusion (or protraction, protruding the jaw) results from the simultaneous contraction of the right and left lateral pterygoid muscles.

5. LATERAL EXCURSION

Lateral excursion (move sideways) results from the contraction of one lateral pterygoid muscle (the mandible is moved bodily to the left by the contraction of the right lateral pterygoid muscle).[8,20]

LEARNING QUESTIONS

Select the one best answer.

1. Which muscle has its origin in the pterygoid fossa?
   a. medial pterygoid muscle
   b. lateral pterygoid muscle
   c. masseter
   d. temporalis muscle

2. The masseter muscle elevates the mandible. Which other muscles are involved in elevating the mandible?
   a. temporalis (anterior fibers) and lateral pterygoid muscles
   b. lateral pterygoid muscles and medial pterygoid muscles
   c. temporalis (posterior and anterior fibers) and medial pterygoid muscles
   d. medial pterygoid muscles and temporalis (anterior fibers)
   e. lateral pterygoid muscles and temporalis (posterior fibers)

3. In which direction do the fibers of the lateral pterygoid muscles travel from their origin to their insertion?
   a. medial and posterior
   b. medial and anterior
   c. lateral and anterior
   d. lateral and posterior

4. Which of the following muscles of facial expression does NOT contribute to moving the lips?
   a. orbicularis oris
   b. risorius
   c. levator labii superioris
   d. depressor labii inferioris
   e. orbicularis oculi

5. Which of the following would you palpate just anterior and superior to the ear?
   a. masseter, the origin
   b. masseter, the insertion
   c. temporalis, posterior fibers
   d. temporalis, anterior fibers
   e. temporalis, the insertion

ANSWERS: 1–a, 2–d, 3–d, 4–e, 5–d.

SECTION V. Nerves of the Oral Cavity

OBJECTIVES

The objectives for this section are to prepare the reader to perform the following:
- List the twelve cranial nerves and briefly describe their function.
- Describe in depth the important branches of the trigeminal nerve and trace the route of each important branch from the brain to the structures that they innervate in the oral cavity.
- Describe the pathway to the oral cavity of the facial nerve and identify the oral structure(s) it innervates (both motor and sensory).
- Describe the pathway to the oral cavity of the glossopharyngeal nerve and identify the oral structure(s) it innervates.
- Describe the pathway to the oral cavity of the hypoglossal nerve and identify the oral structure(s) it innervates.

There are several types of nerve fibers based on their function. **Afferent** [AF er ent] (or **sensory**) fibers convey impulses (such as feeling, touch, pain, taste) from peripheral organs (like the skin or surface of the tongue) to the central nervous system. (*Hint*: Afferent: where "*a*" [as in *a*pproach] means sending impulses *toward* the brain [i.e., from an organ receiving sensory input] so the brain can "feel" it; therefore these impulses are sensory, related to the senses of feeling, touch, pain, taste, etc.)

Efferent [EF er ent] (or **motor**) nerve fibers convey impulses from the central nervous system to the peripheral organs, such as to muscle fibers to initiate contraction. They supply the four pairs of muscles of mastication and other muscles in the region of the mouth. (*Hint*: Efferent: where "*e*" [as in *e*xit] means sending an impulse *from* the brain, often to a muscle, to have a bone move in the intended direction [or to increase force on that bone without movement]; therefore these impulses are motor.)

Secretory fibers are specialized efferent nerve fibers that, upon stimulation, can send messages to glands, like the salivary and lacrimal glands to produce and secrete saliva or tears.

There are **twelve cranial nerves** (indicated by Roman Numerals I-XII) that are responsible for the following functions.[1,21–26]

I	Olfactory [ol FAK toe ree]	Smell
II	Optic	Sight
III	Oculomotor [AHK u lo MO tor]	Orbital muscles for eye movement
IV	Trochlear [TROK le ar]	Orbital muscles for eye movement
V	*Trigeminal [tri JEM i nal]	Movement of the jaws and muscles of mastication; sensation of the face, teeth, and periodontal ligaments
VI	Abducent [ab DOO sent]	Orbital muscles for eye movement
VII	*Facial	Motor to the muscles of facial expression, taste to anterior two-thirds of tongue
VIII	Auditory/(Acoustic)	Sense of hearing, position, and balance
IX	*Glossopharyngeal [GLOSS o feh rin JI al]	Secretory to parotid gland, pharyngeal movements; sensory to pharynx and posterior one-third of tongue; and taste to posterior one-third of tongue
X	Vagus [VAY gus]	Pharyngeal and laryngeal movements: digestive tract
XI	Accessory	Neck movements: sternocleidomastoid and trapezius muscles
XII	*Hypoglossal	Tongue movement (muscles)

*The asterisked nerves are most important when discussing the function of the oral cavity. A detailed discussion of these nerves will include the major branches to structures of the mouth, including teeth, periodontal ligaments and alveolar processes, gingiva (gums), palate and floor of the mouth, muscles of mastication and of facial expression, and tongue (both for muscular action and our sense of taste).

A.   TRIGEMINAL NERVE (FIFTH CRANIAL NERVE)

When discussing the function of the oral cavity, probably the most important nerve is the trigeminal. The trigeminal nerve or fifth cranial nerve is the largest of the cranial nerves and is the major sensory nerve of the face and scalp. It originates in the large semilunar or trigeminal ganglion, a group of nerve cell bodies located on the internal, superior surface of the temporal bone in a small depression within the cranium medial to the foramen ovale. The trigeminal nerve is divided into **three major divisions** (or three nerve branches). (*Hint:* "tri" in *trigeminal* refers to the nerve's three divisions.) **Division I (ophthalmic [ahf THAL mik] nerve)** and **Division II (maxillary nerve)** are only afferent (sensory). **Division III (the mandibular nerve)** is both afferent (sensory) and efferent (motor). Its efferent fibers supply the muscles of mastication.

The maxillary and mandibular divisions of the trigeminal nerve also supply afferent or sensory neurons that provide the brain with information about the position of the teeth and jaws at all times. The interpretation of postural information by the brain (sense of position) is called **proprioception.** Muscles and ligaments have proprioceptive nerve receptors, including the ligaments around the teeth (called periodontal ligaments), and in the lateral aspects of the temporomandibular joints. The periodontal ligament around each tooth is well supplied with proprioceptive (sense of position) neurons from the maxillary and mandibular divisions of the trigeminal nerve. These branches continually send messages to the brain as to the relative position of the mandibular to maxillary teeth. This has a tremendous influence on relative jaw position, movement, and occlusion (the fitting together) of the teeth. Canines are reported to have the richest supply of proprioceptive nerve endings.

The temporomandibular joint also has proprioceptive neurons in the capsule and disc that are innervated by the auriculotemporal branch of the mandibular division of the trigeminal nerve. To a great extent, proprioceptive information, especially from the teeth, determines the subconscious but well-coordinated function of the two complex temporomandibular joints.[24,25] Otherwise, we could experience many unpleasant tooth interferences or frequent joint pain.

Each of the three divisions is divided into many branches. The branches of the maxillary nerve and the mandibular nerve are those that innervate the region of, and around, the oral cavity and will be discussed in the most depth in this section.

1.   DIVISION I (OPHTHALMIC NERVE) OF THE TRIGEMINAL NERVE

The **ophthalmic [of THAL mik] nerve** (see Fig. 1-26) is about 25 mm long and exits from the skull by way of the superior orbital fissure on the superior surface of the orbit (Fig. 1-4). It has three main branches: the smallest lachrymal nerve, the largest frontal nerve (which further divides into supraorbital and supratrochlear), and the nasociliary nerve (with its infratrochlear and nasal branches). The distribution of these and other sensory branches from the trigeminal nerve that supply the skin of the face are shown in Figure 1-25. The ophthalmic nerve and its branches supply sensory innervation (feeling) to the upper third of the face (i.e., the eyeball, the skin of the forehead, scalp, eyelid and nose, part of the nasal mucosa and maxillary sinus, and the secretory fibers to the lacrimal glands). *The ophthalmic nerve does not supply the oral cavity.* (*Hint:* "Ophthal mic" is related to the eye; compare *oph-thal*mologist, a physician who specializes in eyes.)

2.   DIVISION II (MAXILLARY NERVE) OF THE TRIGEMINAL NERVE

The maxillary nerve provides sensory innervation to the middle third of the face, including the palate and maxillary teeth (Fig. 1-25). It exits the brain case of the skull through the **foramen rotundum** (Fig. 1-4). After passing through the foramen rotundum, the maxillary nerve passes into the **pterygopalatine space** and eventually splits into four branches: the pterygopalatine, posterior superior alveolar, infraorbital, and zygomatic nerves. These branches are best viewed in Figures 1-26 and 1-27.

a.   First Branch of the Maxillary Nerve: Pterygopalatine Branch

The first branch of the maxillary nerve, the **pterygopalatine nerve,** splits off closest to the origin of the maxillary nerve, then passes through the pterygopalatine ganglion (Fig. 1-26). A branch of this nerve, called the **descending palatine nerve,** passes through the greater palatine foramen to

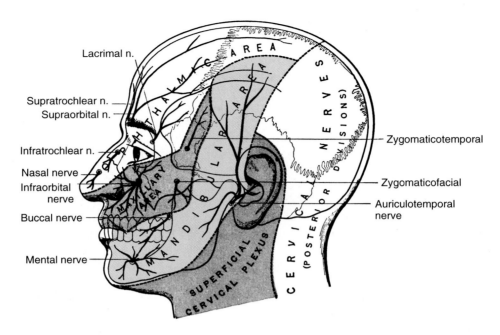

FIGURE 1-25. General distribution to the skin of the three **sensory** divisions of the **trigeminal nerve**. Pain in these areas is felt by impulses sent through the ophthalmic, maxillary, and mandibular branches of this nerve. (Reproduced by permission from Clemente CD, ed. Gray's anatomy of the human body. 30th ed. Philadelphia: Lea & Febiger, 1985:1164.)

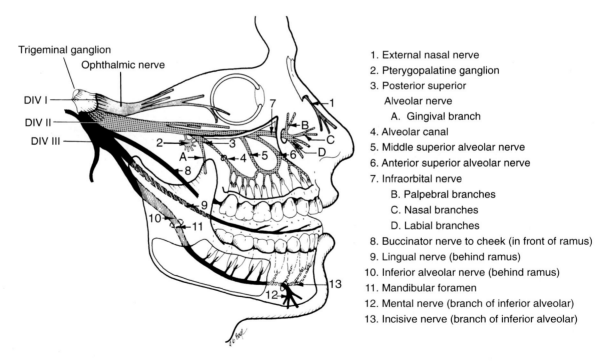

1. External nasal nerve
2. Pterygopalatine ganglion
3. Posterior superior
   Alveolar nerve
      A. Gingival branch
4. Alveolar canal
5. Middle superior alveolar nerve
6. Anterior superior alveolar nerve
7. Infraorbital nerve
      B. Palpebral branches
      C. Nasal branches
      D. Labial branches
8. Buccinator nerve to cheek (in front of ramus)
9. Lingual nerve (behind ramus)
10. Inferior alveolar nerve (behind ramus)
11. Mandibular foramen
12. Mental nerve (branch of inferior alveolar)
13. Incisive nerve (branch of inferior alveolar)

FIGURE 1-26. Trigeminal nerve distribution of the branches of the maxillary and mandibular nerves. Note that the buccinator branch (labeled **#**8) of the mandibular division passes superficial to the ramus to enter the cheek, whereas the lingual nerve (labeled **#**9) and inferior alveolar nerve (labeled **#**10) pass medial to the ramus as they go to the tongue and mandible, respectively. The maxillary nerve and branches are shaded red; the mandibular nerve and branches are black.

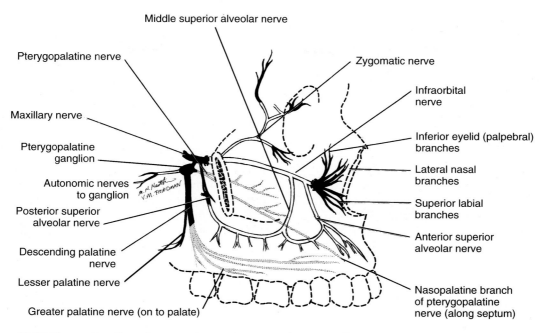

FIGURE 1-27. **Maxillary division of Cranial Nerve V (Trigeminal):** branches that supply the maxillary teeth and surrounding structures. Note that the *black* portions are outside the maxillae, the *white* parts are within the maxillae, and the *red* shaded parts pass through the nasal cavity to enter the palate. (Reproduced by permission from Brand RW, Isselhard DE. Anatomy of oral structures. 2nd ed. St. Louis: C.V. Mosby, 1998, 221.)

become the **greater palatine nerve** as it enters the back of the palate (shaded in Fig. 1-27). The greater palatine nerve spreads anteriorly to supply the mucosa (soft tissue covering) of the posterior portion of the hard palate and the palatal gingiva (gum tissue) next to the posterior teeth (molars and premolars). Just posterior to the greater palatine foramen, the **middle** and **posterior (lesser) palatine nerves** enter the palate through the lesser palatine foramina to spread posteriorly to supply the tonsils and mucosa of the soft palate.

Another long branch of the pterygopalatine nerve, the **nasopalatine nerve** (shaded in Fig. 1-27) runs along the roof of the nasal cavity and diagonally down along the **nasal septum** to emerge onto the anterior palate through the **incisive foramen** (Fig. 1-10). This branch innervates the soft tissue of the nasal septum and gingiva and palatal soft tissue behind the anterior teeth. The right and left nasopalatine nerves communicate with the greater palatine nerves to innervate the entire hard palate.

b. **Second Branch of the Maxillary Nerve: Posterior Superior Alveolar (PSA) Nerve**

Just before the maxillary nerve enters the infraorbital fissure and canal on the floor of the orbit, it gives off its second branch, the **posterior superior alveolar (PSA) nerve**. This branch enters the **alveolar canals** on the infratemporal portion of the maxilla (Fig. 1-26). Once within the trabecular (spongy) bone of the maxilla and the maxillary sinus, its **dental branches** enter small openings in the tooth roots to supply the *maxillary molars* (except for one root, the mesiobuccal root of maxillary first molars). It also innervates the supporting alveolar bone, periodontal ligaments, and facial gingiva next to the maxillary molars, the mucosa of part of the maxillary sinus, and adjacent cheek mucosa.

c. **Third Branch of the Maxillary Nerve: Infraorbital Nerve**

In the pterygopalatine space, a third branch splits off and passes through the inferior orbital fissure on the floor of the orbit and enters the infraorbital canal, where it becomes the **infraorbital** nerve (Fig. 1-26). While within this canal, the infraorbital nerve gives off two branches, the middle superior alveolar and the anterior superior alveolar nerves.

The **middle superior alveolar (MSA)** nerve passes forward along the lining of the maxillary sinus. It gives off small dental branches that enter premolars through their root openings (apical foramina) to supply the *maxillary premolars* (and the mesiobuccal root of the maxillary first molar), supporting alveolar bone, periodontal ligaments, and facial gingiva in the maxillary premolar region and part of the maxillary sinus. It is important to realize that the nerve supplying primary teeth is the same as that to the permanent teeth that replace them. Therefore, the nerve supply to the primary molars is the MSA, the same one that supplies their successors, the permanent premolars.

The second branch given off of the infraorbital nerve while in the infraorbital canal is the **anterior superior alveolar (ASA)** nerve. Its small dental branches supply the pulp, supporting alveolar bone, periodontal ligaments, and facial gingiva of the *maxillary anterior teeth* and part of the maxillary sinus. Comparison of descriptions of the superior alveolar nerves indicates a great lack of uniformity in their distribution. Sometimes, the middle superior alveolar nerve is missing, and the function is taken over by the anterior and posterior alveolar nerves.

After exiting from the infraorbital foramen, the **infraorbital nerve** splits into its end (terminal) branches innervating the skin and mucosa of the side of the nose (**nasal nerve**), skin and mucosa of the lower eyelid (**palpebral** [PAL pe bral] **nerve**), and the skin and mucosa of the upper lip, facial gingiva of maxillary premolars, and anterior teeth (**labial** [LAY bee al] **nerve**) (Fig. 1-26).

d. Fourth Branch of the Maxillary Nerve: Zygomatic Nerve

The **zygomatic nerve** arises in the pterygopalatine fossa, enters the orbit via the inferior orbital fissure, and then divides into the zygomaticotemporal and zygomaticofacial nerves (the upper and lower branches, respectively, of the zygomatic nerve in Fig. 1-27). It supplies the temporal region and the orbit.

3. DIVISION III (MANDIBULAR NERVE) OF THE TRIGEMINAL NERVE

The mandibular nerve is a mixed nerve; that is, it contains both afferent (sensory) and efferent (motor) fibers. It is the only efferent portion of the trigeminal nerve. These motor fibers of the mandibular nerve supply the eight muscles of mastication, plus the mylohyoid muscle and the anterior belly of digastric muscle, which help to retract the mandible. Sensory fibers provide general sensations of touch, pain, pressure and temperature to the skin of the lower third of the face (as seen in Fig. 1-25), as well as the floor of the mouth, anterior two-thirds of the tongue (not taste), and mandibular teeth.

The mandibular nerve exits the neurocranium through the **foramen ovale**. It passes into a space just medial to the zygomatic arch and mandibular ramus, and inferior to the temporal bone, called the **infratemporal space**. As it passes inferiorly toward the mandibular foramen in the mandible, it divides into four sensory branches: the auriculotemporal, buccal, lingual, and inferior alveolar nerves.

a. Auriculotemporal Nerve

The first branch of the mandibular division, the **auriculotemporal** [aw RIK u lo TEM po ral] **nerve** (Fig. 1-28), comes off the main trunk immediately below the base of the skull, turning backwards beneath the lateral pterygoid muscle to supply pain and proprioception fibers to the temporomandibular joint, sensation to the outer ear, the skin of the lateral aspect of the skull and cheek, and other fibers to the parotid gland.

b. Buccinator Nerve

Another branch is the **buccinator** [BUCK sin a tor] (**buccal or long buccal**) **nerve** (Fig. 1-28), which comes off just below the foramen ovale, passes through the infratemporal space between the two heads of the lateral pterygoid muscles, then down and forward, emerging between the anterior border of the masseter and posterior border of the buccinator muscle. It innervates the buccal gingiva in the area of the mandibular molars, and sometimes second premolars. The best place to anesthetize the buccinator nerve is inside the cheek by injecting or depositing the solution into

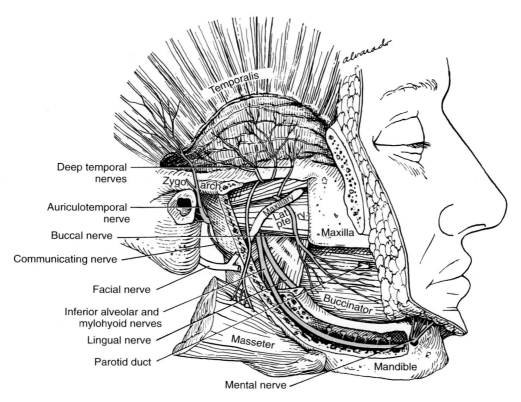

FIGURE 1-28. **Mandibular Division of Cranial Nerve** V, branches. The external wall of the right mandible has been removed to expose the **inferior alveolar nerve** within the mandible, where it gives off the many small branches to each mandibular tooth. (From this view, the teeth are not visible.) Near the premolar area, the inferior alveolar nerve splits into two terminal branches. One branch, the **mental nerve**, exits through the mental foramen to innervate the chin, while the other branch continues within the mandible and is now called the **incisive nerve** (not visible here). Also note the other major branches of the mandibular division: the **lingual nerve**, which is in close proximity to the inferior alveolar nerve posteriorly, but then diverges anteriorly to enter the tongue and the **buccal nerve**, which innervates the cheek and adjacent tissue. Other branches (not shaded) are motor branches of the mandibular nerve supplying the muscles of mastication. (Reproduced by permission from Clemente CD, ed. Gray's anatomy of the human body. 30th ed. Philadelphia: Lea & Febiger, 1985:1166.)

the buccinator muscle near the molars. This nerve also supplies the mucosa and skin of the cheek and corner of the mouth.

c. **Lingual Nerve**

The next branch of the mandibular nerve, given off about 15 mm below the foramen ovale, is the **lingual nerve** branch (Fig. 1-28), which goes to the tongue. It passes downward, medial to the ramus but lateral to the medial pterygoid muscle, to the posterior part of the mylohyoid ridge. It is located closely beneath the mucous membrane near the last molar. The lingual nerve provides general sensation (touch, pain, pressure and temperature, but not taste) to the top (dorsal) and bottom (ventral) surfaces of the anterior two-thirds of the tongue and adjacent tissues. The adjacent tissues include the soft tissue (mucosa) on the floor of the mouth and inner surface of the mandible, and the lingual gum tissue (gingiva) of the entire mandible.

d. **Inferior Alveolar Nerve**

Finally, the **inferior alveolar nerve** (Fig. 1-28) comes off of the mandibular nerve on the medial side of the lateral pterygoid muscle. This large nerve roughly parallels the direction of the lingual nerve to descend between the sphenomandibular ligament and ramus to the mandibular fora-men, where it gives off the **mylohyoid nerve** just before it enters the mandible through the **mandibular foramen** (represented on the medial surface of the mandible in Fig. 1-26). The **my-lohyoid nerve** (efferent) pierces the sphenomandibular ligament and travels forward in the my-lohyoid groove to supply the mylohyoid muscle and the anterior belly of the digastric muscle.

Once the inferior alveolar nerve passes through the mandibular foramen, it is in the **mandibu-lar canal** within the body of the mandible, where it gives off the dental branches that spread

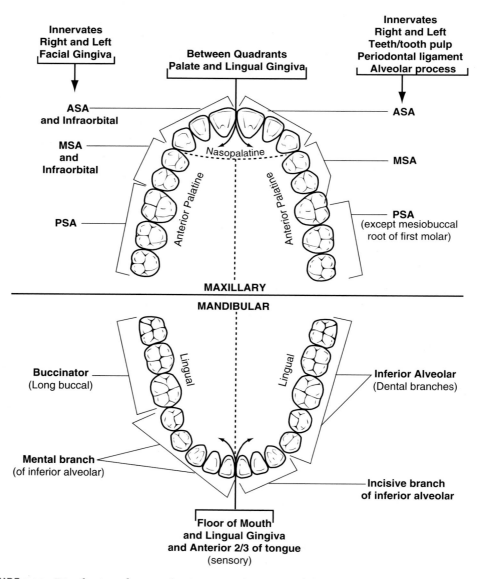

NERVES

FIGURE 1-29. Distribution of nerves that innervate the tissues of the mouth. Nerves listed on the *left* supply facial gingiva on both the right *and* left side of the face; nerves listed on the *right* supply the teeth, tooth pulp, periodontal ligament, and alveolar process on both sides of the face. Regions within the arches are supplied by the nerves listed in those areas.

through trabecular (spongy) bone of the mandible, into the mandibular molar and premolar teeth through the openings into their root tips. It also innervates the periodontal ligaments and alveolar processes of these teeth. In the area of the premolars, the inferior alveolar nerve splits into its two terminal branches: the mental and incisive nerves.

After splitting off of the mandibular nerve, the **mental nerve** (Fig. 1-26) exits from the body of the mandible via the **mental foramen** and supplies the facial gingiva of the mandibular incisors, canines, and premolars and the mucosa and skin of the lower lip and chin on that side up to the midline. The **incisive nerve** (Fig. 1-26) branch can really be considered a continuation of the inferior alveolar nerve, continuing forward within the mandibular canal to supply the mandibular incisor and canine teeth, their periodontal ligaments, and surrounding alveolar process.

Note that if an anesthetic solution is deposited next to the opening of the mandibular foramen, it could *block* the passage of afferent nerve signals from *all* mandibular teeth on that side (by blocking the inferior alveolar and its terminal incisive branch) and on that side of the lower chin and lip area (because another terminal branch, the mental nerve, has also been blocked). Further, since the lingual nerve is in close proximity to the mandibular foramen, its fibers will also be blocked, causing that side of the floor of the mouth, lingual gingiva, and anterior of the tongue to lose feeling. The only part of the mandible that would *not* be numb would be the tissue buccal to the molars, which requires some additional anesthetic solution in the cheek to block the buccinator nerve.

Figure 1-29 and Table 1-3 can be used to help summarize the distribution of the mandibular and maxillary sensory nerve branches to all teeth and surrounding tissues of the mouth.

Other *efferent (motor) branches* of the mandibular nerve supply the muscles of mastication: the **masseteric nerve** to the masseter muscle as well as to the temporomandibular joint, the **posterior and anterior temporal nerves** to the temporalis muscle, the **medial pterygoid nerve** to the medial pterygoid muscle, and the **lateral pterygoid nerve** to the lateral pterygoid muscle.

B. FACIAL NERVE (SEVENTH CRANIAL NERVE)

The **facial nerve** is a mixed nerve (efferent and afferent). From the brain, the facial nerve enters the temporal bone through the **internal acoustic meatus** (Fig. 1-4) and exits from the skull through the **stylomastoid foramen** (Fig. 1-5) between styloid and mastoid processes. It passes through the parotid gland. It then divides into two terminal branches: temporofacial (to the side of forehead) and cervicofacial (to the lower side of the face, orbicularis oris muscle, and chin).

Efferent [EF er ent] **fibers** innervate muscles of facial and visual expression of the face and the scalp. Other muscles supplied by the facial nerve include the posterior belly of the digastric muscle and stylohyoid muscle (Fig. 1-23), the platysma muscle (a broad, thin superficial muscle that covers much of the anterior part of the neck seen in Fig. 1-24), and the stapedius muscle (in middle ear cavity). None of these muscles have any influence on moving the mandible. Efferent **secretory fibers** end in the pterygopalatine and submandibular ganglia and bring about secretions from two pairs of salivary glands: the sublingual glands located just under the mucosa in the floor of the mouth superior to the mylohyoid muscle and the submandibular glands located in the submandibular fossae on the medial surface of the mandible inferior to the mylohyoid muscle.

Afferent [AF er ent] **fibers** of the facial nerve come off superior to the stylomastoid foramen, course through the tympanic cavity, eventually coming out of the skull by way of the **petrotympanic** [PET ro tim PAN ik] **fissure**. They join with the lingual nerve (branch of the mandibular division of the trigeminal nerve) and supply the sense of taste to the anterior two-thirds of the tongue (the body and the tip of the tongue). There are only four primary tastes: sour (acid), sweet, salty, and bitter.[27] Some authors add alkaline and metallic to the taste senses. The tip of the tongue is where one best distinguishes sweet, salty, or alkaline substances. The sides of the tongue are most sensitive to sour (acidic) substances.[27] There are approximately 9000 taste buds in the young adult, more in children, and fewer with advancing age.[27]

Table 1-3

DISTRIBUTION OF BRANCHES OF TRIGEMINAL NERVE TO THE TEETH AND SURROUNDING STRUCTURES

CAREFULLY STUDY THIS COMPREHENSIVE BUT SIMPLE TABLE. THEN, COVERING ONE COLUMN AT A TIME, SEE HOW MANY NERVES YOU CAN RECALL. THESE ARE THE NERVES ANY DENTAL STUDENT, DENTAL HYGIENE STUDENT, OR GRADUATE OF EITHER PROFESSION SHOULD BE MOST FAMILIAR WITH. YOU SHOULD ALSO BE ABLE TO DETERMINE THE LOCATION OF EACH NERVE.

TEETH	TOOTH PULP	GINGIVA	PERIODONTAL LIGAMENT AND ALVEOLAR PROCESS	HARD PALATE
MAXILLARY ARCH				
Anteriors	Anterior superior alveolar N.	Palatal— Nasopalatine N. Labial—infraorbital and anterior superior alveolar N.	Anterior superior alveolar N.*	Nasopalatine N.
Premolars	Middle superior alveolar N.	Palatal—Anterior palatine N. Buccal—Middle superior alveolar and infraorbital N.	Middle superior alveolar N.*	Anterior palatine N.
Molars	Posterior superior alveolar N except MB root of first (supplied by middle superior alveolar N)	Palatal—Anterior palatine N. Buccal—Posterior superior alveolar N.	Posterior superior alveolar N.*	Anterior palatine N. SOFT PALATE: Middle and posterior palatine nerves
MANDIBULAR ARCH				**FLOOR OF MOUTH**
Anteriors	Incisive branch of the inferior alveolar N.	Lingual—Lingual N. Labial—Mental N.	Incisive N.	Lingual N.
Premolars	Dental branch of inferior alveolar N.	Lingual—Lingual N. Buccal—Mental N.	Dental branch of Inferior alveolar N.	Lingual N.
Molars	Dental branch of inferior alveolar N.	Lingual—Lingual N. Buccal—Buccinator N. (Long buccal N.)	Dental branch of Inferior alveolar N.	Lingual N.

* Also supply the maxillary sinus.

C. GLOSSOPHARYNGEAL NERVE (NINTH CRANIAL NERVE)

The **glossopharyngeal** [GLOSS o feh rin JI al] **nerve** exits from the skull via the **jugular** [JUG yoo lar] **foramen** (Fig. 1-4). It then passes down and forward, medial to the styloid process, to enter the tongue. It is a mixed nerve (efferent and afferent) and supplies parts of the tongue and pharynx.

The glossopharyngeal nerves' **efferent** fibers innervate the stylopharyngeus muscle of the pharynx.

Secretory fibers innervate the parotid gland, effecting secretion. This gland is located in front of each ear lobe in the cheek tissues just inferior to the zygomatic arch. The **afferent** fibers of this nerve supply the sense of taste and general sensation to the posterior one-third of the tongue and general sensation to the mucosa of the pharynx and tonsils. (Bitter sensations are noticed on the dorsal (top) surface in the region of the circumvallate papillae on the posterior third of the tongue. One text says that additional taste buds can be found in other structures in the back of the mouth [such as the pillars of the fauces, hard and soft palate, epiglottis, and pharynx].[27,28]) (*Hint*: Glossopharyngeal = glosso [tongue] + pharyngeal [pharynx or throat]).

D. HYPOGLOSSAL NERVE (TWELFTH CRANIAL NERVE)

The **hypoglossal nerve** exits from the skull through the **hypoglossal canal** just above the **occipital condyles** near the anterior border of the large **foramen magnum** (visible just inside the walls of the foramen magnum (Fig. 1-5). It descends steeply, entering the oral cavity at the posterior border of the mylohyoid muscle. This efferent nerve supplies the muscles that move the tongue. These are: genioglossus, styloglossus, hyoglossus, longitudinal, vertical, and transverse. If this nerve becomes damaged from injury or tumor, the tongue will deviate noticeably toward the affected side. (*Hint*: Hypoglossal = hypo [beneath; like a *hypo*dermic needle] + glossal [tongue].)

E. SUMMARY OF NERVE SUPPLY TO THE TONGUE

AFFERENT FIBERS TO THE TONGUE

- Lingual nerve (branch of division III or the mandibular branch of the trigeminal nerve) provides general sensation to the anterior two-thirds (body) of the tongue
- Facial nerve (seventh cranial nerve) provides taste sensation to anterior two-thirds of tongue (body)
- Glossopharyngeal nerve (ninth cranial nerve) is responsible for taste and general sensation in the posterior one-third (or root) of the tongue

EFFERENT FIBERS TO THE TONGUE

- Hypoglossal nerve (twelfth cranial nerve) supplies motor fibers to the muscles of the tongue

LEARNING EXERCISE

- Describe the pathway of the branches of the mandibular division of the fifth cranial nerves as they pass from the brain toward their target organs (especially the maxillary and mandibular teeth and surrounding soft tissue). Name the location where branches split off of the main nerves and name the foramina through which each branch passes. Then, if it is possible on your study skull, take a pipe cleaner and carefully pass it through the foramina to show the passageway of these nerves. Think about where these nerves might be reached by an anesthetic syringe needle and what structures would be anesthetized if anesthetic deposited in that location blocked nerve impulses from all branches of that nerve that are farther away from the brain.
- Repeat the previous exercise for the branches of the maxillary division.
- Sketch the dorsal view of the tongue and label which nerves innervate the anterior two-thirds and posterior one-third for general sensation, taste, and movement (muscles).
- List all twelve cranial nerves in order and their functions.
- Review all words in bold that have phonetic spelling to confirm that your pronunciation is correct.

Select the one best answer.

1. The branches of which nerve cause the masseter muscle fibers to contract, thus squeezing the teeth together?
    a. cranial nerve V: maxillary division
    b. cranial nerve V: mandibular division
    c. cranial nerve V: ophthalmic division
    d. facial nerve
    e. lingual nerve
2. Which of the following nerve branches do NOT need to be anesthetized in order to block the sensation of pain to the pulp and all surrounding bone and gingiva of tooth #27 prior to an extraction?
    a. buccal nerve
    b. mental nerve
    c. incisive nerve
    d. inferior alveolar nerve
    e. lingual nerve
3. Which two nerves branch off of the infraorbital nerve while it is in the infraorbital canal?
    a. MSA and PSA
    b. ASA and MSA
    c. PSA and ASA
    d. MSA and nasopalatine
    e. nasopalatine and greater palatine
4. Anesthetizing nerve fibers of what nerve results in numbness in half of the anterior two-thirds of the tongue?
    a. hypoglossal nerve
    b. glossopharyngeal nerve
    c. lingual nerve branch of the trigeminal nerve
    d. lingual nerve branch of the facial nerve
5. The nerve branch of the trigeminal that provides pain sensation to the mandibular teeth exits the skull through what foramen?
    a. f. ovale
    b. f. rotundum
    c. mandibular f.
    d. mental f.
    e. infraorbital f.

ANSWERS: 1–b, 2–a, 3–b, 4–c, 5–a.

SECTION VI. Vessels Associated with the Oral Cavity

OBJECTIVES

The objectives for this section are to prepare the reader to perform the following:

*   Trace blood through the major blood vessels (arteries) from the heart, to the teeth, and back (through veins) to the heart.
*   Describe the pathway (fossa, spaces, etc.) of the key arteries that supply the teeth and, where possible, feel the pulse.

- **Trace the route of infection from teeth and associated oral structures through the lymph system.**
- **Palpate the location of lymph nodes associated with the spread of infection.**

Nerves and arteries tend to parallel one another, often passing through the same foramen and canals within bones after they meet. Arteries pass up toward the mouth from the heart and nerves come down to the mouth from the brain. Generally, arteries of the face and jaw run a more wiggly or corkscrew course than do veins.

A. ARTERIES

Refer to the pathway of blood from the heart to the teeth in Figure 1-30. Blood courses from the left ventricle of the heart through the aorta to the common carotid artery, which ascends in the neck and divides into the **external carotid** [kah ROT id] **artery** (Fig. 1-31), which gives off the maxillary branches supplying structures in the mouth, and the internal carotid artery (enters the skull; does not supply the mouth). You can feel the pulse of the external carotid just in front of the sternocleidomastoid muscle as required during CPR training.

As the external carotid passes superiorly behind the angle of the mandible, it gives off two important branches to the mouth. First, the **lingual artery** (not seen on Fig. 1-31) comes off near the hyoid bone, then enters the tongue. As with the lingual nerve, this artery supplies the floor of the mouth, adjacent gingiva and the sublingual gland.

Second, the **facial artery** (Fig 1-31) comes off just superior or with the lingual artery. It then passes forward obliquely beneath the submandibular gland, then laterally around the lower border of the mandible. The facial artery and nerve pass together through a shallow notch on the inferior border of the mandible just anterior to the angle. This notch is called the **antegonial** [an ti GO ni al] **notch** (Fig. 1-12). This is an important landmark to be aware of so that you will be able to stop the flow of blood to the face in an emergency. Try to find the facial artery at the antegonial notch with your finger or thumb. You should feel pulsations of the facial artery if you are in the correct spot. From here the facial artery goes upward over the outer surface of the mandible to the face.

Now four branches of the facial artery will be described. Prior to passing onto the face, the **ascending palatine artery** comes off at the highest point of the first bend of the facial artery and ascends to supply structures adjacent to the pharynx (the soft palate, the pharyngeal muscles, the mucosa of the pharynx, and the palatine tonsil). The **submental artery**, which converges with the mylohyoid nerve, supplies structures in the floor of the mouth (the mylohyoid muscle, anterior belly of the digastric muscle, and lymph nodes inferior to the mylohyoid muscle). After passing onto the face, the **inferior** and **superior labial arteries** (Fig. 1-31) surround and supply the lips and the orbicularis oris muscle. **Lateral nasal** and **angular arteries** are the terminal branches of the facial arteries.

There is considerable merging at the midline of the arteries from both sides of the face, rather than the more conventional system, whereby an artery terminates with many small capillaries. This merging of small arteries from opposite sides is called an end-to-end anastomosis. One example is where the right and left superior and inferior labial arteries join at the midline. As one might guess, such an anastomosis can cause problems in arresting hemorrhage about the face.

The **maxillary artery** is probably the most important artery to the dentist and dental hygienist. It arises from the external carotid within the parotid gland (Fig.1-31). The branches of this artery can be considered in *three parts* as shown in Figure 1-32. The branches of the mandibular and pterygopalatine (or first and third) parts are directly involved with the blood supply to the mandibular and maxillary teeth, respectively. The branches of the pterygoid (or middle) part provide blood to the four pairs of muscles of mastication (masseter, temporalis, medial, and lateral pterygoids). Study Figure 1-32 as you read about the following branches of each part of the maxillary artery.

The branch coming off of the *mandibular* (or first) *part* of the maxillary artery (which is of most dental interest) is the **inferior alveolar artery** which, like the inferior alveolar nerve, enters the mandible through the mandibular foramen, supplying branches to the molars and premolars. It then divides into two branches: the **mental artery**, which exits from the mental foramen to the lower lip and chin, and the **incisive artery**, which continues forward within the mandible to supply the anterior teeth (similar to the path of nerves of the same name in Fig. 1-26).

Branches coming off of the *pterygoid* (second) *part* are not involved directly with the teeth but supply blood to the muscles of mastication (posterior and deep temporal, masseteric, and pterygoid branches).

Branches that come off of the *pterygopalatine* (third) *part* of the maxillary artery supply the maxillary teeth and the periodontal ligaments. Note the similarity between the names of the vessels and the names of the nerves that supply the same structures. The **posterior superior alveolar artery** traverses the maxillary sinus,

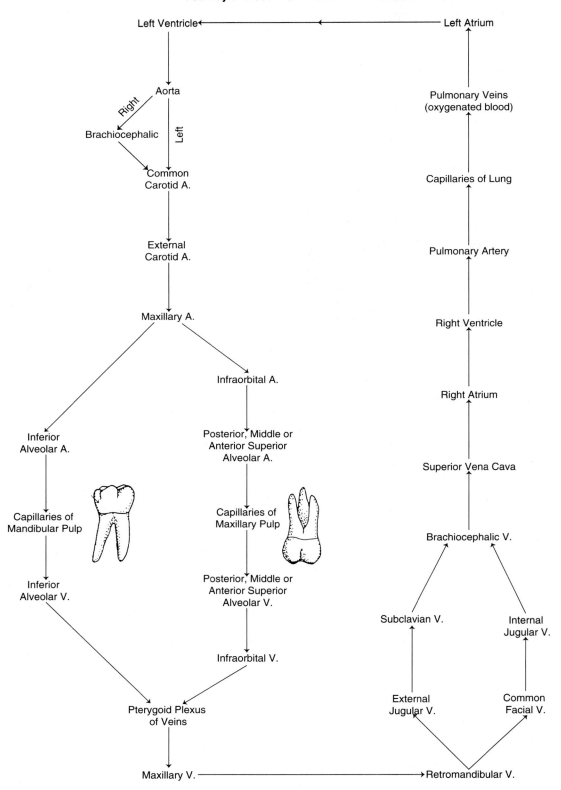

Pathway of Blood From Heart to Tooth and Back to Heart

*(Think in terms of a drop of blood making this round trip)

FIGURE 1-30. Pathway of blood from heart to teeth and back to heart.

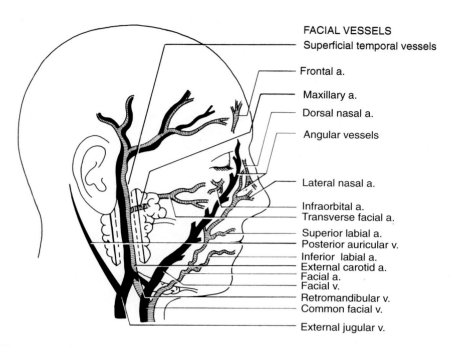

FACIAL VESSELS
- Superficial temporal vessels
- Frontal a.
- Maxillary a.
- Dorsal nasal a.
- Angular vessels
- Lateral nasal a.
- Infraorbital a.
- Transverse facial a.
- Superior labial a.
- Posterior auricular v.
- Inferior labial a.
- External carotid a.
- Facial a.
- Facial v.
- Retromandibular v.
- Common facial v.
- External jugular v.

FIGURE 1-31. Facial vessels. The parotid gland is split apart to show the external carotid artery and vein, with the maxillary artery coming off and passing deep to this gland. Arteries are shaded red; veins are black.

and, like the posterior superior alveolar nerve, supplies the maxillary molars. While within the infraorbital canal, the **infraorbital artery**, like the infraorbital nerve, gives off the **middle superior alveolar artery**, which supplies the premolars, and the **anterior superior alveolar** artery, which supplies the anterior teeth. The **descending palatine** branch of the maxillary artery supplies part of the nasal cavity before it emerges onto the palate through the greater palatine foramina (Fig. 1-10) like the nerves to supply the mucosa of the hard and soft palate and the lingual gingiva. Its terminal part ascends through the incisive canal into the nasal cavity.

The temporomandibular joint is supplied with oxygenated blood from five branches: the ascending pharyngeal and superficial temporal branches of the external carotid artery (Fig. 1-31) and by the anterior tympanic, masseteric, and middle meningeal branches of the maxillary artery (Fig. 1-32).

- Masseteric
- Middle and accessory meningeal
- Anterior tympanic
- Deep auricular
- Superficial temporal
- Maxillary
- Posterior auricular
- External carotid
- Inferior alveolar

- Posterior deep temporalis
- Anterior deep temporalis
- Pterygoid canal
- Sphenopalatine
- Infraorbital
- Pharyngeal
- Descending palatine
- Posterior superior alveolar
- Buccinator
- Pterygoid
- Twig to lingual n.
- Mylohyoid

| Mandibular part | Pterygoid part | Pterygopalatine part |

MAXILLARY ARTERY

FIGURE 1-32. Maxillary artery and the branches of its three major parts. Recall that the *mandibular part* supplies blood to the mandible and teeth, the *pterygoid part* to the muscles of mastication, and the *pterygopalatine part* to the maxillae and teeth.

B. VEINS

Veins tend to be straighter than arteries.[29,30] In many instances, they travel almost the same course as arteries. There are no valves in any of the facial veins. Therefore, an infection in the face can go in either direction through veins. Drainage normally takes place through the veins shown in Figure 1-33.

The **pterygoid** [TER i goid] **plexus of veins** (Fig. 1-33) is a network of veins medial to the upper part of the ramus of the mandible between the temporal and lateral pterygoid muscles or between the lateral and medial pterygoids.[30] The pterygoid plexus collects blood from the upper part of the face, the lips and muscles around the mouth, posterior part of the nasal cavity, the palate, the maxillary alveolar process, and teeth. The pterygoid plexus empties into the **maxillary vein,** which helps drain the plexus. The dense venous plexus surrounds the maxillary *artery* and helps protect it from becoming flattened when the masticatory muscles contract. During muscle contractions, however, blood is driven from the veins.[30]

The **inferior alveolar vein** (not visible in Fig. 1-33) drains the mandible and the mandibular teeth and also empties into the pterygoid plexus of veins. The **facial vein** is formed by the angular and lateral nasal veins. It receives blood from the superior and inferior labial veins and from the muscles of mastication. The course of the facial vein closely parallels that of the facial artery but, of course, the blood flows in opposite directions. The **deep facial vein** connects the pterygoid plexus with the facial vein.

The **lingual veins** (not visible on Fig. 1-33) drain the tongue and empty into either the common facial or internal jugular vein.

The **retromandibular vein** is formed by the union of the superficial temporal and maxillary veins within the parotid gland. It drains the regions supplied by the maxillary and superficial temporal arteries. It drains into the facial vein. The retromandibular and facial veins empty indirectly into the **internal jugular vein** via the **common facial vein.** Blood then passes into the brachiocephalic vein, to the superior vena cava, then through the heart and lungs to become oxygenated before being pumped back to the mouth (Fig. 1-30.)

C. LYMPH

The lymph system is somewhat more complex[31] since it serves to collect tissue fluid that got outside the blood capillary bed and then to return this fluid to the vascular system. In the arterial side of a capillary

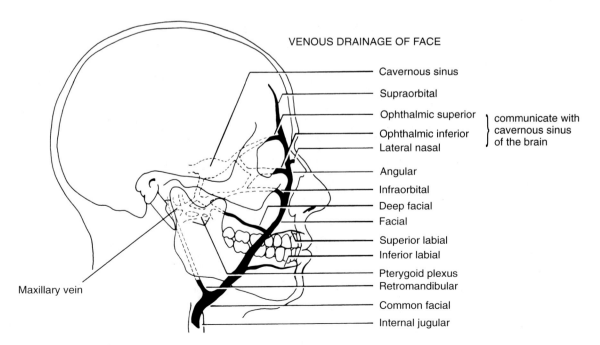

FIGURE 1-33. Venous drainage of the face. The dotted lines represent deeper, less superficial vessels.

LEARNING EXERCISE

Draw the route of a drop of blood from the heart to both a maxillary and mandibular tooth and then back to the heart as shown in Figure 1-30. Name each vessel along the way. Try to visualize this interesting round trip, which takes place about every 10–15 seconds. Remember, the maxillary artery and its branches are probably the most important to the dentist or dental hygienist.

bed, blood pressure exceeds osmotic pressure, so fluid escapes into the tissue spaces. On the venous side of each capillary bed, the blood pressure is lower and the osmotic pressure becomes higher, forcing 90% of the tissue fluid back into the venous capillary bed.[32] The major bulk of the remaining 10% is the lymph, which passes into the lumen of lymph capillaries, is then collected in the nodes (shown in Fig. 1-34), and returned to the blood vascular system.

During times of infection, trauma, or cancerous growth, abnormal amounts of fluids escape (with specialized cells to fight infection, etc.) and result in swollen lymph glands. Since lymph nodes form chains that are then connected by lymph vessels, infection spreads predictably from the site of infection to a specific lymph node, which then drains to another until the lymph system empties back into the veins. The spread pattern is as follows. Refer to Figure 1-34 while reading.

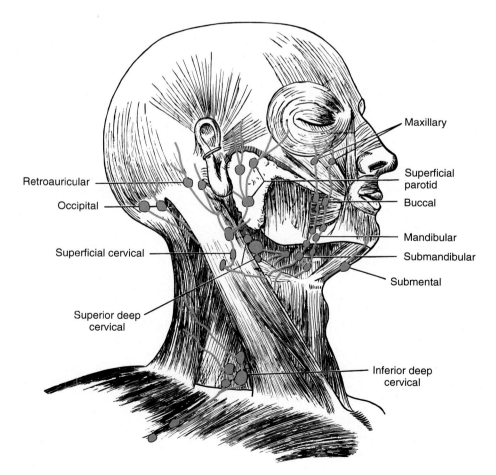

FIGURE 1-34. Lymph nodes of the head and neck. These areas should be palpated during a head and neck examination. (Reproduced by permission from Clemente CD, ed. Gray's anatomy of the human body. 30th ed. Philadelphia: Lea & Febiger, 1985:880.)

Infection in the area of the chin and adjacent structures including the tip of the tongue, anterior floor of the mouth, lower lip and mandibular incisors, and adjacent gingiva (gum tissue) all drain into the **submental nodes** just lingual to the mandibular symphysis area. When enlarged, these nodes can be palpated just posterior to the symphysis area of the mandible.

The submental nodes, as well as most other intraoral structures, including all maxillary and mandibular teeth and facial and palatal gingiva or gum tissue (except around the mandibular anteriors), posterior floor of the mouth, sides of the tongue anteriorly (but not the tip), cheek and side of the nose, upper lip and lateral lower lip, and the maxillary sinus all drain into the **submandibular nodes**. This chain of nodes can be palpated medial but anterior to the angle of the mandible, with the most prominent node in this chain located over the facial artery medial to the antegonial notch.

Parotid [pa ROT id] (or preauricular) **nodes**, located over the parotid gland in front of the ear, receive lymph from the area around the parotid gland, including the adjacent scalp, ear, prominence of the cheek, and eyelids. The parotid and submandibular nodes, as well as excess lymph resulting from a sore throat (inflamed tonsils and pharynx) drain into the **deep and superficial cervical chain of nodes**. These are located along the large sternocleidomastoid neck muscles.

From here, the lymph returns via the venous drainage of the cardiovascular system. On the *left* side, drainage is through the **thoracic** [tho RAS ik] **duct**, which empties into veins at the junction of the **left subclavian** [sub CLAY vi an] and **internal jugular veins**, which ultimately form the **brachiocephalic** [BRAY ki o se FAL ik] **vein**. On the *right* side, lymph empties into the junction of the **right subclavian** and **internal jugular vein**.

LEARNING EXERCISE

1. Describe the pathway by which an infection (or cancer cells) might spread from a maxillary tooth to the neck through the lymph system, then through the venous system.
2. Describe the pathway by which an infection might spread from a mandibular tooth to the neck through the lymph system, then through the venous system.

LEARNING QUESTIONS

Select the one best answer.

1. Which node would first show enlargement from an infection of a mandibular incisor?
   a. submental
   b. submandibular
   c. parotid
   d. cervical
   e. preauricular
2. At what location would you palpate the cervical lymph node chain?
   a. around the sternocleidomastoid muscle
   b. near the symphysis of the mandible
   c. over the submandibular gland
   d. behind the ear
   e. over the parotid gland

3. Branches of what artery supply blood to the mandibular teeth?
   a. maxillary artery
   b. masseteric artery
   c. pterygoid artery
   d. pterygopalatine artery
   e. superficial temporal artery

4. Branches of what artery supply blood to the maxillary teeth?
   a. maxillary artery
   b. masseteric artery
   c. pterygoid artery
   d. pterygopalatine artery
   e. superficial temporal artery

ANSWERS: 1–a, 2–a, 3–a, 4–a.

REFERENCES

1. Clemente CD, ed. Gray's anatomy of the human body. 30th Ed. Philadelphia: Lea & Febiger, 1985.
2. Roman-Ruiz LA. The mental foramen: a study of its positional relationship to the lower incisor and premolar teeth [Masters Thesis]. Columbus, OH: Ohio State University, College of Dentistry, 1970.
3. Sicher H, DuBrul EL. Oral anatomy. 7th ed. St. Louis: C.V. Mosby, 1975:174–209.
4. Edwards LF, Gaughran GRL. Concise anatomy. 3rd ed. New York: McGraw-Hill, 1971.
5. Hickey JC, Allison ML, Woelfel JB, et al. Mandibular movements in three dimensions. J Prosthet Dent 1963;13:72–92.
6. Hickey JC, Woelfel JB, et al. Influence of occlusal schemes on the muscular activity of edentulous patients. J Prosthet Dent 1963;13:444–451.
7. Woelfel JB, Hickey JC, Rinear L. Electromyographic evidence supporting the mandibular hinge axis theory. J Prosthet Dent 1957;7:361–367.
8. Woelfel JB, Hickey JC, Stacy RW. Electromyographic analysis of jaw movements. J Prosthet Dent 1960;10:688–697.
9. Woelfel JB, Hickey JC, Allison ML. Effect of posterior tooth form on jaw and denture movement. J Prosthet Dent 1962;12:922–939.
10. Melfi RC. Permar's oral embryology and microscopic anatomy. 8th ed. Philadelphia: Lea & Febiger, 1988:247–257.
11. Sharry JJ. Complete denture prosthodontics. New York: McGraw-Hill, 1962:45–86.
12. Ricketts RM. Abnormal function of the temporomandibular joint. Am J Orthod 1955;41:425, 435–441.
13. Burch JG. Activity of the accessory ligaments of the temporomandibular joint. J Prosthet Dent 1970;24:621–628.
14. Turell J, Ruiz HG. Normal and abnormal findings in temporomandibular joints in autopsy specimens. J Craniomandibular Disorders: Facial and Oral Pain 1987;1:257–275.
15. Osborn JW, ed., with Armstrong WG, Speirs RL. Anatomy, biochemistry and physiology. Oxford: Blackwell Scientific Publications, 1982:324–343.
16. Haines RW. On muscles of full and of short action. J Anat 1934;69:20–24.
17. Gionhaku N, Lowe AA. Relationship between jaw muscle volume and craniofacial form. J Dent Res 1989;68:805–809.
18. Montgomery RL. Head and neck anatomy with clinical correlations. New York: McGraw-Hill, 1981:202–214.
19. Winter CM, Woelfel JB, Igarashi T. Five-year changes in the edentulous mandible as determined on oblique cephalometric radiographs. J Dent Res 1974;53(6):1455–1467.
20. Kraus B, Jordan R, Abrams L. Dental anatomy and occlusion. Baltimore: Williams & Wilkins, 1969:203–222.
21. Basmajian JV. Grant's medical method of anatomy. 9th ed. Baltimore: Williams & Wilkins, 1975.
22. Edward LF, Gaughran GRL. Concise anatomy. 3rd ed. New York: McGraw-Hill, 1971.
23. Sicher H, DuBrul EL. Oral anatomy. 6th ed. St. Louis: C.V. Mosby, 1975:344–378.
24. Crum RJ, Loiselle RJ. Oral perception and proprioception. A review of the literature and its significance to prosthodontics. J Prosthet Dent 1972;28:215–230.
25. Jerge CR. Organization and function of the trigeminal mesencephalic nucleus. J Neurophysiol 1963;26:379–392.
26. Renner RP. An introduction to dental anatomy and esthetics. Chicago: Quintessence Publishing, 1985:162.

27. Jenkins GN. The physiology of the mouth. 3rd ed. Revised reprint. Oxford: Blackwell Scientific Publications, 1970:310–328.
28. Osborn JW, ed. Anatomy, biochemistry and physiology. Oxford: Blackwell Scientific Publications, 1982:542.
29. Edwards LF, Gaughran GRL. Concise anatomy. 3rd ed. New York: McGraw-Hill, 1971.
30. Sicher H, DuBrul EL. Oral anatomy. 7th ed. St. Louis: C.V. Mosby, 1980:351–376.
31. Montgomery RL. Head anatomy with clinical correlations. New York: McGraw-Hill, 1981:75–82.
32. Paff GH. Anatomy of the head and neck. Philadelphia: W.B. Saunders, 1973.
33. Osborn JR, ed. Dental anatomy and embryology. Oxford: Blackwell Scientific Publications, 1981:133.
34. Palmer RS. Elephants. World Book Encyclopedia 1979;6:178C.
35. Brant, D. Beavers. World Book Encyclopedia 1979;2;147.
36. Melfi RC. Permar's oral embryology and microscopic anatomy. 8th ed. Philadelphia: Lea & Febiger, 1988.
37. Osborn JW, ed. Dental anatomy and embryology. Oxford: Blackwell Scientific Publications, 1981.
38. Montgomery RL. Head and neck anatomy with clinical correlations. New York: McGraw-Hill, 1981.
39. Brand W, Isselhard B. Anatomy of orofacial structures. 5th ed. St. Louis: C.V. Mosby, 1994.
40. Francis CC. Introduction to human anatomy. 6th ed. St. Louis: C.V. Mosby, 1973.
41. Osborn JW, ed. Anatomy, biochemistry and physiology. Oxford: Blackwell Scientific Publications, 1982.
42. Zoo Books: Elephants. Wildlife Education Ltd. San Diego: Frye & Smith, 1980:14.

General References

Reed GM, Sheppard VF. Basic structures of the head and neck. Philadelphia: W.B. Saunders, 1976.
Fehrenbach MJ, Herring SW. Illustrated anatomy of the head and neck. Philadelphia: W.B. Saunders, 1996.
Ash MM. Wheeler's dental anatomy, physiology and occlusion. 7th ed. Philadelphia: W.B. Saunders, 1993.
Dorland's illustrated medical dictionary. 28th ed. Philadelphia: W.B. Saunders, 1985.
Clemente CD, ed. Gray's anatomy of the human body. 30th ed. Philadelphia: Lea & Febiger, 1994.
Clemente CD. Anatomy: a regional atlas of the human body. 4th ed. Baltimore: Williams and Wilkins, 1997.

Oral Examination: Normal Anatomy of the Oral Cavity

2

Topics covered within the two sections of this chapter include the following:
I. Intraoral examination
   A. Examine the lips visually
   B. Examine the vestibule and cheeks
   C. Evaluate the roof of the mouth
   D. Examine the fauces and palatine arches
   E. Examine the tongue
   F. Examine the floor of the mouth
   G. Identify the teeth—count them
   H. Examine the gingiva
II. Location of structures that can be palpated extraorally
   A. Palpate the muscles of mastication
   B. Palpate the temporomandibular joint
   C. Palpate the lymph nodes

OBJECTIVES

This chapter is designed to prepare the learner to perform the following:
- **Identify and describe all normal structures found during an intraoral examination in the following parts of the mouth: lips , vestibule and cheeks, roof of the mouth, fauces area, tongue, floor of the mouth, teeth (count), and gingiva (gums).**
- **Describe the location and palpate (examine by touching) the major muscles of mastication.**
- **Describe the location and palpate the temporomandibular joint posteriorly and laterally.**
- **Describe the location and palpate the lymph nodes that drain the face and neck.**

The following general anatomic terms would be helpful to know before reading this chapter.

circumvallate [sir kum VAL ate]: circum (around), vallate (valley or trench)
filiform: shaped like a thread or filament
fungiform [FUN ji form]: shaped like a fungi or mushroom
fornix: referring to vault-like space
frenum [FREE num] (also frenulum; pl. frena): small fold of tissue that limits movement
linea alba [LIN e a AL ba]: the white (alba) line (linea)
mastication [MAS ti KA shen]: chewing food
vestibule: entrance to the mouth; like an anteroom, known as a vestibule in an old house

During the periodic head and neck cancer screening examination, the dental professional should evaluate all oral and surrounding structures for evidence of pathology. This examination begins with an evaluation of the patient's general health and then includes an assessment of extraoral structures of the head and neck, followed by an intraoral examination that includes an evaluation of all structures from the lips to the throat. The purpose of a complete and thorough extraoral and intraoral examination is to identify areas of pathology that might require follow-up or treatment. The purpose of this chapter is to describe *normal* landmarks that can be identified throughout the mouth so that deviations from normal can more easily be distinguished.

Soft tissue structures cover the bones of the skull and are supplied by the nerves and blood vessels discussed in Chapter 1. As you study this material and examine the mouth, attempt to recall the underlying bones, nerves, and vessels.

SECTION I. Intraoral Examination

The **oral cavity** is bounded anteriorly by the lips, laterally by the cheeks, superiorly by the palate, and inferiorly by the floor of the mouth. The oral cavity can be divided into the outer **oral vestibule**, or space between the teeth (and supporting alveolar processes) and lips, and the **oral cavity proper**, the inner space bounded anteriorly and laterally by the teeth and alveolar processes.

Mucous membrane (mucosa) lines any body cavity opening to the outside of the body. **Oral mucous membrane** lines the oral cavity. It is made up of two layers: outer stratified surface epithelium and underlying connective tissue. It resembles the skin on the outside of the body, except that it is moist. Some areas subjected to the most wear, such as the roof the mouth (over the hard palate) and the gingiva, are covered by a toughened outer tissue called the **keratin** [KER ah tin] **layer**. As wear occurs, it takes on a grayish appearance and is replaced by underlying cells. Other areas of the oral mucous membrane that are protected are more delicate in structure, such as the cheeks and floor of the mouth, and have no keratin layer. This lining mucosa is so thin that the blood vessels located in the underlying connective tissue can easily be seen, giving it a reddish or bluish color.

A. EXAMINE THE LIPS VISUALLY

Use Figure 2-1 as a guide while studying the lips. The lips are the two fleshy borders of the mouth (an upper and a lower) that join at the labial **commissure**. The upper lip is bounded by the cheeks (laterally) at the **nasolabial groove** and by the nose (superiorly). The nasolabial groove runs diagonally downward on each side of the nostril toward the commissure. The lower lip is also bounded laterally by the cheeks, and inferiorly by the chin beginning at the horizontal **labiomental groove**. Recall that the underlying orbicularis oris muscle is the muscle surrounding the opening between the lips that permits us to close our lips

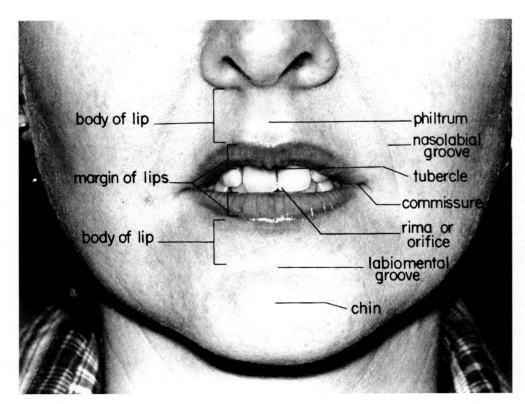

FIGURE 2-1. Surface anatomy of structures in the lips. The margin of the lip is sometimes called the vermilion border. The wet-dry line does not show because the margins were moistened by the tongue in order to photograph well

around a straw. The upper lip and surrounding skin have a **tubercle**, the small rounded nodule of tissue in the center of the lowest part of the upper lip, and a **philtrum** [FIL trum], the depression running from the tubercle to the nostrils.

The **vermilion border** (or zone) is the red border of the lips, representing a transitional zone where the lips merge into mucous membrane. It is the area where females often place lipstick. It is bounded externally on the face by the **mucocutaneous junction**, the junction between skin of the face and vermilion border of the lips. The vermilion border is bounded internally in the mouth by the wet line where labial mucosa begins. A **wet line** (or wet-dry line) is the junction between the outer red portion (vermilion border), which is usually dry , and the inner smooth and moist mucosa. The wet line is located about 10 mm back from the skin. The lips are redder in younger persons than in older persons. In some individuals, the lip color is reddish brown due to the presence of brown melanin pigment. The vermilion border and mucocutaneous junction are important in the head and neck examination, because changes here may be caused by exposure to the sun and could lead to skin cancer.

B. EXAMINE THE VESTIBULE AND CHEEKS

Refer to Figure 2-2 as a guide while studying the vestibule and cheeks. The arch or vault-shaped space between the cheek or lips externally and the teeth and gingiva (gum tissue) of the maxilla or mandible internally is called a **vestibule** (maxillary or mandibular). The **buccal vestibule** is next to the posterior teeth (premolars and molars), whereas the **labial vestibule** is next to the anterior teeth (incisors and

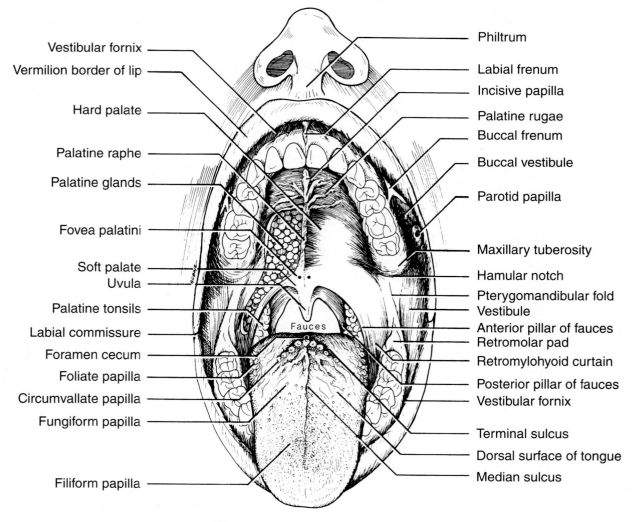

FIGURE 2-2. Structures in the oral cavity.

canines). It is covered with dark pink-colored alveolar mucosa and is rich in blood vessels and minor salivary glands. The tip of your tongue can easily reach into each vestibule to assist in cleaning the facial surfaces of the teeth, and while chewing, to lift food back between the upper and lower teeth. The **vestibular fornix** is the lowest part of the vestibule next to the mandible or highest part next to the maxillae. In the cheeks, the vestibular fornix is where food may collect in patients with nerve damage to the cheek (as with unilateral loss of function of the facial nerve from Bell's palsy or from stroke).

The **labial frenum** [FREE num](plural: frena [FREE nah]) is the thin sheet of tissue that attaches the internal center of the lip (upper and lower) to the mucosa covering the maxillae or mandible near the central incisors. The **buccal frenum** loosely attaches the cheek to the mucosa of the jaw in the area of the premolars (maxillary and mandibular). These frena may be seen by pulling the lower lip and cheek out and inferior and the upper lip and cheek out and superior. Our facial muscles move the buccal frena forward and backward and upward and downward in eating to help, along with the tongue, to place our food back over the chewing surfaces of our teeth while eating. Movement of these frena can also dislodge complete dentures if the denture is designed improperly.

The **buccal mucosa** lining of the inside of the cheeks is shin, but in spots may be rough. Often there is a horizontal white line extending anteroposteriorly on each side at the level where the upper and lower teeth come together, called the **linea alba** [LIN e ah AL ba] buccalis. [*Hint*: "Linea" means line, "alba" means white.] It may extend from the commissural area to the third molar region. This area is often irritated by trauma from biting the cheek. Usually 4–6 mm posterior to the commissure, an elevation of mucous membrane called the **commissural papule** is commonly seen and may be palpated.

The **parotid papilla** [pa ROT id pah PILL e] is a rounded flap of tissue next to the first and second molars at or just superior to the occlusal plane. This papilla covers the duct openings (**Stensen's duct**) from the parotid gland. The large quadrilateral-shaped parotid glands are located in front of each ear and produce 23–33% of our saliva (serous type).[1] These glands may be affected during mumps. [In 1971 and 1972, Dr. Woelfel and Dr. Igarashi supervised 331 dental students as they recorded the position of the right and left parotid papilla on each other. Of 662 parotid papillae, 78% were located between the maxillary first and second molar or by the second molar. Only 22% were by the first molar. In height, 87% of these same papillae were located level with (34%) or above the level (53%) of the occlusal plane. Only 13% were found below the level of the occlusal plane. The widest variation in location among these dental students was in two men, one having his parotid papilla on each side 11 mm above the occlusal plane and the other man with his 8 mm below the level of the occlusal plane. In a similar study of 293 adult men and 114 adult women (258 Caucasian, 11 black, 9 Hispanic), the parotid papilla averaged 3.3 mm above the occlusal plane (right 3.0, left 3.5 mm)[2].]

Fordyce's granules or spots are small, yellowish irregular areas and may be conspicuous inside the lips or buccal mucosa, especially inside the cheeks just posterior to the corner of the mouth. They are really the manifestation of intraoral sebaceous glands—glands normally associated with hair follicles on the skin outside of the mouth. Their presence here may be the result of fusion of the upper and lower parts of the cheek during embryonic development. Such glands have also been found, however, on other parts of the oral mucosa.

C. EVALUATE THE ROOF OF THE MOUTH

The **hard palate** is the firm anterior part of the roof of the mouth with mucosa over the underlying bone (namely, the horizontal plates of the palatine bones and palatine processes of the maxillae). The **soft palate** is the posterior movable part of the roof of the mouth without underlying bony support. The **vibrating line** is the junction between the hard and soft palate.

1. HARD PALATE STRUCTURES

Refer to Figures 2.2 and 2.3 while studying the structures of the hard palate. The hard palate is covered by keratinized grayish red to coral pink tissue. The **incisive papilla** is the small rounded elevation of tissue on the midline of the palate just behind (or lingual to) the central incisors. This papilla is located over the incisive foramen, where the nasopalatine nerve passes from the nasal cavity to innervate the anterior portion of the hard palate. It is the location for injecting anesthetic to numb palatal tissue in this area. [There is a relatively constant 8.5-mm distance from the facial surface of the maxillary central incisors and the center of the incisive papilla. On 326 casts measured by Dr. Woelfel, the average distance was 8.4 mm, with a range of 5.5 to 12 mm.]

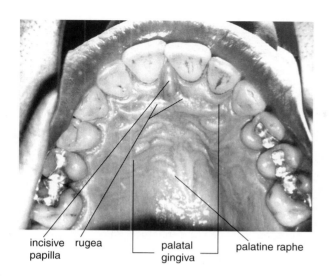

incisive   rugea   palatal   palatine raphe
papilla   gingiva

FIGURE 2-3. The hard palate. Note the prominent palatine rugae and incisive papilla. The palatine raphe is not conspicuous in this subject. In some mouths, this raphe is more distinguishable as a ridge extending anteroposteriorly in the center of the hard palate. Notice the correct universal number on each tooth.

The **palatine raphe** [RAY fee] is the slightly elevated centerline of firm tissue running from front to back (anteroposteriorly) in the hard palate. The intermaxillary suture attachment between right and left maxillae is immediately beneath the surface along this line. The mucosa is firm over the raphe because it is firmly attached to the underlying periosteum and bone without intervening fat or gland cells. The rest of the tissue on both sides of the raphe has fat or salivary gland tissue beneath the surface, so it is softer than the palatine raphe. There are more than 350 very small palatine glands in the posterior third of the hard palate.[3] They secrete thick but slippery saliva.

Palatine rugae [ROO ge] or [ROO je] are a series of palatal tissue elevations, or wrinkles, located just behind the maxillary anterior teeth (Fig. 2-2). They form a pattern like branches on a tree, coming off of the common midline "trunk," the palatine raphe. [Among casts from 939 hygiene students, rugae trees had 3, 4, or 5 branches on each side in 87% of the students. The first main branch was aligned lingual to the canine in 72%. The rugae were well elevated in 85% of the students and flattened in only 14%.]

Rugae are more distinct in young persons than in other persons. However, a longitudinal study of 20 females and 21 males, from age 4 to 22 years, indicated a slight but steady growth in the length of rugae during this period (average: 1.4–2.3 mm). Rugae growth occurred earlier in females, but the males had more branches.[4] Rugae function in two important ways: in tactilely sensing objects or food position and in aiding the tongue's proper placement for the production of certain speech sounds.[5] This part of the palate is often burned by eating pizza when it is too hot or becomes abraded from chewing too much popcorn.

2. STRUCTURES OF THE SOFT PALATE

The soft palate (Fig. 2-2) is found posterior to the hard palate beginning at the vibrating line. Along with the hard palate, it separates the mouth from the nasal passage. It is sometimes redder than the hard palate because of its slightly increased vascularity. Its anterior border extends between the right and left third molars. Unlike the hard palate, there is no bone beneath the surface of the soft palate. Say "ah, ah, ah" forcefully and see the soft palate move or vibrate. The hinged place where you observe the beginning of the soft palate is the **vibrating line**. **Fovea palatini** [FO ve ah pal a TEEN ee] are a pair of pits in the soft palate located on either side of the midline, near but posterior to the vibrating line. They are openings of ducts of minor palatine mucous glands.[5] The **uvula** [YOU view la] is a small fleshy structure hanging from the center of the posterior border of the soft palate.

The soft palate functions during swallowing, and speech. The **pharynx** [FAR inks] is the superior part of the digestive tube between the nose, mouth, and esophagus. During swallowing, the soft palate moves to close off the nasal pharynx from the oral pharynx to prevent regurgitation of food into the nasal cavity. The soft palate is raised to seal the oral cavity from the nasal cavity during blowing or when producing explosive consonants (like "b" and "p").

D. EXAMINE THE FAUCES AND PALATINE ARCHES

Refer to Figure 2-2 while studying the fauces and surrounding structures. The **fauces** [FAW seez] is the posterior boundary of the oral cavity. It is the opening from the mouth into the oropharynx (throat) for air when breathing through the mouth and for food, since the oropharynx leads to the esophagus and stomach. The fauces is bounded inferiorly by the dorsum of the tongue, laterally by a palatal arch or pillars, and superiorly by the soft palate. Examine the fauces and palatine arches (Fig. 2-2) by having the patient open and say "ahhh . . . . ." You may have to gently push the tongue down with a tongue depressor. *Be careful;* patients may gag.

Identify the anterior and posterior palatine pillars or arches that descend from the soft palate. The **anterior arch** is also named the **glossopalatine** [GLOSS o PAL a tine] arch, and the **posterior arch** is named the **pharyngopalatine** [fah RING go PAL a tine] arch, after the muscles beneath them. [*Hint:* The arch from the tongue (*glosso*) to the palate (*glosso*palatine anterior arch) is more anterior than the arch from the pharynx or throat behind it (*pharyngo*palatine posterior arch).] The **palatine tonsils** are located between the anterior and posterior pillars. These tonsils may become enlarged and inflamed during infections of the respiratory system. Patients may have had these surgically removed.

The **pterygomandibular** [TER i go mand DIB you lar] **fold** is a fold of tissue that appears to connect the mandible and the maxilla. This is easy to see when the mouth is opened wide, as this action stretches this fold, extending from the **retromolar pad** on the mandible to the pterygoid process of the sphenoid bone just behind the **maxillary tuberosity**. This fold is an important landmark for the anesthetic syringe needle to enter when aiming toward the mandibular foramen, where the inferior alveolar nerve can best be anesthetized before entering the mandibular canal and going into the body of the mandible. The **retromylohyoid** [REH tro my lo HI oid] **curtain** (Fig. 2-2) is a curtain of mucous membrane in the back of the mouth near the floor, extending between the anterior pillar of the fauces and the pterygomandibular fold. It is an important limiting structure in forming the lingual flange (edge) of a mandibular complete denture.

E. EXAMINE THE TONGUE

The tongue is a broad, flat organ largely composed of muscle fibers and glands. It rests in the floor of the mouth within the curved body of the mandible. The tongue changes its shape with each functional movement. The anterior two-thirds is called the **body**, and the posterior one-third is the tongue **base** or **root**. Examine the tongue by wrapping it in a damp gauze square and gently pulling it first to one side, then to the other.

1. DORSUM OF THE TONGUE

Use Figure 2-2 as a guide for landmarks on the dorsum (top) of the tongue. However, most people are unable to stick their tongue as far forward as in this illustration. The **dorsum** (dorsal or superior surface) of the tongue is the principle organ of taste and is invaluable during speech, mastication, and deglutition (swallowing). The dorsum of the tongue is grayish-red and is rough. It is covered by two kinds of papillae. The fine hair-like **filiform papillae**, which are quite numerous, cover the anterior two-thirds of the dorsal surface of the tongue. They are arranged in lines somewhat parallel to the terminal sulcus.[3] The more sparse, scattered, and shorter **fungiform papillae** are easy to identify because of their round mushroom cap shape and deep red color. Fungiform papillae are most concentrated near the tip of the tongue.[3]

Two other papillae types are also found on or near the posterior one-third of the tongue. The first are large, red, leaf-like projections on the lateral surface known as **foliate papillae** [FO li ate pah PILL e]. They contain some taste buds. The **circumvallate** [ser kum VAL ate] **papillae** are 8 to 12 large, flat, mushroom-shaped papillae forming a V-shaped row on the dorsum near the posterior third of the tongue. Their walls contain numerous taste buds. The **foramen cecum** [SEE kum] is a small circular opening immediately posterior to the center of the "V," formed by the circumvallate papilla. This foramen is the remnant of the thyroglossal duct from which the thyroid gland developed. The **terminal sulcus** is a shallow groove running laterally and forward on either side of the foramen cecum but posterior to the circumvallate papillae. It is usually necessary to hold the tongue quite firmly with gauze and pull it forward in order to see the circumvallate papillae and their neighboring structures because of their extremely posterior location. The smoother posterior third of the dorsum contains numerous mucous producing glands and lymph follicles (or nodules) referred to as the lingual tonsil (not visible on Fig. 2-2).

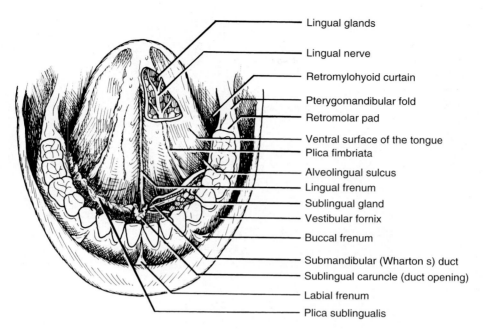

- Lingual glands
- Lingual nerve
- Retromylohyoid curtain
- Pterygomandibular fold
- Retromolar pad
- Ventral surface of the tongue
- Plica fimbriata
- Alveolingual sulcus
- Lingual frenum
- Sublingual gland
- Vestibular fornix
- Buccal frenum
- Submandibular (Wharton s) duct
- Sublingual caruncle (duct opening)
- Labial frenum
- Plica sublingualis

FIGURE 2-4. Structures of the under surface of the tongue (ventral surface) and floor of the mouth.

2. VENTRAL SURFACE OF THE TONGUE

The **ventral** or undersurface of the tongue is shiny, and blood vessels are visible. Refer to Figure 2-4. The **lingual frenum** is a thin sheet of tissue that attaches the center of the undersurface of the tongue to the floor of the mouth. Raise your tongue and watch how this tissue fold limits the amount of tongue movement. [Measurements on 333 casts by Dr. Woelfel indicated the frenum attachment to be 8.03 $\pm$ 1.5 mm below the gingival sulcus of the mandibular central incisors; range 5.4 to 11 mm. Assuming an average length mandibular central incisor (8.8 mm), the lingual frenum attaches about 17 mm below the incisal edge of these teeth.] In a person who is tongue-tied, the lingual frenum is firmly attached perhaps only 3 or 4 mm below the gingival margins of the central incisors and may severely limit tongue movement. Further, as the tongue moves, this type of frenum could pull on the attached gingiva contributing to periodontal problems. A simple surgical procedure corrects this type of situation.

  Plica fimbriata [PLY kah fim bri AH tah] (fimbriated folds) are delicate fringes of mucous membrane on each side of the frenum on the ventral surface of the tongue. The free edge of this fold may have a series of fringe-like processes. These are very delicate and often difficult to see unless gently moved by the tongue blade or mirror. In some animals, these fringes of tissue serve to keep the teeth clean.

F. EXAMINE THE FLOOR OF THE MOUTH

Visually examine the floor of the mouth by having the patient raise the tongue. Also, feel for unusual lumps by palpating the floor of the mouth with the forefinger of one hand pressing against the floor and opposed outside of the mouth by the fingers of the other hand.

  Like the ventral surface of the tongue, the tissues of the floor of the mouth are shiny, and some large blood vessels may be seen near the surface. The **alveolingual sulcus** (Fig. 2-4) is the broad, valley-shaped space between the tongue and mandibular alveolar bone. You can gently place your finger in this broad sulcus and press laterally to confirm whether there are any bony ridges on the medial surface of the mandible. A prominent bump in this area might be a relatively common occurrence: a mandibular torus.

  A **mandibular torus** (plural tori) (Fig. 2-5A) is a bulbous protuberance of bone beneath a thin mucous membrane covering on the medial side of the mandible often found in the premolar region. Mandibular tori are probably inherited as a genetic trait, and are not uncommon. They usually cause no problems, but may be irritated during chewing of coarse foods, or when mandibular dental impressions are made. After several or all lower teeth have been lost and removable dentures are to be made, mandibular tori must

A

B

FIGURE 2-5. A. Mandibular tori (three large bulbous elevations of bone) on the lingual surface of a stone cast of the mandible. (Note: the mandibular first molars have six, instead of the usual five, cusps.). B. A maxillary torus palatinus.

be surgically excised. (A similar torus may also occur in the middle of the palate and is called a **torus palatinus**) (Fig. 2-5B). **Exostosis** is the general term used to describe any hyperplastic bony growth projecting outward from the bone surface, such as a torus palatinus or mandibular torus, but can also be used to describe bony ridges that may form on the facial (cheek) surface of the mandible or maxillae.

Refer to Figure 2-4 while studying these landmarks on the floor of the mouth. On the floor, the overlying sublingual folds, called the **plica sublingualis**, extend anteriorly on each side of the floor of the mouth from the first molar region to the lingual frenum. Along these folds are many small openings of ducts from underlying **sublingual salivary glands** located in this region. These sublingual glands secrete purely mucous (ropy-type) saliva, producing only 5–8% of our saliva.[1]

In the center line at the junction between the right and left sublingual folds, on either side of the lingual frenum, is a pair of bulges called **sublingual caruncles**, each with an opening from ducts of salivary glands (**Wharton's ducts**). Wharton's ducts drain the large submandibular glands located posteriorly on either side in the submandibular fossae of the internal surface of the mandible. These glands produce about two-thirds of our saliva.[1] Their secretions are primarily serous (two-thirds serous cells, one-third mucous cells[6]). If you gently move your finger from posterior to anterior over the sublingual folds, saliva should come out of the caruncles. A person normally secretes over a pint of saliva during 24 hours (300 ml between meals, 300 ml while eating, and only 20 ml while sleeping), based on averages from 600 people.[1]

G. IDENTIFY THE TEETH—COUNT THEM

An important part of the oral examination is to determine which teeth are erupted in the mouth, identify them by name or universal number, and determine which teeth are missing. When the number of teeth is fewer than expected for a patient, a careful history can confirm tooth loss by disease or accident or teeth removed for orthodontic treatment. When history does not confirm such reasons for tooth loss, radiographs are recommended to rule out the possibility of unerupted teeth beneath the mucosa or surrounded by bone (impacted teeth) or to confirm that a tooth never formed. It is also possible for the patient to have extra (supernumerary) teeth or unexpected teeth (such as primary teeth in a 30-year-old). These factors impact on treatment planning decisions and should be documented.

The total number of teeth depends on the age of the individual and the stage of development of the teeth. As stated in the first section in this text, the complete **primary dentition** consists of 20 teeth. Children between 2 1/2 and 5 3/4 years of age will usually have all 20 teeth present in the mouth. For the next 6 years, there is normally a mix of some primary and some permanent teeth (called **mixed dentition**) until about 12 years of age, when all primary teeth have been exfoliated and only permanent teeth are present. At age 12, there would normally be 28 permanent teeth (all but the unerupted third molars). Eventually (by the late teens or early 20's), the complete **permanent** (or secondary) **dentition** consists of 32 teeth, including the four third molars that erupt (become visible) into the mouth.

H. EXAMINE THE GINGIVA

The **periodontium** is defined as the supporting tissues of the teeth, including surrounding alveolar bone (already discussed), the gingiva, the periodontal ligament, and the outer layer of the tooth roots (covered with cementum). The **periodontal ligament** is the thin ligament of many fibers that connects the outer layer of the tooth root (which is covered with cementum) with the thin layer of dense bone (lamina dura) lining each alveolus or tooth socket (See Fig. 2-10). The **gingiva** is that part of the masticatory (keratinized) oral mucous membrane that covers the alveolar process of the jaws and surrounds the cervical portions of the teeth. It is firmly attached to the teeth and to the surrounding bone. The gingiva is the visible part of the periodontium that is evaluated in the initial oral examination.

Healthy gingiva is stippled (that is, textured with many small depressions, like an orange peel) and coral pink in persons with light pigmentation (Fig. 2-6)). In persons with dark coloring of the hair and skin and in those of Mediterranean origin the gingiva may be brown or spotted with brown (**melanin pigmentation**) (Fig. 2-7). This pigmentation may occur up to the mucogingival junction. It is a common occurrence in people with darkly colored and black skin, Asians, people from India, and people of Mediterranean origins (Italians, Arabs, Yemenites, Turks, and some Jewish people).

Healthy gingiva varies in appearance from individual to individual and in different areas of the same mouth. It is usually pink (or pigmented), with thin margins just covering the junction of the tooth crown and root (cementoenamel junction). The margins of gingiva follow around each tooth parallel the cervical line, so there is a repeated parabolic arch pattern evident in Figure 2-7. Healthy interdental papillae are pointed and fill the interproximal spaces between teeth.

Gingiva can be visually divided into zones as shown in Figure 2-8. The most incisal (or most occlusal) part is *un*attached gingiva which includes the free gingiva and the interproximal papillae. **Free gingiva** (or marginal gingiva) is the tissue that is not attached to the tooth or alveolar bone. It surrounds each tooth to form a collar of tissue with a space or gingival sulcus (crevice) hidden between it and the tooth. Free gingiva extends from the **free gingival margin** (the edge of gingiva closest to the chewing or incising sur-

FIGURE 2-6. Healthy gingiva, close up. Note the ideal contours and stippled (orange peel) surface texture, usually most noticeable on the maxillary labial attached gingiva.

FIGURE 2-7. Healthy teeth, gingiva, and mouth with several patches of melanin pigmentation in the attached gingiva (especially evident near the maxillary incisors and mandibular canines). (Courtesy of Lewis J. Claman, D.D.S., M.S.)

FIGURE 2-8. Clinical components or zones of the gingiva. Note that the interdental papillae should, but do not completely, fill the interproximal spaces between the mandibular incisors. The tissues are otherwise healthy. (Courtesy of Lewis J. Claman, D.D.S., M.S.)

faces of the teeth) to the **free gingival groove** (visible in about 1/3 of adults) that separates attached gingiva from free gingiva. The **interdental (interproximal) papilla** is that part of the unattached gingiva between the teeth. It fills the interproximal space and also has the hidden sulcus, where dental floss can fit once it is passed between the teeth. An interdental papilla conforms to the shape of the contact area between adjacent teeth.

Attached gingiva is a band or zone of gray to light or coral pink keratinized masticatory mucosa that is firmly bound to the underlying bone (Fig. 2-8). It extends between the free gingiva (at the free gingival groove if present) and the more movable alveolar mucosa. The amount or width of attached gingiva varies normally from 3 to 12 mm.

The **mucogingival line** (junction) (Fig. 2-8) is a scalloped junction between attached gingiva and the looser, redder alveolar mucosa. **Alveolar mucosa** is movable mucosa, dark pink to red, due to increased vascularity and more delicate nonkeratinized tissue just apical to the mucogingival line. It is more delicate and less firmly attached to the underlying bone than the attached gingiva and is more displaceable as well, because of the underlying vessels and connective tissue. Palpate these two types of tissues and you will feel the difference in firmness. This alveolar mucosa is found in three places: maxillary and mandibular facial and mandibular lingual aspects but not on the palate, which has firm keratinized tissue for almost the entire surface. Therefore, the mucogingival line is present on the *facial* aspects of the maxillary and mandibular gingiva but only on the *lingual* aspect of mandibular gingiva.

Keratinized gingiva is the general term used to describe both the free and attached gingiva. It is widest on the facial (vestibular) aspect of maxillary anterior teeth and the lingual aspect of mandibular molars. It is narrowest on the facial aspect of mandibular premolars.[7]

The **gingival sulcus** (Fig. 2-9) is not seen visually but can be evaluated with a periodontal probe, since it is actually a space (or potential space) between the tooth surface and the narrow unattached cervical collar of free gingiva. The gingival sulcus is lined with the sulcular epithelium. It extends from the free gingival margin to the junctional epithelium [averaging 0.69 mm in depth].[8] **Junctional** (or attached) **epithelium** (seen in cross section in Figure 2-10) is a band of tissue at the most apical portion of the gingival sulcus that attaches the gingiva to the tooth. It is about 1 mm in width.[8] Then there is a 1–1.5 mm connective tissue attachment to the root above the osseous (bony) crest of bone. It is usually recommended that the margins of artificial crowns and inlays be kept 3 mm from this osseous crest.

Clinically, the gingival sulcus ranges in probing depth from about 1–3 mm and should not bleed when correctly probed. The periodontal probe usually penetrates into the junctional epithelium, hence the difference between the depth determined through clinical probing and the depth seen on a microscopic cross-section.[9] [In a survey by Dr. Woelfel, 267 dental hygiene students measured their gingival sulcus depth

FIGURE 2-9. Periodontal probe in place in the gingival sulcus. A. Interproximal probing in sulcus bounded by interdental papilla. B. Facial probing in gingival sulcus bounded by free gingiva.

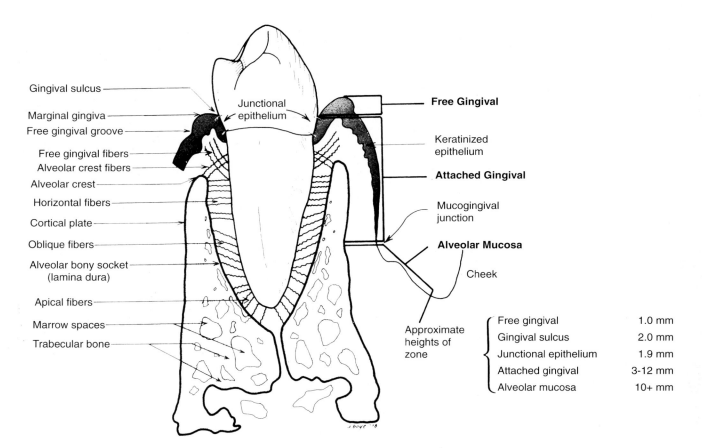

Gingival sulcus

Marginal gingiva

Free gingival groove

Free gingival fibers
Alveolar crest fibers

Alveolar crest

Horizontal fibers

Cortical plate

Oblique fibers

Alveolar bony socket
(lamina dura)

Apical fibers

Marrow spaces

Trabecular bone

Junctional
epithelium

Free Gingival

Keratinized
epithelium

Attached Gingival

Mucogingival
junction

Alveolar Mucosa

Cheek

Approximate
heights of
zone

Free gingival	1.0 mm
Gingival sulcus	2.0 mm
Junctional epithelium	1.9 mm
Attached gingival	3-12 mm
Alveolar mucosa	10+ mm

FIGURE 2-10. Periodontium including zones of gingiva and periodontal fiber groups. Mesial side of a mandibular left first premolar is suspended in its alveolus by the five groups of periodontal ligament fibers: apical, oblique, horizontal, alveolar crest, and free gingival fibers are visible. A sixth group, called transseptal fibers, not visible in this drawing, attaches from the cementum of one tooth to the cementum of the adjacent tooth at a level between the free gingival and alveolar crest fibers. The fibers of the periodontal ligament are much shorter than depicted here, averaging only 0.2 mm long (see actual size in Fig. 1.9).

with a calibrated periodontal probe. The average gingival sulcus depths for mandibular first molars midbuccal were: 1.5 ± 0.5 mm; midlingual: 1.7 ± 0.6 mm; mesiolingual and distolingual: 2.5 ± 0.5 mm. These measurements indicate that the gingival sulcus is usually deeper interproximally. Similar measurements made on the mesiofacial aspect of mandibular canines (1.9 ± 0.8 mm), maxillary canines (1.8 mm), maxillary first premolars (1.9 ± 0.7 mm), and maxillary first molars (2.1 ± 0.7 mm) indicate sulci slightly deeper on posterior teeth than those on anterior teeth.]

Note in Figure 2-10 that the periodontal ligament is made up of four groups of tiny fibers with differing directions and attachments and different names. The **apical, oblique, horizontal,** and **alveolar crest fibers** connect different parts of the tooth root (cementum) to the lamina dura of the tooth socket. **Free gingival fibers** are directed from tooth root (cementum) into free gingiva. A sixth group, the **transseptal fibers,** are not seen on Figure 2-10 since they run directly from the root (cementum) of one tooth to the cementum of the adjacent tooth at a level between the free gingival and alveolar crest fibers.

Although not gingiva, there are two soft tissue landmarks just behind the last molars that will be presented here. Immediately posterior to the maxillary last molar is a firm tissue bulge over bone of the alveolar ridge called the **maxillary tuberosity** (Fig. 2-2). A similar, less prominent, pear-shaped elevation of movable tissue distal to the mandibular last molar is the **retromolar pad** (Fig. 2-2) [*Hint:* "Retro" means behind or distal, to the last molar]. When a person has fully erupted third molars, the maxillary tuberosities and retromolar pads are small, because these teeth occupy these regions.

SECTION II. Location of Structures That Can Be Palpated Extraorally

A. PALPATE THE MUSCLES OF MASTICATION

Muscles of the head and neck can be palpated to identify pain or tenderness that could be related to problems in the temporomandibular joint or to an imbalance in the occlusion. For this reason, it is important to be able to locate these muscles extraorally. Each muscle pair can be palpated bilaterally with the middle finger of each hand while using the index and fourth finger to palpate surrounding soft tissue. Palpate these muscles on a partner while using Figure 2-11 as a guide.

- **Masseter:** Feel the body of the masseter by palpating the bulge over the angle of the mandible when your partner clenches. Move your finger down toward the angle of the mandible to feel the insertion and up toward the zygomatic arch (inferior border of the zygomatic bone and zygomatic process of the temporal bone) to feel the origin.
- **Medial pterygoid:** Feel the bulge when your partner clenches while palpating the medial surface of the angle of the mandible at the insertion. It may help to have your partner lean the head forward as you gently palpate inward and upward. This may cause some discomfort.
- **Temporalis, anterior fibers:** Palpate the origin of the anterior fibers just above a line between the eyebrow and superior border of the ear. Feel the bulge when your partner clenches.
- **Temporalis, posterior fibers:** Palpate the origin of the posterior fibers of the temporalis just above and distal to the superior border of the ear. Since this muscle is involved in retruding the mandible, see if you can feel a bulge when the partner retrudes (pulls back) the mandible.
- **Lateral pterygoid** (intraoral palpation): The lateral pterygoid can only be palpated intraorally. Feel this muscle by placing your index finger in the vestibule behind the maxillary tuberosity. (Use a skull to see how to reach the lateral plate of the pterygoid process of the sphenoid bone.) With your partner's mouth slightly open and the mandible moved slightly toward the side being palpated, slide your finger back toward the lateral pterygoid plate for the origin of the lateral pterygoid muscle. The anterior border of the condyloid process is the location of part of the insertion of this muscle. This may be uncomfortable to a patient even if the muscle is not sore.

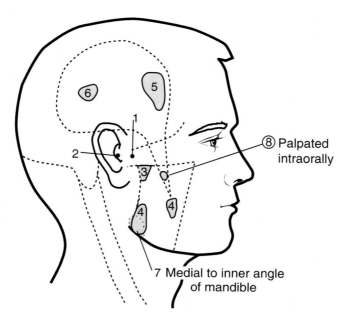

FIGURE 2-11. Sites for palpation of temporomandibular joint and muscles of mastication (origin and insertion locations). 1. Lateral surface of mandibular condyle; 2. Posterior surface of mandibular condyle; 3. Masseter (origin); 4. Masseter (insertion); 5. Temporalis (anterior fibers that close mandible); 6. Temporalis (posterior fibers that retract mandible); 7. Medial pterygoid; 8. Lateral pterygoid (palpated intraorally)

B.   PALPATE THE TEMPOROMANDIBULAR JOINT

Palpate the lateral aspect of the mandibular condyle by pressing directly over the joint just anterior to the external opening of the ear and inferior to the zygomatic arch (Fig. 2-12). Feel the head of the condyle move as your partner opens and closes the mandible and as your partner slides the mandible from side to side. You should feel the most movement over the right condyle when opening and moving the mandible to the left and feel the most movement over the left condyle when opening or moving to the right.

Palpate the dorsal or posterior surface of the mandibular condyle by placing your little finger into the external auditory meatus (ear canal opening) and press anteriorly forward. Feel the condyle when your partner opens, closes, and moves the mandible laterally from side to side.

C.   PALPATE THE LYMPH NODES

The evaluation of lymph nodes during a dental exam is important, since swollen nodes may indicate infection from sites that drain into them, or they may be indicators of the spread of cancer. Nodes, when swollen, can be felt by passing the fingers over the location of each node group. Using Figure 1-34 as your guide, palpate the *submental* nodes (just below the chin), the *submandibular* nodes (inside the angle of the mandible and over the submandibular gland), the *retroauricular* and *superficial parotid* nodes (anterior and posterior to the ear), and the *cervical* nodes (surrounding the large sternocleidomastoid neck muscle).

1. Nasolabial groove
2. Philtrum
3. Tubercle (upper lip)
4. Labiomental groove
5. Hyoid bone
6. Laryngeal prominence
    (Adam's apple)
7. Sternum
8. Clavicle
9. Carotid artery (dotted lines)
10. Sternocleidomastoid muscle
11. Submandibular gland
12. Masseter muscle
13. Parotid gland
14. Head of condyle
15. Zygomatic process
16. Temporalis muscle
17. Thyroid gland

FIGURE 2-12. Structures described in the first two chapters that relate to oral function.

LEARNING EXERCISE

Examine a partner (using infection control procedures) and identify each of the structures listed here. (The order of structures on this list is the same as that encountered within the chapter so it should be easy to follow the text as you perform the exam.) Use a tongue depressor or a mouth mirror to retract the lips and cheeks. A good light is needed, and a mouth mirror is useful for reflecting light into remote areas, and for holding the tongue or cheek out of the way during your examination. Also, study the location of the other landmarks that may be palpable in the face and neck shown in Figure 2-12, such as the parotid gland, the submandibular gland, the hyoid bone, the laryngeal prominence, the sternocleidomastoid muscle, and the thyroid gland.

I. INTRAORAL EXAM

A. Lips
___ 1. Commissure
___ 2. Nasolabial fold
___ 3. Labiomental groove
___ 4. Tubercle
___ 5. Philtrum
___ 6. Vermilion zone
___ 7. Mucocutaneous junction
___ 8. Wet line

B. Vestibule (and cheeks)
___ 1. Fornix
___ 2. Labial frenum
___ 3. Buccal frenum
___ 4. Buccal mucosa (possibly with linea alba)
___ 5. Commissural papule
___ 6. Parotid papilla (drains Stensen's duct, see if saliva drains by gently milking the cheek from posterior toward the duct)
___ 7. Fordyce spots

C. Roof of mouth
1. Hard palate
___ a. Incisive papilla
___ b. Palatine raphe
___ c. Rugae
___ d. Torus palatinus (if present)
2. Soft palate
___ a. Vibrating line (have partner say "Ah, ah, ah")
___ b. Fovea palatini
___ c. Uvula (in front of pharynx)

D. Fauces Area
___ 1. Glossopalatine arch
___ 2. Pharyngopalatine arch
___ 3. Palatine tonsils (if present)
___ 4. Pterygomandibular fold (an important landmark for future injections)
___ 5. Retromylohyoid curtain

E. Tongue

    1. Dorsum (top) and lateral borders with papillae that have taste buds

       __ Filiform papilla

       __ Fungiform papilla

       __ Foliate papilla

       __ Circumvallate papilla (difficult to see; way back)

       __ Foramen cecum and terminal sulcus (probably not visible)

    2. Ventral (underneath) surface

       __ Lingual frenum

       __ Plica fimbriata

F. Floor of mouth

__ 1. Alveolingual sulcus

__ 2. Are the following present?

    __ Mandibular torus

    __ Buccal exostosis

__ 3. Sublingual folds (plica sublingualis) over sublingual glands and sublingual caruncles (draining Wharton's duct). Try to milk out saliva with your finger pressing gently from posterior to anterior)

G. Teeth—maxillary and mandibular

    How many in each arch? Maxillary _____   Mandibular _____

H. Gingiva

    What is the color? _____

    Is it stippled? _____

__ 1. Free gingiva (is keratinized) with free gingival margin. (Recall that the gingival sulcus and junctional epithelium are hidden by this free gingiva and must be evaluated with a probe.)

__ 2. Free gingival groove

__ 3. Interdental papilla

__ 4. Attached gingiva (is keratinized)

__ 5. Mucogingival junction

__ 6. Alveolar mucosa

__ 7. Maxillary tuberosity

__ 8. Retromolar pad

II. STRUCTURES TO PALPATE EXTRAORALLY

A. Muscles

__ 1. Masseter: origin and insertion

__ 2. Medial pterygoid: insertion

__ 3. Temporalis

    __ Anterior fibers (origin and intraoral insertion)

    __ Posterior fibers (origin and intraoral insertion)

__ 4. Lateral pterygoid (palpate intraorally for origin)

B. Temporomandibular Joint (palpate during movements)
___ Lateral surface
___ Posterior surface

C. Lymph Nodes
___ Submental
___ Submandibular
___ Cervical
___ Parotid

LEARNING QUESTIONS

Test your newly acquired knowledge by matching the landmarks with their description. Place appropriate letter or letters on line on left.

___ 1. Dorsum of tongue

___ 2. Hard palate

___ 3. Pharynx

___ 4. Elevated midline of hard palate

___ 5. Stensen's duct

___ 6. Alveolar mucosa

___ 7. Fordyce's spots

___ 8. Melanin

___ 9. Gingiva between teeth

___ 10. Palatal tissue bump between teeth #8, 9

___ 11. Vibrating line

___ 12. Wharton's duct openings

___ 13. Labial frenum

___ 14. Ventral surface of tongue

___ 15. Oral cavity

___ 16. Retromolar pad

___ 17. Maxillary tuberosity

___ 18. Filiform papillae

(continued)

a. Mouth

b. Dark pigment on attached gingiva

c. Anteriorly in floor of mouth where the plica sublingualis meet

d. Underside of tongue

e. Hair-like papillae covering two-thirds of dorsum of tongue

f. Top side of tongue

g. Sebaceous glands on inside of cheek

h. Interdental papillae

i. Opens on inside of cheek near maxillary molars

j. Palatine raphe

k. Attaches lip to mucosa covering jaw (upper and lower)

l. Behind soft palate

m. Incisive papilla

n. Lines floor of vestibule

o. Firm, covered by gingiva, has rugae

p. Ridge of bone lingual to mandibular premolars

q. Elevation of tissue distal to mandibular last molar

r. Elevation of tissue distal to maxillary last molar

(continued)

___ 19. Torus mandibularis

___ 20. Attached gingiva

___ 21. Fauces

___ 22. Nasolabial groove

___ 23. Labiomental groove

___ 24. Sublingual gland

___ 25. Submandibular gland

___ 26. Plica sublingualis

___ 27. Uvula

___ 28. Plica fimbriata

___ 29. Foliate papilla

___ 30. Circumvallate papillae

___ 31. Alveololingual sulcus

___ 32. Palatine tonsils

___ 33. Retromylohyoid curtain

___ 34. Fungiform papillae

___ 35. Alveolar mucosa

___ 36. Fovea palatini

___ 37. Parotid gland

___ 38. Philtrum

___ 39. Commissure

___ 40. Exostosis

s. Junction of hard and soft palate

t. Tightly attached—pink color

u. Mucous salivary glands beneath anterior third of tongue

v. Large serous salivary gland beneath posterior third of tongue

w. At corners of mouth where lips join

x. Diagonal grooves from nostrils to corner of mouth

y. Horizontal depression below lower lip

z. Vertical depression on upper lip

aa. Opening from oral cavity to pharynx

bb. Serous salivary gland just in front of ear

cc. loosely attached

dd. Fold in floor of mouth beneath tongue

ee. Slight fold on each side of ventral surface of tongue

ff. Hangs downward in center of soft palate

gg. On lateral surfaces of posterior third of tongue

hh. Space between mandibular teeth and tongue

ii. 8 to 12 circular papillae arranged in a V-shape

jj. Pocket of mucous membrane between anterior pillar and pterygomandibular fold

kk. Located between anterior and posterior pillars in throat

ll. Bulbous protuberance on facial side of mandible in premolar region

mm. Sparse round mushroom-shaped papillae on dorsum of tongue

nn. Located just posterior to vibrating line

Answers: 1–f, 2–o, 3–l, 4–j, 5–i, 6–n or cc, 7–g, 8–b, 9–h, 10–m, 11–s, 12–c, 13–k, 14–d, 15–a, 16–q, 17–r, 18–e, 19–p , 20–t, 21–aa, 22–x, 23–y, 24–u, 25–v, 26–dd, 27–ff, 28–ee, 29–gg, 30–ii, 31–hh, 32–kk, 33–jj, 34–mm, 35–n or cc, 36–nn, 37–bb, 38–z, 39–w, 40–ll

REFERENCES

1. Jenkins GN. The physiology of the mouth. 3rd ed. Revised reprint. Oxford: Blackwell Scientific, 1970:310–328.
2. Foley PF, Latta GH. A study of the position of the parotid papillae relative to the occlusal plane. J Prosthet Dent 1985;53:124–126.
3. Osborn JW, Armstrong WG, Speirs RL, eds. Anatomy, biochemistry and physiology. Oxford: Blackwell Scientific, 1982:535.
4. Simmons JD, Moore RN, Errickson LC. A longitudinal study of anteroposterior growth changes in the palatine rugae. J Dent Res 1987;66:1512–15.
5. Renner RP. An introduction to dental anatomy and esthetics. Chicago: Quintessence Publishing, 1985.
6. Brand RW, Isselhard DE. Anatomy of orofacial structures. 5th ed. St. Louis: C.V. Mosby, 1994.
7. Lang N, Loe H. The relationship between the width of keratinized gingiva and gingival health. J Periodontol 1972;43:623.
8. Gargiulo A, Wentz F, Orban B. Dimensions and relationships of the dentogingival junction in humans. J Periodontol 1961;32:261.
9. Polson A, Caton J, Yeaple R, Zander H. Histological determination of probe tip penetration into gingival sulcus of humans using an electronic pressure-sensitive probe. J Clin Periodontol 1980;7:479.

Other General References

Clemente CD, ed. Gray's anatomy of the human body. 30th ed. Philadelphia: Lea & Febiger, 1985.
Clemente CD, Anatomy:a regional atlas of the human body. 4th ed. Baltimore, Williams & Wilkins,1997.
DuBrul EL. Sicher and duBrul's oral anatomy. St. Louis: C.V. Mosby, 1988.
Beck EW. Mosby's atlas of functional human anatomy. St. Louis: C.V. Mosby, 1982.
Dunn MJ, Shapiro CZ. Dental anatomy/head and neck anatomy. Baltimore: Williams & Wilkins, 1975.
Montgomery RL. Head and neck anatomy with clinical correlations. New York: McGraw-Hill, 1981:236–240.

3 Basic Terminology for Understanding Tooth Morphology

Prior to reading this chapter, be sure to master the terms used to identify teeth in Chapter 1, Section I.

The background terminology and concepts presented in this chapter are divided into seven sections as follows:

I. Tooth identification systems: Universal, Palmer, and International Numbering Systems
II. Terminology used to describe the parts of a tooth
   A. Four tissues of a tooth
   B. Anatomic versus clinical crown and root
III. Terminology used to define tooth surfaces
   A. Terms that identify outer surfaces of anterior versus posterior teeth
   B. Terms that identify inner surfaces (toward the tongue) of maxillary versus mandibular teeth
   C. Terms that differentiate biting surfaces of anterior versus posterior teeth
   D. Terms that differentiate approximating surfaces of teeth
   E. Divisions of the crown or root of a tooth (for purposes of description)
   F. Terms to denote tooth surface junctions or dimensions
   G. Root-to-crown ratio
IV. Terminology used to describe the morphology of a tooth
   A. Morphology of an anatomic crown
   B. External morphology of the anatomic root
   C. Relative size
V. Terminology related to the ideal tooth alignment of teeth in dental arches
   A. Root axis line
   B. Height of contour (crest of curvature)
   C. Contact areas (or proximal heights of contour)
   D. Embrasure spaces
VI. Ideal occlusion: Inter (between) arch relationship of teeth
VII. Tooth development from lobes

OBJECTIVES

This chapter is designed to prepare the learner to perform the following:

- Use the Universal Numbering System to identify permanent and primary teeth.
- Recognize the Palmer and International System and "translate" it to the Universal System.
- Identify and describe the four tissues of a tooth, their location, mineral content, and function.
- Differentiate an anatomic crown and root from a clinical crown and root.
- Name each tooth surface for anterior and posterior teeth.
- From all views, divide a tooth crown and root into thirds and label each third.

- **Define terms used to denote a specific dimension of a tooth.**
- **Describe and identify (by name) common tooth bumps, ridges, depressions, and grooves for each type of tooth.**
- **Describe and recognize the parts of a root.**
- **Describe and identify the attributes of ideal tooth alignment relative to other teeth within the arch, including the cusp or incisal edge position relative to the tooth's midroot axis line, location of heights of contour and proximal contacts, and relative sizes of embrasure spaces.**
- **Describe and identify the ideal interarch relationship of teeth in Class I occlusion, especially the relationship of first molars and canines.**
- **Identify the number of developmental lobes that form each tooth and recognize the anatomic landmarks of a tooth that may result from these lobe divisions.**

When we enter into any new field of study, it is initially necessary to learn the particular language of that field. Without an adequate vocabulary, we can neither understand nor make ourselves understood. Definitions and explanations of terms used in descriptive tooth morphology are the basic foundation for understanding subject matter presented in subsequent chapters. You must learn a few basics, similar to learning a foreign language. You will soon become nearly as familiar with these dental terms as you are with your name, and you will continue to use the majority of them throughout your professional dental career.

SECTION I. Tooth Identification Systems: Universal, Palmer, and International Numbering Systems

The making and filing of accurate dental records is an important task in any dental practice. To do so expeditiously, it is necessary to adopt a type of code or numbering system for teeth. Otherwise, for each tooth being charted, one must write something like "maxillary right second molar mesio-occlusodistal amalgam restoration with a buccal extension" (11 words, or 81 letters). Simplified by using the Universal Numbering System (and other standard abbreviations to denote tooth surfaces described later in chapter 12), this same information would be "2MODBA" (only six symbols). There are also two other numbering systems, the Palmer and the International Systems. As can be seen in Table 3-1, the tooth in the previous example (Universal number 2), using the Palmer Notation System, would be number 7| , and when using the International System the tooth would be number 17.

The **Universal Numbering System**, first suggested by Parreidt in 1882, was officially adopted by the American Dental Association in 1975. It is accepted by third party providers and is endorsed by the American Society of Forensic Odontology. Basically, the Universal Numbering System uses numbers 1 through 32 for the **permanent dentition**, starting with 1 for the maxillary right third molar, going around the arch to the maxillary left third molar as 16; dropping down on the same side, the left mandibular third molar becomes 17, and then the numbers increase clockwise around the lower arch to 32, which is the lower right third molar. This numbering system is used for each permanent tooth in the illustration in Figure 3-1.

For the 20 teeth in the **primary dentition**, letters of the alphabet are used from A through T. The letter A represents the maxillary right second molar, sequentially around the arch and through the alphabet to J for the maxillary left second molar, then dropping down on the same side to K for the mandibular left second molar, and then clockwise around the lower arch to T for the lower right second molar.

The **Palmer Notation System** utilizes four brackets (to denote each quadrant) which surround a number (denoting the tooth in that quadrant). The specific brackets are designed to represent each of the four quadrants of the dentition, as if you are facing the patient:

_| is upper right
|_ is upper left
¯| is lower right
|¯ is lower left

The **permanent teeth** in each quadrant are numbered from 1 (nearest to the arch midline) to 8 (farthest from the midline). For example, 1 is a central incisor, 2 is a lateral incisor, 3 is a canine, etc. This number is placed within the bracket that indicates its quadrant. For example, the lower left central incisor, lower left second pre-

Table 3-1

MAJOR TOOTH IDENTIFICATION SYSTEMS

	Tooth	UNIVERSAL Right	UNIVERSAL Left	PALMER NOTATION Right	PALMER NOTATION Left	INTERNATIONAL (F.D.I.) Right	INTERNATIONAL (F.D.I.) Left
DECIDUOUS DENTITION — MAXILLARY TEETH	Central incisor	E	F	A|	|A	51	61
	Lateral incisor	D	G	B|	|B	52	62
	Canine	C	H	C|	|C	53	63
	First molar	B	I	D|	|D	54	64
	Second molar	A	J	E|	|E	55	65
DECIDUOUS DENTITION — MANDIBULAR TEETH	Central incisor	P	O	A̅|	|A̅	81	71
	Lateral incisor	Q	N	B̅|	|B̅	82	72
	Canine	R	M	C̅|	|C̅	83	73
	First molar	S	L	D̅|	|D̅	84	74
	Second molar	T	K	E̅|	|E̅	85	75
PERMANENT DENTITION — MAXILLARY TEETH	Central incisor	8	9	1|	|1	11	21
	Lateral incisor	7	10	2|	|2	12	22
	Canine	6	11	3|	|3	13	23
	First premolar	5	12	4|	|4	14	24
	Second premolar	4	13	5|	|5	15	25
	First molar	3	14	6|	|6	16	26
	Second molar	2	15	7|	|7	17	27
	Third molar	1	16	8|	|8	18	28
PERMANENT DENTITION — MANDIBULAR TEETH	Central incisor	25	24	1̅|	|1̅	41	31
	Lateral incisor	26	23	2̅|	|2̅	42	32
	Canine	27	22	3̅|	|3̅	43	33
	First premolar	28	21	4̅|	|4̅	44	34
	Second premolar	29	20	5̅|	|5̅	45	35
	First molar	30	19	6̅|	|6̅	46	36
	Second molar	31	18	7̅|	|7̅	47	37
	Third molar	32	17	8̅|	|8̅	48	38

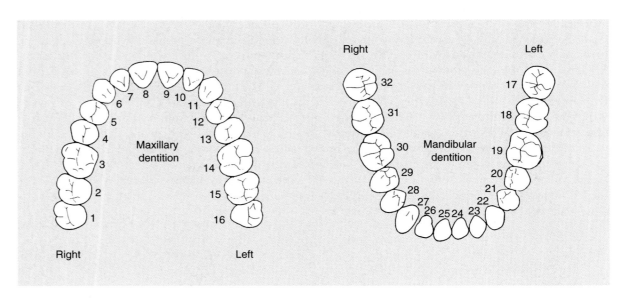

FIGURE 3-1. A drawing of the occlusal and incisal surfaces of the maxillary and mandibular adult dentitions. The numerals 1 to 32 inside the arches give the *Universal numbering code* commonly used for record keeping.

molar, and upper right canine would be shown as ⌐T, ⌐5, and 3⌐, respectively. For **primary teeth**, the same four brackets are used to denote the quadrants, but letters of the alphabet A through E represent the primary teeth (with A being a central incisor, B a lateral incisor, C a canine, etc.). If you are confused, refer to Table 3-1 for clarification.

The **International Numbering System** (Federation Dentaire Internationale [FDI]) uses two digits for each tooth, permanent or primary. The *first digit* denotes the quadrant (right or left) *and* arch (maxillary or mandibular) *and* dentition (permanent or primary) as follows:

1 = Permanent dentition, maxillary, right side.
2 = Permanent dentition, maxillary, left side.
3 = Permanent dentition, mandibular, left side.
4 = Permanent dentition, mandibular, right side.
5 = Primary dentition, maxillary, right side.
6 = Primary dentition, maxillary, left side.
7 = Primary dentition, mandibular, left side.
8 = Primary dentition, mandibular, right side.

The *second digit* denotes the tooth position relative to the midline, from closest to farthest away. Therefore, the second digits 1 through 8 stand for the permanent central incisor through the third molar and 1 through 5 stand for the primary central incisor through the primary second molar. Combining the first and second digits using the International System, all numbers within the range 11 through 48 represent permanent teeth. For example, 48 is a permanent mandibular right third molar, since the first digit, 4, indicates the mandibular right quadrant for a permanent tooth, and the second digit, 8, indicates the eighth tooth from the midline in that quadrant, namely, the third molar. Numbers within the range 51 through 85 represent primary teeth. For example, 51 is a primary maxillary right central incisor since the first digit, 5, indicates the maxillary right quadrant for a primary tooth, and the second digit, 1, indicates the first tooth from the midline in that quadrant, namely, the central incisor. All of the tooth numbers are shown in Table 3-1. You will find it easy to become familiar with any system by first learning (memorizing) the number or letters for key teeth, possibly the central incisors, canines, and first molars. **NOTE: Unless otherwise stated, the Universal System of tooth numbering is used throughout this text.**

SECTION II. Terminology Used to Describe the Parts of a Tooth

A. FOUR TISSUES OF A TOOTH

The tooth is made up of four tissues: enamel, dentin, cementum, and pulp. The first three of these are mostly inorganic or calcified (containing considerable mineral content) and surround the pulpal tissue where the nerves and blood supply are found. Only two tissues are visible in an intact extracted tooth: enamel and cementum. The other two tissues (dentin and pulp) are usually not visible unless the tooth is badly decayed, sectioned, or prepared with a bur, removing the outer layers. Refer to Figure 3-2 while reading about each tissue.

Enamel [ee NAM el] is the white, protective external surface of the anatomic *crown*. It is highly calcified or mineralized and is the hardest substance in the body. The mineral content is 95% calcium hydroxyapatite (which is calcified and inorganic). The remaining substances include 4% water and 1% enamel matrix (organic matter). It develops from the enamel organ (ectoderm) and is a product of a specialized type of epithelial cell called **ameloblasts** [ah MEL o blasts].

Cementum [se MEN tum] is the dull yellow external layer of the tooth *root*. The cementum is very thin next to the cervical line, no thicker than a page in this text (only 50-100 μm thick). It is composed of 65% calcium hydroxyapatite (calcified and inorganic), 23% organic matter (collagen fibers), and 12% water and is about as hard as bone. It develops from the dental sac (mesoderm), and it is produced by cells called **cementoblasts** [se MEN toe blasts].

The **cementoenamel** [se MEN toe ehn AM el] **junction** separates the enamel of the anatomic crown from the cementum of the anatomic root. This junction is also known as the **cervical** [SER vi kal] **line**, denoting that it surrounds the neck or **cervix** [SER viks] of the tooth.

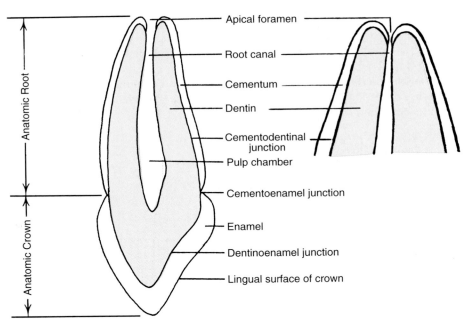

FIGURE 3-2. A maxillary anterior tooth sectioned longitudinally through the center to show the distribution of the *tooth tissues* and the shape of the pulp cavity (made up of pulp chamber and root canal). On the right is a close-up of the apical portion depicting the usual expected constriction of the root canal near the apical foramen. The layer of cementum covering the root of an actual tooth is proportionately much *thinner* than seen in these drawings.

Dentin [DEN tin] is the hard, yellowish tissue underlying the enamel and cementum making up the major bulk of the inner portion of each tooth crown and root. It extends internally from the pulp cavity in the center of the tooth outward to the inner surface of the enamel (on the crown) or cementum (on the root). Dentin is not normally visible except on a dental radiograph, on a sectioned tooth, or on a badly worn tooth. Dentin is composed of 70% calcium hydroxyapatite (calcified and inorganic), 18% organic matter (collagen fibers), and 12% water, making it harder than cementum but softer than enamel. Dentin develops from the embryonic dental papilla (mesoderm). The cells that form dentin are called **odontoblasts** [o DON toe blasts] located at the junction between pulp and dentin.

The **dentinoenamel** [DEN tin o ehn AM el] **junction** is the inner surface of the enamel cap where enamel joins dentin (only visible on a cross-section or when preparing a tooth for a restoration). The **cementodentinal** [se MEN toe DEN tin al] or **dentinocemental junction** is the inner surface of cementum lining the root (also only visible on teeth in cross-section).

Pulp is the soft (not calcified) tissue in the cavity or space in the center of the crown and root called the **pulp cavity**. The pulp cavity has a coronal portion (**pulp chamber**) and a root portion (**pulp canal[s]**). The pulp cavity is surrounded by dentin, except at a hole (or holes) near the root tip (apex) called an **apical** [APE i kal] **foramen**, plural foramina. Like dentin, the pulp is normally not visible, except on a dental radiograph (x-ray) or sectioned tooth. It develops from the dental papilla (mesoderm). Pulp is soft connective tissue containing a rich supply of blood vessels and nerves. Functions of the dental pulp are:

- *Formative*: Dentin-producing cells (odontoblasts) produce dentin throughout the life of a tooth. This is called secondary dentin.
- *Sensory*: Nerve endings permit the sense of pain from heat, cold, drilling, sweet, decay, trauma, or infection. However, the nerve fibers in a dental pulp are unable to distinguish the cause of the pain.
- *Nutritive*: Pulp transports nutrients from the bloodstream to cells of the pulp that reach the osteoblasts in the dentin. Surprisingly, blood in the tooth pulp had passed through the heart only 6 seconds previously.
- *Defensive or protective*: Pulp responds to injury or decay by forming reparative dentin (by the odontoblasts). Undifferentiated mesenchymal cells serve to replace injured or destroyed odontoblasts.

B. *ANATOMIC* VERSUS *CLINICAL* CROWN AND ROOT

1. ANATOMIC CROWN AND ROOT DEFINITION

The **anatomic crown** is that part of the tooth (in the mouth or hand held) normally covered by an enamel surface (Fig. 3-2), and the **anatomic root** is the part of a tooth covered by a cementum surface. A cervical line (or cementoenamel junction) separates the anatomic crown from the anatomic root. This relationship does not change over a patient's lifetime.

2. CLINICAL CROWN AND ROOT (ONLY APPLIES WHEN THE TOOTH IS IN THE MOUTH AND AT LEAST PARTIALLY ERUPTED)

The **clinical crown** refers specifically to the amount of tooth visible in the oral cavity, and the **clinical root** refers to the amount of tooth that is *not* visible since it is beneath the gingiva. Clinically, the gingival margin in a 25-year-old patient with healthy gingiva approximately follows the curvature of the cervical line, and under these conditions the clinical crown is essentially the same as the anatomic crown. However, the gingiva or gingival margin is not always at the level of the cervical line because of the eruption process early in life or due to recession of the gingiva later in life. For example, the gingival margin on a partially erupted tooth of a 10-year-old covers much of the enamel of the anatomic crown of the tooth, resulting in a clinical crown (exposed in the mouth) which is much shorter than the anatomic crown. The clinical root (not visible in the mouth) would be longer than the anatomic root (consisting of the anatomic root plus the part of the anatomic crown covered with gingiva).

In contrast, the gingival margin in a 60-year-old person may exhibit gingival recession, especially after having periodontal disease or periodontal therapy, exposing more of the anatomic root, and result in a clinical crown that is longer than the anatomic crown (made up of all of the anatomic crown and part of the anatomic root that is exposed). In this situation, the clinical root is shorter than the anatomic root.

LEARNING EXERCISE

Examine the mouths of several persons of different ages to see if the cervical line is visible or hidden. As the individual grows older, the location of the margin of the gingiva may recede toward the root tip (apically) because of periodontal disease or injury (such as from the faulty use of oral hygiene aids). Of course, the location of the cervical line on the tooth remains the same. In other words, the distinction between the anatomic crown and root does not change over a lifetime.

SECTION III. Terminology Used to Define Tooth Surfaces

A. TERMS THAT IDENTIFY OUTER SURFACES OF ANTERIOR VERSUS POSTERIOR TEETH

All teeth have surfaces that are named according to their usual alignment within the dental arch. Refer to Figure 3-3 when studying the terms to denote tooth surfaces. The **facial surface** of a tooth is the surface toward the face, that is, the outer surface of a tooth in the mouth resting against or next to the cheeks or lips. Facial may be used to designate this portion of any tooth, anterior or posterior. Another name for the facial surface of *posterior* teeth is **buccal** [BUCK k'l], located next to the cheek (labeled on tooth **#**3 in Fig. 3-3). It is incorrect to use this term when speaking about the incisors or canines because they do not approximate the cheeks. The facial surface of *anterior* teeth are properly called **labial** [LAY bee al] **surfaces**, located next to the lip (labeled on tooth **#**6 in Fig. 3-3). This term should not be used when referring to the premolars or the molars.

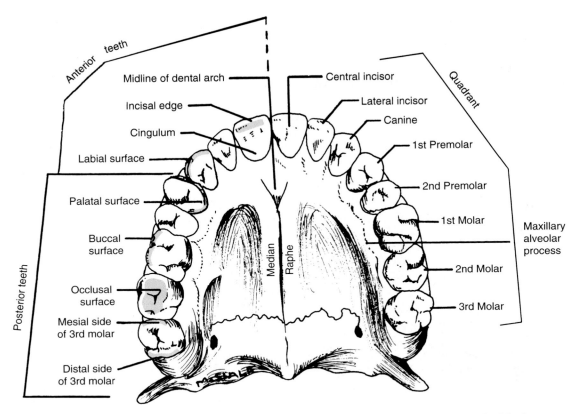

FIGURE 3-3. Maxillary dental arch of teeth with the *tooth surfaces* labeled. Remember that the labial surface of an anterior tooth and the buccal surface of a posterior tooth are both referred to as facial surfaces. Also, the mesial and distal sides or surfaces are correctly called proximal surfaces.

B. TERMS THAT IDENTIFY INNER SURFACES (TOWARD THE TONGUE) OF MAXILLARY VERSUS MANDIBULAR TEETH

The **lingual** [LIN gwal] **surface** is the surface of a maxillary or mandibular tooth nearest the tongue. In the maxillary arch, this surface can also be called **palatal surface** due to its proximity with the palate (labeled on tooth **#5** in Fig. 3-3).

C. TERMS THAT DIFFERENTIATE BITING SURFACES OF ANTERIOR VERSUS POSTERIOR TEETH

The **occlusal** [ahk KLOO zal] **surface** is the chewing surface of a posterior tooth (labeled on tooth **#2** in Figure 3-3). Anterior teeth (incisors and canines) do not have an occlusal surface but do have an **incisal edge**, which is the cutting edge, ridge, or surface (labeled on tooth **#8** on Figure 3-3).

D. TERMS THAT DIFFERENTIATE APPROXIMATING SURFACES OF TEETH

The **proximal** [PROCK se mal] **surfaces** are the sides of a tooth generally next to an adjacent tooth. Depending on whether the tooth surface faces toward the arch midline between the central incisors or away from the midline, it is either a **mesial** [MEE zi al] **surface** (closer to the midline) or a **distal** [DIS tal] **surface** (farther from the midline). These surfaces are labeled on tooth **#1** in Figure 3-3. Note that the mesial surface of all teeth touch, or are closest to, the distal of the adjacent tooth except between the central incisors where the mesial surface of one central incisor faces another mesial surface. Also, the distal surface of the last molar in each arch does not approximate another tooth. Proximal surfaces are generally not considered to be self-cleansing (by the action of the cheeks and lips and tongue), when compared to the facial, lingual, and occlusal surfaces, which are more self-cleansing.

E. DIVISIONS OF THE CROWN OR ROOT OF A TOOTH (FOR PURPOSES OF DESCRIPTION)

A tooth can be divided into thirds in order to define more precisely the location of its specific landmarks. When viewing a tooth from the facial, lingual, mesial, or distal surface, *horizontal* lines can divide the tooth *crown* into thirds: cervical, middle, and occlusal (or incisal). Similarly, *horizontal* lines can divide the *root* into thirds: cervical, middle, and apical (toward the root tip or apex) (Fig. 3-4).

When viewing the tooth from the *facial (or lingual)* surface, *vertical* lines can be used to divide the crown or root into mesial, middle, and distal thirds. When viewing the tooth from the *proximal* (mesial or distal) surface, *vertical* lines can be used to divide the crown or root into facial, middle, and lingual thirds.

F. TERMS TO DENOTE TOOTH SURFACE JUNCTIONS OR DIMENSIONS

To describe the junction (line) where two surfaces meet (called an external **line-angle**), the names for the two surfaces are combined by changing the "al" ending in the first surface to an "o." Examples of external line-angles of a molar crown include mesio-occlusal, mesiolingual, mesiofacial, disto-occlusal, distolingual, distofacial, bucco-occlusal, and linguo-occlusal. Examples of these external line angles are seen in Figure 3-5. **Point angles** are the junctions of three tooth surfaces at a point, such as a mesiobucco-occlusal point angle.

To describe a dimension of a tooth, combined terms can be used to denote the direction over which the dimension was taken. For example, the length of an incisor crown from the incisal edge to the cervical line could be called the incisocervical dimension or the dimension incisocervically (Fig. 3-5). Other similar terms used to describe a crown dimension include faciolingual or buccolingual, mesiodistal, and cervico-occlusal. Root dimensions could also be described as cervicoapical.

G. ROOT-TO-CROWN RATIO

If we know the length of a tooth root (from the cervical line to the tip of the longest root) and the length of the crown (from the cervical line to the tip of the longest cusp or highest part of the incisal edge), we can calculate a **root-to-crown ratio**. For example, the average root length of a maxillary central incisor is only 13.0 mm, and the crown length is 11.2 mm, which are really close to the same size. The root-to-crown ratio is 13 divided by 11.2, which equals 1.16. This ratio of *close to one* indicates that the root is not much longer than the crown. Contrast this with a maxillary canine, where the average root is much longer, at 16.5 mm, but the crown is only 10.6 mm for a much larger root-to-crown ratio of 1.56. A larger ratio like this indicates that the root is over one and a half times longer than the crown. The ratio becomes clinically significant, since a tooth with a *small* root-to-crown ratio (closer to one) is not a good candidate for attaching and supporting false teeth because the additional attached teeth would apply even more forces on a tooth that already has a short root, compared to its crown length.

Arbitrary division of teeth

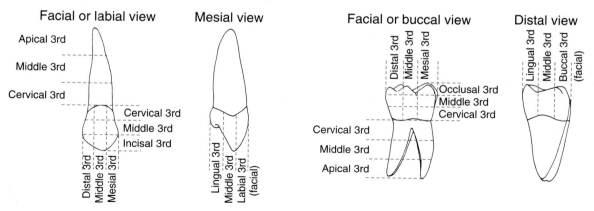

FIGURE 3-4. Diagram of a maxillary canine and a mandibular first molar to show the manner in which the parts of a tooth may be divided into *thirds* from each view for purposes of description, location of anatomic landmarks, contact areas, and so forth.

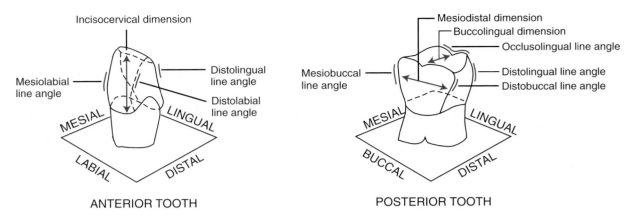

FIGURE 3-5. Diagrammatic representation of an incisor and molar crown showing the surfaces and external tooth *line angles* and *indications for dimensions.*

SECTION IV. Terminology Used to Describe the Morphology of a Tooth

A. MORPHOLOGY OF AN ANATOMIC CROWN

Teeth are made up of many bumps, ridges, depressions and grooves. Specific tooth structures that occur with some frequency on teeth within a class have been assigned specific names. To identify the following anatomic structures, reference will be made primarily to representative drawings of a canine (See Fig. 3-8) and a premolar (See Fig. 3-9).

1. BULGES (ROUNDED) AND RIDGES (LINEAR)

A **cusp** (with a **cusp tip**) is a pointed part, or peak, located on the occlusal surfaces of molar and premolar teeth and on the incisal edges of canines. Each cusp is named according to its location on the tooth. For example, on a two-cusped premolar, the two cusps are named buccal and lingual. On a four-cusped molar, the four cusps are named mesiobuccal, distobuccal, mesiolingual, and distolingual. Refer to Figure 3-6 for a sampling of cusp names on various teeth in the mouth.

Each cusp tip has four **cusp ridges** (linear prominences) of enamel converging toward it. These four ridges form the shape of a four-sided, somewhat rounded pyramid. If you were to draw a line along the greatest linear bulge of each of these four ridges, the lines would intersect at the cusp tip, forming a + shape seen by the dotted lines on the buccal cusp of the tooth in Figure 3-7. On this cusp, three of the ridges are named after the circumferential tooth surface they extend toward: the *facial* (buccal or labial) ridge actually extends onto the facial surface, the *mesial* cusp ridge extends from the cusp tip toward the mesial surface, and the *distal* cusp ridge extends from the cusp tip toward the distal surface. The fourth ridge from the cusp tip to the faciolingual center of the tooth is called a *triangular* ridge.

The **mesial and distal cusp ridges** are also known as **cusp slopes** or cusp arms. They are the inclined surfaces or slopes that converge at the cusp tip to form an angle when viewed from the facial or lingual aspect (seen on the facial view of a canine in Fig. 3-8A and on the lingual cusp of a premolar from the occlusal view in Fig. 3-9). Seen from the facial or lingual views, this cusp angle (how sharp or how blunt) is an important trait for certain classes or types of teeth.

On incisor and canine teeth (Fig. 3-8B), **marginal ridges** are located on the mesial and distal border of the lingual surface and converge toward the cingulum. On posterior teeth, they are located on the mesial and distal borders of the occlusal surface (Fig. 3-9A).

Triangular ridges are located on each major cusp of *posterior* teeth. Each triangular ridge extends from a cusp tip generally toward the middle of the occlusal surface faciolingually (Fig. 3-9A). Each cusp on all posterior teeth has one triangular ridge, except the mesiolingual cusp on maxillary molars, which has two triangular ridges (Fig. 3-10). When one triangular ridge from a facial cusp tip joins with a triangular ridge from a lingual cusp tip, the two ridges together form a longer ridge called

CUSPS

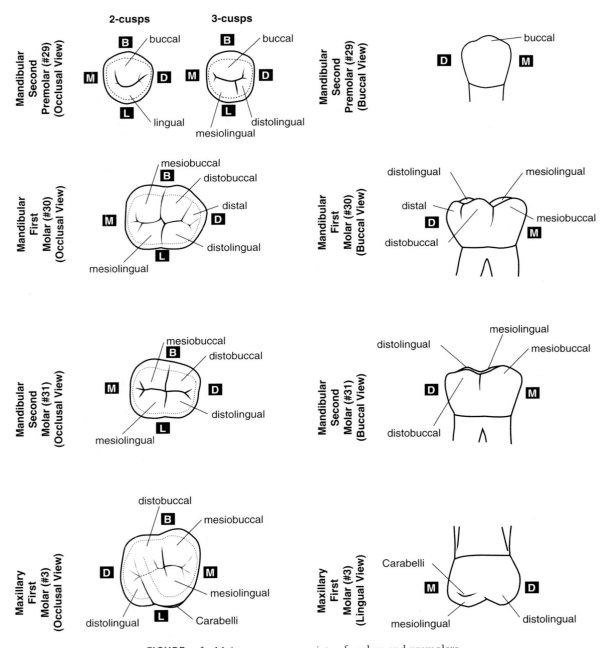

FIGURE 3-6. Major *cusps* on a variety of molars and premolars.

All cusps are basically a gothic pyramid

The cuspal gothic pyramid produces 4 ridges:
1. Mesial cusp ridge
2. Distal cusp ridge
3. Buccal cusp ridge (labial ridge on canines)
4. Triangular ridge on posterior teeth (lingual ridge on canines)

FIGURE 3-7. Buccal cusp showing the pyramidal design (actually the pyramid with rounded sides is called a gothic pyramid) of the *four cusp ridges* that make up each cusp. These are numbered 1-4 around the cusp tip (X) on a maxillary right first premolar. (Courtesy of Drs. Richard W. Huffman and Ruth Paulson).

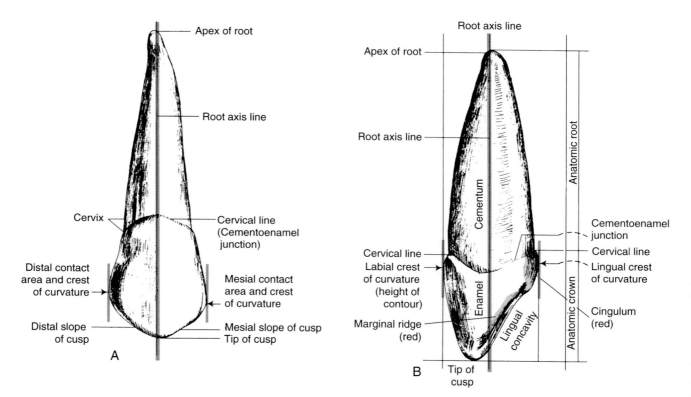

FIGURE 3-8. A. Labial surface of the maxillary right canine showing the location of proximal contacts (crests of curvature). The *root axis* is determined by bisecting the root at the cervix. B. Mesial side of the same maxillary right canine. The root axis line bisects the root in the cervical area. Customarily, other parts of the tooth are located or described relative to this line. For instance, the cusp tip of this canine is labial to the root axis line.

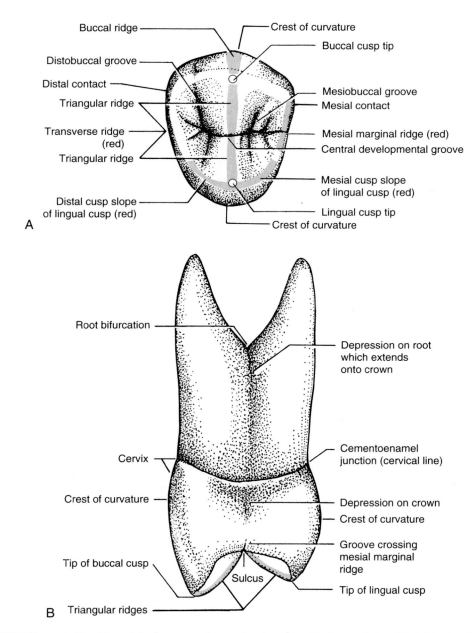

FIGURE 3-9. A. Maxillary right first premolar, occlusal surface. Notice *mesial and distal contact* locations and facial and lingual *height of contour (crests of curvature)*. **B**. Maxillary right first premolar, mesial surface. The *sulcus* is the occlusal depression between cusps (like a valley) that is seen on all posterior teeth. The *height of contour* (crest of curvature) from this view is in the cervical third on the buccal and in the middle third on the lingual (as on all posterior teeth).

RIDGES

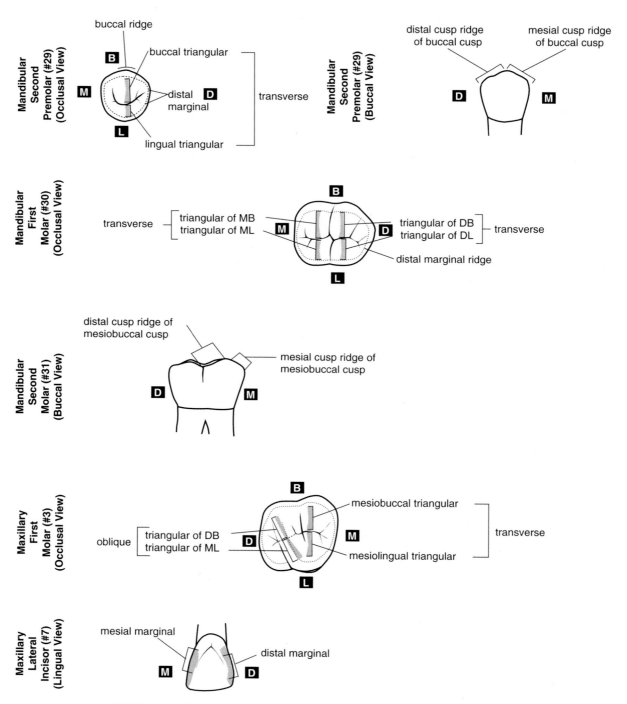

FIGURE 3-10. Examples of a variety of *ridges* on molars, premolars, and incisors.

either a transverse or oblique ridge. A **transverse ridge** crosses the occlusal surface of posterior teeth in a more or less buccolingual direction (e.g., running between the buccal and lingual cusp on a premolar [Fig. 3-9A] or between the mesiolingual and mesiobuccal cusps on a molar [seen on the premolar and mandibular first molar in Fig. 3-10]). An **oblique ridge** is a ridge found only on maxillary molars. It crosses the occlusal surface obliquely (diagonally) and is made up of the triangular ridges of the mesiolingual and the distobuccal cusps (seen on the maxillary first molar in Fig. 3-10).

Perhaps the subtlest ridge coming off of the cusp tip is the facial (labial or buccal) ridge. The **buccal (cusp) ridge** is a subtle ridge running cervico-occlusally in approximately the center of the buccal surface of premolars, more pronounced on the first premolars than on the second premolars (Fig. 3-9A). Similar in appearance on canines, the **labial ridge** runs cervicoincisally and is most prominent in the center of the maxillary canines.

LEARNING EXERCISE

The diagram in Figure 3-11 represents the ridges seen from the occlusal view that bound the occlusal table of a premolar. Name each ridge next to its corresponding number.

Other bulges or ridges can be seen on the cervical third of a tooth facially and lingually. On the lingual of all anterior teeth, the **cingulum** [SING gyoo lum] is the enlargement or bulge on the cervical third of the lingual surface of the crown on anterior teeth (incisors and canines) (Fig. 3-8B). Finally, found on the facial surface of permanent molars and all primary teeth, the **cervical ridge** is a subtle ridge running *mesiodistally* in the cervical one-third of the buccal surface of the crown (seen later in Chapter 7 in Fig. 7-23).

Mamelons are three small tubercles or scallops, each formed from one of the three facial developmental lobes on the incisal edges of newly erupted incisors (Fig. 3-12). (Lobes will be described in more detail in Section VII of this chapter.) Usually mamelons are not evident on adult dentition since they are worn off after the tooth comes into functional contacts with its opposing tooth. If you have the opportunity, observe a 7-year-old smile to see these mamelons on newly erupted incisors. When mamelons remain on an adult, it is because these teeth do not contact opposing teeth in function, as may occur with an anterior open-bite relationship. When a patient desires, the dentist can reduce the mamelons to make the incisal edge more uniformly curved.

Finally, **perikymata** [pear i KY mah tah] are the numerous, minute horizontal ridges on the enamel of newly erupted permanent teeth (Figs. 3-13 and 3-14). They form from the overlapping of layers of enamel laid down during tooth formation. These lines are closer together in the cervical part of the crown than they are nearer the incisal edge. They are most easily seen on the labial surfaces of the anterior teeth because of their accessible location. Perikymata are more prominent on the teeth of young people than on the teeth of older persons because perikymata, like mamelons, wear away from ongoing abrasion due to eating and even tooth brushing with abrasive tooth pastes.

2. DEPRESSIONS AND GROOVES

The **sulcus** is the broad depression or valley on the occlusal surfaces of posterior teeth, the inclines of which are formed by triangular ridges that often converge at the depth of the sulcus in a developmental **groove** (see Fig. 3-9. B). Grooves and their sulcuses are important escapeways for opposing upper and lower cusps and food morsels when the mandible moves from side-to-side (lateral movements) and protrudes forward (protrusive movements). Partially chewed food squirts out toward the tongue and cheeks.

Developmental grooves are sharply defined narrow linear depressions, short or long, formed during tooth development and usually separating the lobes or major portions of a tooth (described in Sec-

Figure 3.11

1. _____

2. _____

3. _____

4. _____

5. _____

6. _____

7. _____

8. _____

9. _____

10. Transverse

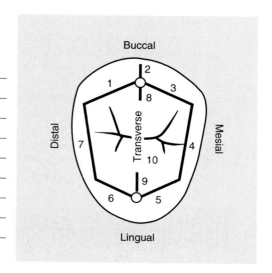

FIGURE 3-11. List ridges on this maxillary premolar.

Answers: 1. distal cusp ridge of buccal (cusp) ridge; 2. buccal (cusp) ridge; 3. mesial cusp ridge of buccal cusp; 4. mesial marginal ridge; 5. mesial cusp ridge of lingual cusp; 6. distal cusp ridge of lingual cusp; 7. distal marginal ridge; 8. triangular ridge of buccal cusp; 9. triangular ridge of lingual cusp.

tion VII of this chapter). Like cusps, the major grooves are named according to their location. For example, on the premolar in Figure 3-15, the *central* groove is located in the buccolingual center of the tooth and runs mesiodistally. At each end of the central groove both mesially and distally, *fossa developmental grooves (or triangular fossa grooves)* may be found splitting off toward the corners of the tooth. These grooves can be named for the corner of the tooth toward which they aim, for example, the mesiobuccal fossa developmental groove (sometimes just called mesiobuccal groove). On many molars, a *buccal* groove runs from the central groove onto the buccal surface, and a *lingual* groove extends from the central groove onto the lingual surface (Fig. 3-16).

Additional grooves that are not developmental grooves are called **supplemental grooves**. These small irregularly placed grooves on the occlusal surface do *not* occur at the junction of the lobes or major portions of the tooth. Supplemental grooves are named for the surface or corner of the tooth where they are located (e.g., a mesiolingual supplemental groove) (Fig. 3-15).

FIGURE 3-12. Example of three distinct unworn *mamelons* present on the incisal edge of a mandibular right central incisor, labial view.

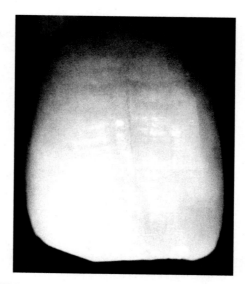

FIGURE 3-13. *Perikymata* on the labial surface of a maxillary right central incisor.

Perikymata

FIGURE 3-14. **A.** Magnified view of *perikymata* (imbrication lines) near the cementoenamel junction, where they are closest together. Notice their wave-like pattern. The cervical line is quite irregular at this magnification, and the cementum is thin, not necessarily extending to the enamel at every point. **B.** Cross-section of enamel showing perikymata waves on the right and the long enamel rods packed tightly and extending inward from the surface on the left. **C.** Higher magnification (x220) of enamel surface shows enamel rod ends on the perikymata waves. Enamel rods are about 4 μm in diameter. (These scanning electron micrographs were kindly provided by Dr. Ruth B. Paulson, Associate Professor Emeritus, Division of Oral Biology, Ohio State University.)

Central developmental groove (**C**)

Fossa developmental grooves (**F**)

Supplemental grooves (**S**)

Marginal ridge groove (**M**)

FIGURE 3-15. An occlusal surface of a maxillary right first premolar depicting various *occlusal grooves*. Some texts consider the fossa grooves as supplemental grooves. (Courtesy of Drs. Richard W. Huffman and Ruth Paulson.)

GROOVES

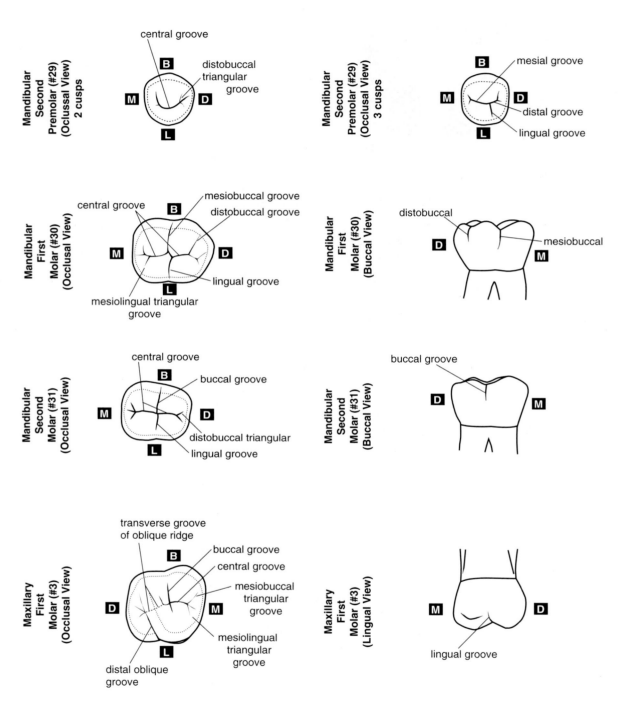

FIGURE 3-16. Examples of developmental *grooves* on molars and premolars.

A **fissure** is a very narrow cleft or crevice at the depth of any groove, caused by the incomplete fusion of enamel during tooth development (Fig. 12.1). Decay (dental **caries** [CARE eez]) often begins in a deep fissure (described in more detail in Chapter 12).

A **fossa** [FAH sah] (plural, fossae) is a small hollow or depression found between the marginal ridges on the lingual surfaces of anterior teeth (particularly maxillary incisors) and on the occlusal surfaces of all posterior teeth. **Pits** often occur at the depth of a fossa where two or more grooves join. For example, within the mesial fossa on a premolar there is a mesial pit at the junction of the central groove with the mesiobuccal and mesiolingual fossa grooves (Fig. 3-17A). Like fissures that are found at the depth of grooves, pits are enamel defects where dental decay may begin. Examples of the names assigned to fossae and pits for various teeth are seen in Figure 3-18.

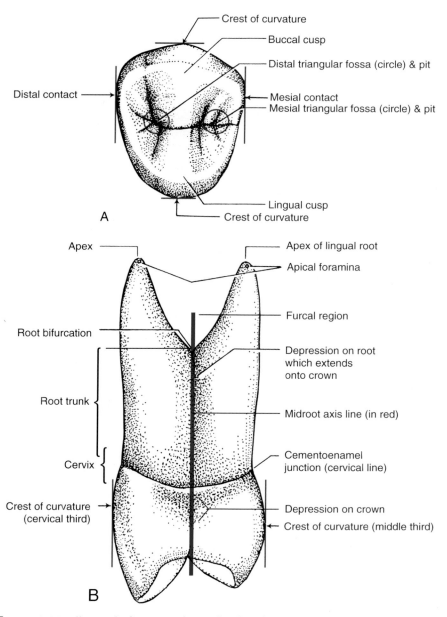

FIGURE 3-17. **A**. Maxillary right first premolar, occlusal surface. Notice the *mesial and distal triangular fossae*. **B**. Maxillary right first premolar, mesial surface. The space between the two roots is the *furcal region*, and the root area between the cervical line and root bifurcation is the *root trunk*.

FOSSAE AND PITS

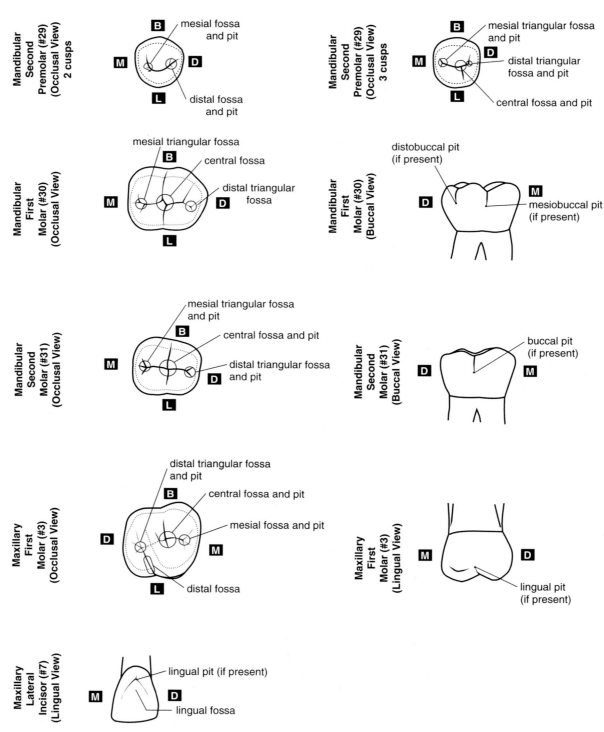

FIGURE 3-18. Examples of various *fossae* (often with associated *pits*) on molars, premolars, and incisors.

Table 3-2

AVERAGE MEASUREMENTS ON 4,572 EXTRACTED TEETH FROM OHIO FROM A STUDY BY DR. WOELFEL AND HIS FIRST-YEAR DENTAL HYGIENE STUDENTS OF THE OHIO STATE UNIVERSITY COLLEGE OF DENTISTRY, 1974–1979. SIZE RANGES ARE SHOWN IN TABLES IN EACH CHAPTER.

MAXILLARY TEETH	CROWN LENGTH (MM)		ROOT LENGTH (MM)	ROOT TO CROWN RATIO	OVERALL LENGTH (MM)	CROWN WIDTH M-D (MM)	CERVIX WIDTH M-D (MM)	CROWN WIDTH F-L (MM)	CERVIX WIDTH F-L (MM)	MESIAL CERVICAL CURVE (MM)	DISTAL CERVICAL CURVE (MM)
Central incisor (398)	11.2		13.0	1.16	23.6	8.6	6.4	7.1	6.3	2.8	2.3
Lateral incisor (295)	9.8		13.4	1.37	22.5	6.6	4.7	6.2	5.8	2.5	1.9
Canine (321)	10.6		16.5	1.56	26.3	7.6	5.6	8.1	7.6	2.1	1.4
First premolar (234)	8.6		13.4	1.56	21.5	7.1	4.8	9.2	8.2	1.1	0.7
Second premolar (224)	7.7		14.0	1.82	21.2	6.6	4.7	9.0	8.1	0.9	0.6
First molar (308)	7.5	MB	12.9	1.72	20.1	10.4	7.9	11.5	10.7	0.7	0.3
		DB	12.2								
		L	13.7								
Second molar (309)	7.6	MB	12.9	1.70	20.0	9.8	7.6	11.4	10.7	0.6	0.2
		DB	12.1								
		L	13.5								
Third molar (305)	7.2	MB	10.8	1.49	17.5	9.2	7.2	11.1	10.4	0.5	0.2
		DB	10.1								
		L	11.2								
Avg. 2,392 Upper teeth	8.77		13.36	1.55	21.59	8.23	6.11	9.20	8.48	1.40	0.97
MANDIBULAR TEETH											
Central incisor (226)	8.8		12.6	1.43	20.8	5.3	3.5	5.7	5.4	2.0	1.6
Lateral incisor (234)	9.4		13.5	1.43	22.1	5.7	3.8	6.1	5.8	2.1	1.5
Canine (316)	11.0		15.9	1.45	25.9	6.8	5.2	7.7	7.5	2.4	1.6
First premolar (238)	8.8		14.4	1.64	22.4	7.0	4.8	7.7	7.0	0.9	0.6
Second premolar (227)	8.2		14.7	1.80	22.1	7.1	5.0	8.2	7.3	0.8	0.5
First molar (281)	7.7	M	14.0	1.83	20.9	11.4	9.2	10.2	9.0	0.5	0.2
		D	13.0								
Second molar (296)	7.7	M	13.9	1.82	20.6	10.8	9.1	9.9	8.8	0.5	0.2
		D	13.0								
Third molar (262)	7.5	M	11.8	1.57	18.2	11.3	9.2	10.1	8.9	0.4	0.2
		D	10.8								
Avg. 2,180 Lower teeth	8.62		13.85	1.62	21.61	8.17	6.24	8.22	7.44	1.20	0.80

Hint: In summary, if you compare tooth morphology to a mountain range, the mountain peak would be the cusp tip. Ridges emanating from the mountain peak are like the cusp ridges and triangular ridges. The depression between the height of the mountains (or cusps) is a valley, like the tooth sulcus. The dried riverbed at the bottom of the valley (sulcus) is like a groove (and if cracked open, it is like a fissure). Where riverbeds converge, the whirlpools and eddies may have formed a depression, like a fossa, possibly with a pit at its depth. Needless to say, it is hard to define exactly where a mountain stops and a valley starts, just as it would be hard to point to exactly where a tooth cusp stops and a sulcus begins. Just realize that these terms are not precise but that they are helpful when learning how to reproduce tooth form during construction of crowns and placement of fillings or when learning to finish and polish an existing filling.

B. EXTERNAL MORPHOLOGY OF THE ANATOMIC ROOT

Refer to Figure 3-17 while studying the external morphology of tooth roots. Recall that the anatomic root is the part of a tooth that has a cementum surface. The **apex** of the root is the tip or peak at the end of the root, often with visible openings called **apical foramina**, where the nerves and blood vessels enter into the tooth pulp. The **cervix** [SUR viks] or neck of the tooth is the slightly constricted region of union of the crown and the root.

Some new terms apply to multirooted teeth. The **root trunk** or trunk base is the part of the root of a multirooted molar or two-rooted premolar next to the cementoenamel junction that has not yet split (like a stubby tree trunk before it gives off branches) (Fig. 3-17B). The **furcation** [fur CAY shun] is the place on multirooted teeth where the root trunk divides into separate roots (called a **bifurcation** on two-rooted teeth and a **trifurcation** on three-rooted teeth). The **furcal region** or interradicular space is the region or *space* between two or more roots, apical to the place where the roots divide from the root trunk.

C. RELATIVE SIZE

Using a sample size of 4,572 extracted teeth, the average dimensions of each type of tooth have been determined and serve as the basis for many statements made within this textbook. These data are presented in Table 3-2 and are useful for determining the tooth with the longest crown, the longest overall length, the shortest root, and so forth.

SECTION V. Terminology Related to the Ideal Alignment of Teeth in Dental Arches

---

When viewed from the occlusal aspect, each dental arch is somewhat U-shaped or parabolic like the famous arch in St. Louis (recall Fig. 3-1). The incisal edges and the buccal cusp tips follow a curved line around the outer edge of the dental arch; the lingual cusp tips of the posterior teeth follow a curved line nearly parallel to the buccal cusp tips. Between the buccal and lingual cusps is the **sulcular groove**, which runs anteroposteriorly the length of the posterior teeth.

When the arches are viewed *from the buccal aspect*, an **anteroposterior curve** (curve of Spee) is evident where the cusp tips of posterior teeth follow a gradual curve anteroposteriorly (see Fig. 3-20). The curve in the maxillary arch of teeth is convex, while that in the mandibular arch of teeth that fit together against the maxillary teeth is concave. A **mediolateral curve** (Curve of Wilson) is a side-to-side curve (represented by the dotted line in Fig. 10-8). When viewed from the anterior aspect with the mouth slightly open, you can see that the lingual cusps of the posterior teeth are aligned at a more inferior level than the buccal cusps on both sides and in both arches. When the buccal and lingual cusps of the molars or premolars on either side of the arch are connected forming one line from the left side to the right side, this curve is evident. The mediolateral curve of the maxillary arch is convex, whereas that of the mandibular arch is concave.

A. ROOT AXIS LINE

The **root axis line** is an imaginary line through the center of the tooth root. It can be visualized on the facial or lingual surface as a line that divides the tooth at the cervix into mesial and distal halves (Fig. 3-8A). When viewing the mesial or distal surface, it divides the tooth at the cervix into facial and lingual halves (Fig. 3-8B). It is an important reference line for describing the location of tooth landmarks. For example, you will learn that the incisal cusp ridge of many mandibular incisors is more likely to be lingual to the root axis line, whereas for many maxillary incisors it is more likely to be labial to the root axis line.

B. HEIGHT OF CONTOUR (CREST OF CURVATURE)

The shape and height of the greatest curvature or convex bulge on tooth surfaces helps determines the direction of food particles as they are pushed cervically over the tooth surfaces during mastication. When we are chewing food, these natural tooth convexities divert food away from the collar of tissue (gingiva) surrounding the neck of the tooth and toward the buccal vestibule and toward the palate or tongue, thus preventing trauma to the gingiva. If teeth were flat in their middle and cervical thirds, a great deal of food would lodge and remain near the gingival margin and sulcus until removed by a toothpick or toothbrush or by dental floss. Needless to say, it would behoove the dentist, dental hygienist, and/or dental technician to reproduce and maintain these natural concavities when restoring a tooth, when finishing and polishing fillings near the gum line, or when replacing a tooth with a bridge or dental implant. Thus the restored or replaced tooth will be more self-cleansing and protect the adjacent gingiva.

Refer to Figure 3-17 while reading the following. The **height of contour (crest of curvature)** is the highest point of a curve or greatest convexity or bulge farthest from the root axis line. The height of contour on the facial and lingual surfaces of the crown is where this greatest bulge would be touched by a tangent line drawn parallel to the root axis line (Fig. 3-17). The location of the height of contour on the facial and lingual surfaces of the crowns of teeth can be best seen from the mesial or distal views and is usually located in either the cervical third or the middle third (never the occlusal or incisal third) (Fig. 3-17B).

The location of the height of contour on the *facial* surface of *all* crowns is located in the cervical third. The location of the lingual height of contour differs, depending on whether the tooth is anterior or posterior. The *lingual* height of contour on *anterior* teeth is on the cingulum, which is in the cervical third. The *lingual* height of contour on *posterior* teeth is more likely to be located in the middle third. Refer to Table 3-3 for a summary of the location of the facial and lingual heights of contour when moving from anterior teeth to posterior teeth.

C. CONTACT AREAS (OR PROXIMAL HEIGHTS OF CONTOUR)

When the teeth are in normal alignment within an arch, the location of the mesial and distal heights of contour (when viewed directly from the facial or lingual sides) is essentially the same location as contact areas (seen from the facial view in Fig. 3-19 and from the occlusal view in Fig. 3-17A). **Contact areas** are the greatest heights of contour on the proximal surfaces of tooth crowns, where one tooth touches an adjacent tooth. Floss must pass through contact areas to clean the proximal surfaces, which are otherwise inaccessible to the toothbrush.

In a young person, contact areas on teeth start off on recently approximating teeth as contact *points*. Then, as the teeth rub together in function, these points become somewhat flattened and truly become contact *areas*. It has been shown by careful measurements that, by age 40 in a healthy mouth with a complete dentition, 10 mm of enamel has been worn off the contact areas of the teeth in an entire arch. This averages 0.38 mm per contact area on each tooth and certainly emphasizes the amount of proximal attrition that occurs. Therefore, we would expect contact areas on teeth of older people to be large and somewhat flattened.

Contact areas viewed from the facial are characteristically located in the incisal or occlusal third, in the middle third, or at the junction of the incisal and middle (or occlusal and middle) thirds. Contact points are not normally cervical to the middle of the tooth crown and are therefore never located in the cervical third (Fig 3-19). The contact of each tooth with the adjacent teeth has important functions:

- The combined anchorage of all teeth within each arch making positive contact with each other *stabilizes* the position of teeth within the dental arches.
- Contact helps *prevent food impaction*, which can contribute to decay and gum and bone disease (periodontal disease).
- Contact *protects the interdental papillae* of the gingiva by shunting food toward the buccal and lingual areas.

Table 3-3

SUMMARY OF TOOTH CHARACTERISTICS FOR ANTERIOR AND POSTERIOR TEETH

Proximal Contacts (Proximal crest of curvature) viewed from the facial aspect

All teeth: Distal contacts are more cervical than mesial contacts except mandibular first premolars (where the mesial is more cervical) and mandibular central incisors (mesial and distal contacts are at the same level).

All anterior teeth: Mesial contacts are in the incisal third (or for the maxillary canine, at the junction of the incisal and middle thirds). Contact areas become more cervical when moving from the midline (where they are almost at the incisal edge) to the distal of the canine.

All posterior teeth: Mesial contacts are at or near the junction of the middle and occlusal thirds. Mesial and distal contact areas become more cervical toward the distal of the arch (accentuated by shorter and slightly tilted crowns), but mesial and distal contacts are more nearly at the same level than for anterior teeth.

Contact Location viewed from the occlusal or incisal

Anterior: Tooth contacts are nearly centered faciolingually.

Posterior: Contacts are larger than anterior contact areas and tend to be slightly buccal to the middle third buccolingually.

Proximal Cervical Line (Cementoenamel junction) Curvatures

All teeth: Generally have greater proximal cervical line curvature on the mesial than the distal. Proximal cervical line curvatures are greater on the incisors and tend to get smaller when moving toward the last molar, where there may be no curvature at all. On many posterior teeth, the cervical line is in a more occlusal position on the lingual.

Facial and Lingual Crest of Curvatures

All teeth have the *facial* crest of curvature in the cervical third.

Anterior teeth have the *lingual* crest of curvature in the cervical third (on the bulge of the cingulum).

Posterior teeth have the *lingual* crest of curvature at or near the middle third of the crown.

Facial embrasure
Lingual embrasure
Interproximal space
Occlusal embrasure

Refer to Table 3-3 for a summary of the relative position of proximal contacts when moving from anterior teeth to posterior teeth. A **diastema** [di ah STEE mah] is a space between two adjacent teeth that do not contact each other (See Fig. 3-21).

D. EMBRASURE SPACES

When adjacent teeth contact, the continuous space which surrounds each contact area can be divided into four separate triangular **embrasure** spaces (Fig. 3-19. These spaces are narrowest closest to the contact area where the teeth are in tight contact, and widen facially to form a **buccal or labial embrasure**, widen lingually to form a **lingual embrasure**, and widen occlusally (or incisally) to form an **occlusal or incisal embrasure**. The fourth space, cervical to the contact area and between two adjacent teeth, is properly called the interproximal space.

The **interproximal space**, when viewed from the facial or lingual, is a triangular embrasure space between adjacent teeth located cervical to their contact area. The sides of the triangle are formed by the proximal surfaces of adjacent teeth, with the apex of the triangle at the contact between two teeth. This space is occupied in periodontally healthy persons by the interdental papilla (see Figs. 3-21 and 3-22). Sometimes this interproximal space is referred to as the **cervical or gingival embrasure**.

The **lingual embrasure** is ordinarily *larger* than the **facial embrasure**, because most teeth are narrower on the lingual side than on the facial side and because their contact points are located facial to the faciolingual midline of the crown. These contact area locations and the buccal and lingual embrasures are seen when the dental arch is examined from the occlusal view in Figure 3-19.

The **occlusal or incisal embrasure** is usually shallow from the occlusal surface or incisal edge to the contact areas and is narrow faciolingually on anterior teeth but broad on posterior teeth. The occlusal embrasure is the area between the marginal ridges on two adjacent teeth and occlusal to their contact area. This is where we place the dental floss before passing it through the contact area to clean tooth surfaces in the interproximal space.

Embrasures surrounding good proximal contact areas serve as spillways to direct food away from the gingiva. When the occlusal embrasure is incorrectly shaped in a dental restoration (amalgam, composite, or gold), fibrous food will readily lodge in the interproximal spaces and can be removed only with dental floss. This food impaction is not only an annoyance, but it can contribute to the formation of dental decay and periodontal disease (bone loss).

SECTION VI. Ideal Occlusion: Inter (Between) Arch Relationships of Teeth

It is important to learn the relationships of teeth in ideal occlusion in order to identify malocclusions that could contribute to dental problems. **Occlusion** [ah KLOO zhun] is contacting of occlusal and incising surfaces of opposing maxillary and mandibular teeth. To occlude literally means to close, as in shutting your mouth and closing your teeth together. The importance of proper occlusion cannot be overestimated. It is essential to both general and dental health and to a patient's comfort and ability to speak, chew, and enjoy food. Understanding occlusion requires not only a knowledge of the relation of the mandible to the maxillae but also of the temporomandibular joints, their complexities, and the muscles, nerves, ligaments, and soft tissues that affect the position of the mandible. These topics were briefly covered in Chapters 1 and 2. The arrangement of teeth within the dental arches (alignment, proximal contacts, and embrasure spaces) was discussed in the last section, and the *ideal* relationship of the mandibular dental arch of teeth to the maxillary dental arch of teeth will be presented in this section.

Ideal tooth relationships were described and classified in the early 1900s by Edward H. Angle. He classified ideal occlusion as Class I and defined it based on the relationship between the maxillary and mandibular dental arches. When closed together the teeth are in their **maximal intercuspal position**, or *best fitting together* of the teeth, as shown in Figures 3-20, 3-21, and 3-22. This is achieved on hand-held models when the maxil-

FIGURE 3-19. These photographs are of large plastic tooth models and give an indication of the location of *contact points* between adjacent teeth. The quadrant of teeth on the left are the occlusal and incisal surfaces of the permanent maxillary dentition; on the right are the mandibular dentition. Also shown are *embrasure spaces*.

Anterioposterior curve
(curve of Spee)

FIGURE 3-20. Dental stone casts fitting together in the maximum intercuspal position (tightest fit). Notice that, from this view, each tooth has the potential for contacting two opposing teeth except the maxillary third molar. The vertical white line marks the *relationship of first molars in Class I occlusion*; the mesiobuccal cusp of the maxillary first molar occludes in the mesial buccal groove of the mandibular first molar. The curved arrows denote the *curve of Spee.*

FIGURE 3-21. Maxillary and mandibular teeth of the permanent dentition are in the maximum intercuspal position. Observe the *interproximal spaces* filled with the *interdental papillae* between each pair of teeth. Notice how each tooth is in contact with adjacent teeth, except between tooth numbers 24 and 25, and between tooth numbers 23 and 24. Spaces are called *diastematas*. Note how the incisal edges and cusp tips of maxillary teeth *overlap* the mandibular teeth and how the greater width of the maxillary central incisors causes each of them to overlap not only the mandibular central incisor but also half of the mandibular lateral incisor. The numbers depict the Universal Tooth Identification System.

FIGURE 3-22. The subject is the same as in Figure 3-21, but here the right cheek is drawn back. Notice how each maxillary tooth overlaps two mandibular teeth, and the mesiobuccal cusp of the maxillary first molar (just visible on tooth 3) appears to be in occlusion with the mesiobuccal area (groove) on tooth #30.

lary teeth fit as tightly as possible against the mandibular teeth (i.e., are most stable). The following specific tooth relationships define Class I occlusion.

- **Horizontal overlap of anterior teeth**: The incisal edges of maxillary anterior teeth overlap the mandibular teeth such that the incisal edges of maxillary teeth are labial to the incisal edges of mandibular teeth (Fig. 3-20).
- **Vertical overlap of anterior teeth**: The incisal edges of the maxillary anterior teeth extend below the incisal edges of the mandibular teeth so that, when viewed from the facial, the incisal edges of mandibular incisors are hidden from view by the overlapping maxillary incisors (Fig. 3-21).
- **Relationship of posterior teeth**: The maxillary *posterior* teeth are slightly buccal to the mandibular posterior teeth (Figs. 3-21 and 3-22) so that:
- The buccal cusps and buccal surfaces of the maxillary teeth are buccal to those in the mandibular arch.
- The lingual cusps of maxillary teeth rest in occlusal fossae of the mandibular teeth.
- The buccal cusps of the mandibular teeth rest in the occlusal fossae of the maxillary teeth.
- The lingual cusps and lingual surfaces of the mandibular teeth are lingual to those in the maxillary arch.
- **Relative Alignment**: The vertical (long) axis midline of each maxillary tooth is slightly distal to the vertical axis of the corresponding mandibular tooth (Figs. 3-21 and 3-22) so that:
- The tip of the mesiobuccal cusp of the maxillary first molar is aligned directly over the mesiobuccal groove on the mandibular first molar (Fig. 3-20). This relationship of first molars (the first permanent teeth to erupt) is a *key factor* in the definition of Class I occlusion. Further, the maxillary canine fits into the facial embrasure between the mandibular canine and first premolar.
- Each tooth in a dental arch has the potential for contacting with two teeth in the opposing arch, except the mandibular central incisor (which is narrower than the maxillary central incisor) and the maxillary last molar. Subsequently, the distal surface of the maxillary first molar is posterior to the distal surface of the mandibular first molar (Fig. 3-20).

To summarize, *ideal occlusion* involves a Class I relationship between the maxillary and mandibular first molars in maximum intercuspation. Also, only the canines touch when the mandible moves to either side, without molar and premolar contacts. Finally, ideally there should be *no* large facets and/or bruxing habits, bone loss, crooked teeth, loose teeth, or joint pain.[1]

SECTION VII. Tooth Development from Lobes

In terms of the evolution of the dentition, tooth crowns are said to have developed from **lobes** or primary growth centers (Fig. 3-23). All *normal* teeth show evidence of having developed from three or more lobes. As a general rule, the facial portion of incisors and canines and premolars forms from three lobes, and the cingulum area and lingual cusp(s) each form from one lobe. Therefore, incisors develop from four lobes: *three facial* lobes forming three incisally located mamelons and *one lingual* lobe forming the cingulum area. Canines and most premolars also develop from four lobes: *three facial* lobes forming the facial portion and *one lingual* lobe forming the cingulum area on the canine and the one lingual cusp. An EXCEPTION is the *three-cusp* type premolar, which has one buccal and two lingual cusps, and therefore forms from five lobes: three forming the facial cusp and two (one each) forming the two lingual cusps. The three lobes of the facial surface of anterior teeth and premolars are usually evidenced by the three very subtle vertical ridges separated by two depressions.

As a general rule, each molar *cusp* forms from *one* lobe. For example, the mandibular first molar has five cusps (three buccal and two lingual) and develops from five lobes. Only some maxillary third molars have as few as three lobes forming three cusps. Two types of tooth anomalies, peg-shaped maxillary lateral incisors and some extra teeth (also called supernumerary teeth), form from less that three lobes.

LEARNING EXERCISE

Sketch a tooth and adjacent gingiva in cross section (as in Fig. 3-2) and label the following structures: enamel, dentin, cementum, pulp cavity, pulp chamber, apical foramen location, dentinoenamel junction, cementoenamel junction, dentinocemental junction, periodontal ligament space, alveolar bone, gingiva, gingival sulcus, anatomic crown, and anatomic root.

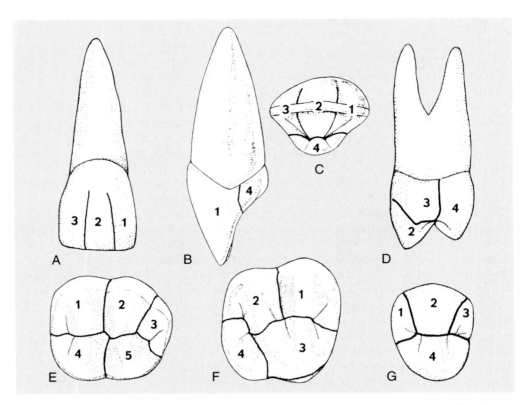

FIGURE 3-23. *Lobes* or primary anatomic divisions on teeth. Drawings **A**, **B** and **C** are the facial, mesial and incisal views, respectively, of a maxillary central incisor which, like all anterior teeth, has *four* lobes. The lingual cingulum develops from one lobe (labeled 4) seen in view B and C. Mamelons may appear on the incisal edge of newly erupted incisors, an indication of the three labial lobes. Drawings **D** and **G** are the mesial and occlusal views, respectively, of a maxillary first premolar that also forms from *four* lobes. Here the lingual lobe forms the lingual cusp. The divisions between the facial and lingual lobes are evidenced by the marginal ridge developmental grooves. Drawing **E** is a mandibular first molar with five lobes, three buccal and two lingual, which is one lobe per cusp. Drawing **F** is a maxillary first molar with three larger lobes and one smaller lobe, or one per cusp. The Carabelli cusp, when present, is a part of the large mesiolingual lobe.

LEARNING QUESTIONS

These questions were designed to help you confirm that you understand the terms and concepts presented in this chapter. Answer each question by circling the letter(s) of the correct answer (or answers). More than one answer may be correct.

1. If you read an article in a British dental journal that refers to tooth #48, you would suspect they were using the International Numbering System. What universal number (or letter) would they be talking about?

    a. 25
    b. J
    c. 30
    d. T
    e. 32

2. Using the Universal Numbering System, what numbers are used to identify maxillary canines?
    a. 6
    b. 8
    c. 10
    d. 11
    e. 27

3. Which tooth junctions are NOT normally visible on a hand-held intact tooth?
    a. cementoenamel junction
    b. dentinoenamel junction
    c. dentinocemental junction
    d. dentinopulpal junction

4. Which statement(s) is(are) likely to be true on a person with a barely erupted tooth #9?
    a. The clinical crown is larger than the anatomic crown.
    b. The clinical crown is smaller than the anatomic crown.
    c. The clinical root is larger than the anatomic root.
    d. The clinical root is smaller than the anatomic root.

5. Which tooth surface(s) face(s) the lips or cheeks?
    a. facial
    b. distal
    c. buccal
    d. occlusal
    e. labial

6. Which pairs of teeth have a mesial surface touching a mesial surface?
    a. 25 and 26
    b. 16 and 17
    c. 7 and 8
    d. 1 and 32
    e. 8 and 9

7. When viewing tooth #8 from the distal view, it can be divided into thirds from the incisal to the cervical and from the facial to the lingual. Which third is NOT possible to see from the distal view?
    a. facial
    b. cervical
    c. middle
    d. mesial
    e. incisal

8. If you were observing the *faciolingual* length of a tooth, what surface(s) could you be viewing?
    a. mesial
    b. occlusal
    c. proximal
    d. labial
    e. distal

9. If the root-to-crown ratio of a maxillary molar (#14) is 1.72, and that of another molar, #16, is 1.49, which tooth has the longest *root* relative to its shorter *crown*?
   a. #14
   b. #16
   c. More information is required in order to answer this question.

10. Which of the following bumps or ridges is NOT likely to be found on a maxillary premolar?
    a. oblique ridge
    b. cingulum
    c. mesial marginal ridge
    d. transverse ridge
    e. triangular ridge

11. Which ridges may help *surround* the perimeter of the occlusal surface of a premolar?
    a. mesial marginal ridge
    b. distal marginal ridge
    c. mesial cusp ridge of the buccal cusp
    d. distal cusp ridge of the lingual cusp
    e. transverse ridge

12. What is the correct order of anatomic landmarks of a tooth with two roots from the cemento-enamel junction to the root tip?
    a. cervix, trunk, furcation, apex
    b. trunk, cervix, furcation, apex
    c. trunk, furcation, cervix, apex
    d. cervix, trunk, apex, furcation
    e. furcation, trunk, cervix, apex

13. When viewed from the proximal views, what is the location of the greatest bulge (crest of curvature or height of contour) on the *facial* surface of *all* teeth?
    a. occlusal third
    b. lingual third
    c. buccal third
    d. middle third
    e. cervical third

14. Which space(s) contain the part of the gingiva known as the interdental papilla?
    a. the buccal embrasure
    b. occlusal embrasure
    c. lingual embrasure
    d. cervical embrasure
    e. interproximal space

15. Ideal Class I occlusion involves an important first permanent molar relationship where the mesiobuccal cusp of the maxillary first molar is located within the:
    a. mesiobuccal groove of the mandibular first molar
    b. distobuccal groove of the mandibular first molar
    c. buccal groove of the mandibular second molar
    d. mesiobuccal groove of the mandibular second molar
    e. distobuccal groove of the mandibular second molar

16. Where do *lingual* cusps of *maxillary* teeth occlude in ideal class I occlusion?
    a. in the buccal embrasure space between mandibular teeth
    b. in the lingual embrasure space between mandibular teeth
    c. in the occlusal embrasure space between mandibular teeth
    d. in occlusal fossae of mandibular teeth

17. How many developmental lobes form a premolar with two cusps (one buccal cusp and one lingual cusp)?
    a. 1
    b. 2
    c. 3
    d. 4
    e. 5

Answers to learning questions: 1–e; 2–a, d; 3–b, c, d; 4–b, c; 5–a, c, e; 6–e; 7–d; 8–a, b, c, e; 9–a; 10–a, b; 11–a, b, c, d; 12–a; 13–e; 14–d, e; 15–a; 16–d; 17–d.

REFERENCES

1. Ash MM. Wheeler's dental anatomy, physiology, and occlusion. 7th ed. Philadelphia: W.B. Saunders, 1993.

General References

Jordan R, Abrams L, Kraus B. Kraus' dental anatomy and occlusion. St. Louis: Mosby Year Book, 1992.
Renner RP. An introduction to dental anatomy and esthetics. Chicago: Quintessence Publishing, 1985.

4 Morphology of the Permanent Incisors

This chapter is divided into the following three sections, each with its own learning objectives.

I. General description of incisors
  A. Functions of incisors
  B. Morphology of incisors
  C. Class traits for all incisors
  D. Arch traits that distinguish maxillary from mandibular incisors
II. Maxillary incisor type traits: similarities and differences useful to distinguish maxillary central incisors from maxillary lateral incisors (from all views)
  A. Maxillary incisors from the labial view
  B. Maxillary incisors from the lingual view
  C. Maxillary incisors from the proximal views
  D. Maxillary incisors from the incisal view
  E. Variations in maxillary incisors
III. Mandibular incisor type traits: similarities and differences useful to distinguish mandibular central incisors from mandibular lateral incisors (from all views)
  A. Mandibular incisors from the labial view
  B. Mandibular incisors from the lingual view
  C. Mandibular incisors from the proximal views
  D. Mandibular incisors from the incisal view
  E. Variations in mandibular incisors

Using the maxillary right lateral incisor as a representative example for all incisors, refer to the Appendix, page 1, while reading Section I of this chapter. Within this text, the word "Appendix" followed by a number and letter (e.g., Appendix 1a) is used to denote the appendix page (number 1) and item (letter a) being referred to. The appendix pages are designed to be torn out to facilitate study and minimize page turns as you read the main text. Other appendix pages will be referred to throughout this and several chapters that follow.

SECTION I. General Description of Incisors

OBJECTIVES

The reader should be able to perform the following:
- Describe the functions of incisors.
- List class traits common to all incisors.
- List arch traits that can be used to distinguish maxillary from mandibular incisors.
- From a selection of all teeth, select and separate out the incisors.
- Divide a selection of all incisors into maxillary and mandibular.

Refer to Figure 1.2 or, better yet, to a model of the complete set of permanent teeth while becoming familiar with the location and universal number of each incisor. There are four maxillary incisors: two central incisors (first maxillary incisors: universal numbers 8 and 9) and two lateral incisors (second maxillary incisors: numbers 7 and 10). There are four mandibular incisors: two central incisors (first mandibular incisors: numbers 24 and 25) and two lateral incisors (second mandibular incisors: numbers 23 and 26).

Central incisors are located on either side in their respective arch (maxillary or mandibular) with their mesial surfaces next to one another at the midline, usually in contact. (A space between these or other teeth is called a **diastema** [die a STEE mah].) Their distal surfaces contact the mesial surfaces of the lateral incisors. Lateral incisors are therefore, just distal to central incisors, with their mesial surfaces in contact with the distal surfaces of the adjacent central incisors. Their distal surfaces contact the canines. (Did you know that the tusks on an elephant are maxillary central incisors? [recall Table 1-1] They have the largest diastema in the world, large enough for the massive trunk between their central incisors.)

A. FUNCTIONS OF INCISORS

The mandibular incisors function with the maxillary incisors to (a) cut food (mandibular incisors are moving blades against the stationary maxillary incisors), (b) enable articulate speech (consider the enunciation of a toothless person), and (c) help to support the lip and maintain an esthetic appearance. By current standards, a person lacking one or more incisors has an undesirable appearance (Did you ever hear the song, "All I want for Christmas are my two front teeth"?). Their fourth function, by fitting the incisal edges of the mandibular incisors against the lingual surfaces of the maxillary incisors, is (d) to help guide the mandible posteriorly during the final phase of closing just before the posterior teeth contact.

B. MORPHOLOGY OF INCISORS

The morphology, or anatomy, of a tooth can best be studied by considering the shape (outline) and contours (ridges and grooves) visible on each tooth surface. All tooth crowns have five surfaces, that is, four side surfaces plus a chewing or cutting surface or edge, depending on whether it is a posterior tooth (chewing in the back part of the mouth) or an anterior tooth (cutting in the front of the mouth). In the study of tooth morphology, the description and location of the ridges, grooves, convexities, and concavities on each tooth surface should be well fixed in your mind in order to describe and identify teeth by arch, type, class, and side of the mouth; to reproduce tooth contours when constructing crowns, bridges, and fillings; and to remove deposits (tartar and calculus) skillfully from crowns and roots or when finishing and polishing existing restorations.

When discussing traits, the external morphology of an incisor is customarily described from each of five views: (a) **facial** (or **labial**), (b) **lingual** (tongue side), (c) **mesial**, (d) **distal**, and (e) **incisal**. Due to similarities between the mesial and distal, these surfaces will be discussed together in this text under the heading of **proximal** surface.

In the study of any single type of human tooth, such as the maxillary central incisor, it is necessary to realize that this tooth varies in form in different people as much as facial features vary from one person to another. One study of a collection of 100 maxillary central incisors showed considerable difference in such characteristics as size, relative proportions, and color.[1] Information in this text on crown length, crown width, and root length is taken from measurements of extracted teeth by Dr. Woelfel and by his dental hygiene students at Ohio State University between 1974 and 1979. Teeth were collected from dentists in Ohio. The ranges indicate how greatly the same tooth can vary in size. See Tables 4-1A and B. For example, among the 398 maxillary central incisors measured, one central incisor was 16 mm longer than the shortest one. There was a lesser, but still considerable, range in crown length (6 mm) and in crown width (3 mm) from the smallest to the largest tooth found in this sample. *Specific data collected from Dr. Woelfel's studies are presented throughout the text in brackets* [like this].

C. CLASS TRAITS FOR ALL INCISORS

First, consider the class traits of incisors, that is, traits that apply to *all* incisors. Recall from Chapter 3 that the facial surface of all anterior teeth forms from the three labial portions called the mesial, middle, and distal lobes. Therefore, incisors usually have two shallow vertical developmental depressions separating the parts of the facial surface formed by these three lobes (These depressions are denoted by the subtle shading on the drawings in Fig. 4-3). The three lobes also contribute to three **mamelons**, which are seen

Table 4-1A

SIZE OF MAXILLARY INCISORS (MILLIMETERS)

Dimension Measured	398 CENTRALS		295 LATERALS	
	Average	Range	Average	Range
Crown length	11.2	8.6–14.7	9.8	7.4–11.9
Rooth length	13.0	6.3–20.3	13.4	9.6–19.4
Overall length	23.6	16.5–32.6	22.5	17.7–28.9
Crown width M-D	8.6	7.1–10.5	6.6	5.0–9.0
Rooth width (cervix)	6.4	5.0–8.0	4.7	3.4–6.4
Faciolingual crown size	7.1	6.0–8.5	6.2	5.3–7.3
Faciolingual root (cervix)	6.4	5.1–7.8	5.8	4.5–7.0
Mesial cervical curve	2.8	1.4–4.8	2.5	1.3–4.0
Distal cervical curve	2.3	0.7–4.0	1.9	0.8–3.7

Table 4-1B

SIZE OF MANDIBULAR INCISORS (MILLIMETERS)

Dimension Measured	226 CENTRALS		234 LATERALS	
	Average	Range	Average	Range
Crown length	8.8	6.3–11.6	9.4	7.3–12.6
Root length	12.6	7.7–17.9	13.5	9.4–18.1
Overall length	20.8	16.9–26.7	22.1	18.5–26.6
Crown width M-D	5.3	4.4–6.7	5.7	4.6–8.2
Root width (cervix)	3.5	2.7–4.6	3.8	3.0–4.9
Faciolingual crown size	5.7	4.8–6.8	6.1	5.2–7.4
Faciolingual root (cervix)	5.4	4.3–6.5	5.8	4.3–6.8
Mesial cervical curve	2.0	1.0–3.3	2.1	1.0–3.6
Distal cervical curve	1.6	0.6–2.8	1.5	0.8–2.4

FIGURE 4-1. Left and right maxillary central incisors, *lingual views.* Both teeth are *"shovel shaped"* due to their deep lingual fossae along with pronounced lingual marginal ridges and cingula. Both teeth have three rounded protuberances on their incisal edge called *mamelons* (arrows). The right tooth has a *pit* on the incisal border of the cingulum where caries can penetrate without being easily noticed.

on the incisal edges of newly emerged incisor teeth (Fig. 4-1). Finally, remember that a fourth (lingual) lobe forms the cingulum.

1. CHARACTERISTICS OF *ALL* INCISORS FROM THE *FACIAL VIEW*

Refer to Appendix page 1 while studying the similarities of *all* incisors. (Note that there are exceptions to the general incisor traits presented here, and they are noted in capital letters.)

All incisor *crowns*, when viewed from the *facial*, have a relatively straight or slightly curved incisal edge (versus all other teeth that have one or more pointed cusp tip.) Their crowns are relatively rectangular, longer incisogingivally than wide mesiodistally (Appendix 1a). They taper from the widest mesiodistal areas of proximal contact toward the cervical line and are therefore narrowest in the cervical third and broader toward the incisal third (Appendix 1b). Incisor crown outlines are more convex on the distal than on the mesial sides (EXCEPT the mandibular central which is symmetrical) (Appendix 1c). Incisor mesioincisal angles are more acute (sharper) than distoincisal angles EXCEPT on the symmetrical mandibular central incisors where the angles are not noticeably different (Appendix 1d). Incisor crown contact areas (greatest height of contour proximally) on the mesial surface are located in the incisal third. On the distal surface the contact areas are more cervical than the mesial EXCEPT on the distal of the mandibular central, which is at the same level as the mesial due to its symmetry (Appendix 1e). The incisal edge of all incisors (EXCEPT the mandibular central) slopes cervically toward the distal. Finally, the cervical line on the facial curves toward the apex in the middle of the facial (and lingual) sides (Appendix 1-l).

Incisor *roots*, when viewed from the *facial*, taper (become more narrow) from the cervical line to the apex (Appendix 1f). They are wider faciolingually than mesiodistally (EXCEPT maxillary central incisors, where the mesiodistal width is approximately the same as the faciolingual thickness) (compare root views in Appendix 1g). Incisor roots may bend in the apical one-third (EXCEPT maxillary central incisor roots, which are not as likely to bend); this bend is more often toward the distal (Appendix 1h). Incisor roots are longer than the crowns (Appendix 1i).

2. CHARACTERISTICS OF *ALL* INCISORS FROM THE *LINGUAL VIEW*

Incisor *crowns*, when viewed from the *lingual*, have a narrower lingual surface because the mesial and distal sides converge lingually (best appreciated from the incisal view, Appendix 1j). The mesial and distal marginal ridges converge toward the cingulum (Appendix 1k).

3. CHARACTERISTICS OF *ALL* INCISORS FROM THE *PROXIMAL VIEWS*

Incisor *crowns*, when viewed from the *proximal* are wedge-shaped (Appendix 1m). They have a *facial* height of contour (greatest bulge) that is in the cervical third just incisal to the cervical line and are therefore more convex cervically than incisally on their labial surfaces (Appendix 1n). The *lingual* height of contour is also in the cervical third on the cingulum, but the contour of the incisal two-thirds of the lingual surface is concave from cingulum area to the incisal edge. Therefore, the lingual outline is S-shaped, being convex over the cingulum and concave from the cingulum nearly to the incisal edge (Appendix 1p). The lingual concavity on the maxillary anterior teeth is a most important guiding factor in the closing movements of the lower jaw, because the mandibular incisors fit into this concavity and against marginal ridges of the maxillary incisors as maximum closure or occlusion is approached. The cervical line proximally curves toward the incisal edge. The resultant curve is greater on the mesial surface than on the distal (compare the mesial and distal views in Appendix 1o).

The incisor *roots*, when viewed from the *proximal* are widest at the cervical and gradually taper to a rounded apex (Appendix 1f). Normally, all have a longitudinal depression in middle third of the *mesial* root surface. (Only the mandibular central and lateral incisors also have a prominent longitudinal depression on the *distal* surface.)

4. CHARACTERISTICS OF *ALL* INCISORS FROM THE *INCISAL VIEW*

The *crowns* when viewed from the *incisal* have a lingual fossa that is concave just incisal to the cingulum. They have an incisal ridge that terminates mesiodistally at the widest portion of the crown (Appendix 1q). The labial outline is broader and less curved than the convex lingual outline (Appendix 1r). Marginal ridges converge toward the cingulum (Appendix 1k), and the crown outline tapers from proximal contact toward the cingulum (Appendix 1j), resulting in a narrower lingual than labial side.

D. ARCH TRAITS THAT DISTINGUISH MAXILLARY FROM MANDIBULAR INCISORS

Refer to Appendix page 2 while reading about these arch traits that can be used to distinguish mandibular incisors from maxillary incisors.

The **mandibular incisors** (relative to the maxillary incisors) are generally smaller than maxillary incisors. Mandibular central and lateral incisors look more alike and are more nearly the same size in the same mouth, compared to greater differences between maxillary central and lateral incisors. *Mandibular* incisor crowns are flatter on the mesial and distal sides (Appendix 2q) and have contact areas located nearer the incisal ridge than maxillary incisors (Appendix 2r and 2i). *Mandibular* incisor crowns are relatively wider faciolingually than mesiodistally compared to maxillary incisors, which are wider mesiodistally (Appendix 2n). *Mandibular* incisor crowns also have smoother lingual surfaces with less prominent anatomy than maxillary crowns, which have deeper fossae and more pronounced marginal ridges (Appendix 2m). Finally, *mandibular* incisor roots are longer in proportion to their crowns than are maxillary incisors.

Incisal edges of *mandibular incisors* are usually positioned lingual to the root axis line, whereas the incisal edges of *maxillary incisors* are more often on or labial to the root axis line (best seen from the proximal views on Appendix 2o). Attrition on the incisal edges of incisors that occurs when shearing or incising food results in a wear pattern that is different on maxillary incisors compared to mandibular incisors (Fig. 4-2). This wear pattern occurs when the labial part of the incisal edges of mandibular incisors slides forward and downward while contacting the lingual surface and part of the incisal edge of opposing maxillary incisors. The wear results in a shiny flat, polished surface of enamel on the incisal edge called a **facet** [FAS it]. Assuming a normal tooth relationship, facets that commonly form on mandibular incisors are more on the labial slope of the incisal edge, sloping cervically toward the labial. In contrast, facets on *maxillary incisors* occur more on the lingual slope of the incisal edge, sloping cervically toward the lingual fossa or lingual marginal ridges.

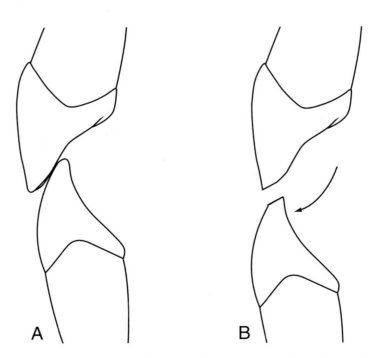

FIGURE 4-2. **A.** The normal relationship of incisors when posterior teeth are biting tightly together. **B.** The arrow indicates the direction of movement of the mandibular incisor moving forward with the mandible (protruding) so the incisors work edge to edge during incision. The resultant *wear pattern* or facets on the incisal edges of maxillary incisors occurs more onto the lingual surface (wear facets slope cervically toward the lingual) whereas wear occurs primarily on the facial surface on the mandibular incisor (wear facets slope cervically toward the labial).

LEARNING EXERCISE

Refer to Table 4-2 for a summary of the noticeable arch traits that distinguish maxillary from mandibular incisors, and see how many of them can be used to differentiate the maxillary and mandibular incisors in Figures 4-3 through 4-6 and 4-8 through 4-11.

Table 4-2

VIEWS OF THE MAXILLARY AND MANDIBULAR INCISORS

MAXILLARY INCISORS	MANDIBULAR INCISORS
LABIAL VIEW	
Wider crowns mesiodistally	Narrower crowns mesiodistally
Less symmetrical crown	More symmetrical crowns
More rounded M and D incisal angles	More square M and D incisal angles
Contact areas more cervical	Contact areas very incisal
LINGUAL VIEW	
Lingual anatomy more distinct:	Lingual surface smoother:
Pronounced marginal ridges	Almost no marginal ridges
Deeper lingual fossa	Shallower lingual fossa
Sometimes lingual pits	No pits
Larger cingulum	Smaller cingulum
PROXIMAL VIEWS	
Incisal edge on or labial to root axis line	Incisal edge on or lingual to root axis line
Facets on lingual slope of incisal edge	Facets on labial slope of incisal edge
Mesial root surfaces are more convex	Mesial root surfaces have depressions
INCISAL VIEW	
Crowns wider M-D than F-L	Crowns wider F-L than M-D
plus the four traits seen from lingual view can also be seen from the incisal view	

SECTION II. Maxillary Incisor Type Traits: Similarities and Differences Useful to Distinguish Maxillary Central Incisors from Lateral Incisors (from All Views)

OBJECTIVES

This section is designed to prepare the learner to perform the following:

- Describe the type traits that can be used to distinguish the permanent maxillary central incisor from the maxillary lateral incisor.
- Describe and identify the labial, lingual, mesial, distal, and incisal surfaces for all maxillary incisors.
- Assign a universal number to maxillary incisors present in a mouth (or on a model) with complete dentition. If possible, repeat this on a model with one or more maxillary incisors missing.
- Select and separate maxillary incisors from a selection of all teeth on a bench top.
- Holding a maxillary incisor, determine whether it is a central or a lateral and right or left. Then assign a universal number to it.

Within this section, the maxillary central and lateral incisors will be compared for similarities and differences. These differences are presented for each view of the tooth: facial, lingual, proximal (mesial and distal), and incisal.

A. MAXILLARY INCISORS FROM THE *LABIAL VIEW*

LEARNING EXERCISE

Examine several extracted maxillary central and lateral incisors and/or tooth models as you read. Hold these teeth root up and crown down, as they are positioned in the mouth. Also, tear out and refer to Appendix page 2 and refer to Figure 4-3 as you study about the labial traits of incisors.

1. CROWN SHAPE OF MAXILLARY INCISORS FROM THE *LABIAL VIEW*

The *crown* of the **maxillary central incisor** is the longest [average: 11.2 mm] of all human tooth crowns (although canines may be longer overall) and is also the widest of all incisors. The crown is usually longer (incisogingivally) than wide (mesiodistally) [averaging 2.6 mm longer] (Appendix 2a). The crown is narrowest in the cervical third and becomes broader toward the incisal third.

There is great morphologic variation in the **maxillary lateral incisor**. It may be missing altogether, it may resemble a small slender version of a maxillary central incisor; it may be quite asymmetrical; or it may be peg shaped (as seen later in Chapter 11). Normally, the labial surface of the maxillary lateral incisor is much like that of the central incisor, but it is more convex or less flat mesiodistally and overall it appears narrower mesiodistally. Mamelons, and particularly labial depressions, are less prominent and less common than on the central incisor.

The crown of the average *maxillary lateral incisor* is narrower [about 2 mm] than the crown of the central incisor, and the root is longer [about 0.5 mm], giving this entire tooth a long slender look (Appendix 2a and 2d). The crown outline is less symmetrical than the central incisor.

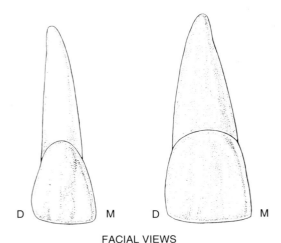

D   M D   M

FACIAL VIEWS

Right maxillary   Right maxillary
lateral incisor   central incisor

FIGURE 4-3. Maxillary central and lateral incisors, *labial views*, with traits that distinguish maxillary central from lateral incisors and traits that distinguish right and left sides.

TRAITS TO DISTINGUISH MAXILLARY CENTRAL FROM LATERAL INCISOR: LABIAL VIEW

CENTRAL INCISOR	LATERAL INCISOR
Larger crown, wider cervically	Smaller crown; narrower cervically
More symmetrical	Less symmetrical; tipped distally at cervix
Mesial incisal angle is a right angle	Mesial incisal is rounder and less acute
Distal contact closer to incisal ridge	Distal contact is near middle third
Less root tip bend to distal	Root tip often bends to distal
Incisal edge straighter, more horizontal	Incisal edge slopes cervically to distal

MAXILLARY INCISORS(Labial)

TRAITS TO DIFFERENT MAXILLARY RIGHT FROM LEFT INCISOR: LABIAL VIEW	
CENTRAL INCISOR	LATERAL INCISOR

Mesial crown outline flatter; distal more rounded
Mesioincisal angle more acute (sharper) than distoincisal angle
Distoincisal angle more rounded than mesioincisal angle
Distal contact more cervical than mesial contact

2. MAXILLARY INCISOR INCISAL-PROXIMAL CROWN ANGLE FROM THE *LABIAL VIEW*

On **maxillary central incisors**, the corner or angle formed by the mesial and incisal surfaces (called the mesioincisal angle) forms nearly a right angle. The distoincisal corner is more rounded and the angle is slightly obtuse or greater than a right angle (Appendix 2b).

On **maxillary lateral incisors**, both the mesioincisal and distoincisal angles are more rounded than on the central incisor (Appendix 2b). The mesioincisal angle is more acute and the distoincisal angle is even wider or more obtuse than on the central incisors, accentuated by the incisal edge sloping cervically toward the distal (more so than on the maxillary central incisor) (Appendix 2c).

3. PROXIMAL CONTACT AREA OF MAXILLARY INCISORS FROM THE *LABIAL VIEW*

For all human teeth, contact areas are located in one of three places: in the incisal (occlusal) third, at the junction of the incisal and middle thirds, or in the middle third of the crown. Tooth contact areas are never located in the cervical third of teeth. The *mesial* contacts of *both* a maxillary central and lateral incisor are in the incisal third, very near the incisal edge for the central and slightly more cervical for the lateral. The *distal* contacts of *both* incisors are more cervical than the mesial: for a **maxillary central incisor** it is near the junction of the incisal and the middle thirds; for the **maxillary lateral incisor** it is even more cervical, sometimes in the middle third (making this contact the most cervical for any incisor).

4. ROOT-TO-CROWN PROPORTIONS OF MAXILLARY INCISORS FROM THE *LABIAL VIEW*

On a **maxillary central incisor**, the root is only slightly longer than the crown [root-to-crown ratio is 1.16:1] (Appendix 2d). The **maxillary lateral incisor** root is longer than on the central [by 0.4 mm, comparing measurements of 398 maxillary central incisors and 295 lateral incisors]. This results in a root that appears longer in proportion to the crown than on the maxillary central incisor (Appendix 2d).

5. **ROOT SHAPE OF MAXILLARY INCISORS FROM THE *LABIAL VIEW***

The root of the **maxillary central incisor** is thick in the cervical third and narrows through the middle to a blunt apex. Its outline and shape is much like an ice cream cone. An apical bend is *not* common in the maxillary central incisor. The central incisor root is the only maxillary tooth that is as thick at the cervix mesiodistally as faciolingually [6.4 mm]. The seven other maxillary tooth roots are thicker faciolingually than mesiodistally [ranging from 1.1 to 3.4 mm thicker for the lateral incisors and premolars, respectively]. Because of its shortness and conical shape, the maxillary central incisor root may be a poor risk to support a replacement tooth as part of a dental bridge (that is, a replacement tooth crown attached to, and supported by, two adjacent teeth).

The root of a **maxillary lateral incisor** tapers evenly toward the rounded apex, and the apical end is commonly bent distally [12 of the 14 maxillary lateral incisors in Fig. 4-3, lower row).

B. **MAXILLARY INCISORS FROM THE *LINGUAL VIEW***

Refer to Figure 4-4 while studying about the lingual traits of maxillary incisors.

1. **LINGUAL FOSSA OF MAXILLARY INCISORS FROM THE *LINGUAL VIEW***

The large lingual fossa is located immediately incisal to the cingulum and bounded by two marginal ridges. The fossa of both maxillary incisors may be either shallow or deep, but either way they are usually deeper than fossae in *mandibular* incisors. Maxillary incisors with a deep lingual fossa and prominent mesial and distal marginal ridges are called "shovel-shaped incisors" (Fig. 4-1).[2–6] [Dr. Woelfel examined the maxillary incisors on casts of 715 dental hygiene students and found that 32% of the central incisors and 27% of the lateral incisors have some degree of shoveling. The rest had smooth concave lingual surfaces without prominent marginal ridges or deep fossae.] The lingual fossa of the *maxillary lateral incisor*, although smaller in area, is often even more pronounced than on the central incisor. Note this difference on many teeth in Figure 4-4.

2. **CINGULUM OF MAXILLARY INCISORS FROM THE *LINGUAL VIEW***

The cingulum on the **maxillary central incisor** is usually well developed and is located off-center, distal to the root axis line that bisects the root longitudinally. (This can also be seen from the incisal view.) The cingulum of the **maxillary lateral incisor** is narrower than on the central, and it is almost centered on the root axis line (Appendix 2e).

3. **MARGINAL RIDGES OF MAXILLARY INCISORS FROM THE *LINGUAL VIEW***

The mesial and distal marginal ridges vary in prominence on *all maxillary incisors* from one person to another. They may be prominent or inconspicuous. They may also have been worn smooth (forming facets) from attrition or chewing by the mandibular incisors. Due to the distal placement of the cingulum and incisal edge slope cervically toward the distal, the mesial marginal ridge of the **maxillary central incisor** (from proximal contact area to cingulum) is longer than its distal marginal ridge. On the **maxillary lateral incisor**, the distal marginal ridge is also shorter than the mesial, because the incisal edge slopes cervically from mesial to distal, even more so than on the central (Appendix 2f). The longer mesial marginal ridge of the maxillary lateral incisor outline is nearly straight, while the shorter distal marginal ridge outline is curved cervicoincisally, as on the central incisor. Note this difference in many lateral incisors in Figure 4-4.

4. **MAXILLARY INCISOR PITS AND ACCESSORY RIDGES FROM THE *LINGUAL***

The lingual anatomy of the **maxillary central incisor** is variable. Its fossa may be deep but smooth, that is, with no lingual ridges bordering the fossa. Accessory lingual ridges, if present, are small or narrow and extend vertically from the cingulum toward the center of the fossa. Accessory ridges may be 1, 2, 3, or 4 in number (on Fig. 2-3, tooth **#9** shows these accessory ridges most clearly). Tiny grooves separate these ridges. [Inspection of 506 maxillary central incisors by Dr. Woelfel revealed 36% with none of these ridges, 27% with one small ridge, 28% with two accessory ridges, 9% with three ridges, and only three teeth with four small ridges.]

Maxillary Incisors (Lingual)

TRAITS TO DISTINGUISH MAXILLARY CENTRAL FROM LATERAL INCISOR: LINGUAL VIEW

CENTRAL INCISOR	LATERAL INCISOR
Larger shallow lingual fossa	Deep but small fossa
Cingulum distally positioned	Cingulum centered
Less frequent lingual pits	More common lingual pits
Plus six outline characteristics seen from facial apply to lingual outline	

TRAITS TO DIFFERENTIATE MAXILLARY RIGHT FROM LEFT INCISOR: LINGUAL VIEW

CENTRAL INCISOR	LATERAL INCISOR
Cingulum toward distal	Longer and straighter M marginal ridge
	Distal marginal ridge more curved than M
Longer mesiolingual marginal ridge	
Plus four outline characteristics from facial also apply to lingual outline	

FIGURE 4-4. Maxillary central and lateral incisors, *Lingual views*, with traits that distinguish maxillary central from lateral incisors, and traits that distinguish right and left sides.

The **maxillary lateral incisor** may also have small vertical accessory lingual ridges on and incisal to the cingulum, only they are fewer in number and less common. [Inspection of 488 maxillary lateral incisors by Dr. Woelfel revealed 64% with none of these small ridges, 32% with one small accessory ridge, and only 4% with two ridges.]

On *both* maxillary incisors, a lingual pit is frequently detectable at the incisal border of the cingulum where the mesial and distal marginal ridges converge. This pit may need to be restored or filled by the dentist to arrest decay, especially on maxillary lateral incisors. (Notice the deep lingual pits in many maxillary lateral incisors in Fig. 4-4.)

5. **ROOT SHAPE OF MAXILLARY INCISORS FROM THE *LINGUAL VIEW***

The root contour of *all maxillary incisors*, like all anterior teeth, is convex and tapers, becoming narrower toward the lingual side (Fig. 4-4).

C.   MAXILLARY INCISORS FROM THE *PROXIMAL VIEWS*

Refer to Figure 4-5 while studying about the proximal traits of maxillary incisors.

1. **INCISAL EDGE OF MAXILLARY INCISORS FROM THE *PROXIMAL VIEWS***

On *both* maxillary incisors, the incisal edge is commonly just labial to the root axis line or may be on the root axis line. When viewed from the distal, the distoincisal edge of the **maxillary central incisor** is on or just lingual to the axis line because of a slight distolingual twist of the incisal edge (seen incisally in Appendix 2g).

2. **CERVICAL LINE OF MAXILLARY INCISORS FROM THE *PROXIMAL VIEWS***

As on all anterior teeth, the cervical line of all maxillary incisors curves incisally on the mesial and distal tooth surfaces, and this curvature is greater on the mesial surface than on the distal surface. This difference is most pronounced on the anterior teeth. The *mesial* curvature of the cervical line of the **maxillary central incisor** is larger than for any other tooth [average: 2.8 mm] extending incisally one-fourth of the crown length, whereas the *distal* cervical line curves less [on the average 2.3 mm]. The curvature of the *mesial* cervical line of the **maxillary lateral incisor** is also considerable but slightly less than on the central [averaging 2.5 mm or one-fourth of the crown length].

3. **HEIGHT (CREST) OF CONTOUR OF MAXILLARY INCISORS FROM THE *PROXIMAL VIEWS***

On the labial outline, the height of contour on *all* maxillary incisors is in the cervical third, just incisal to the cervical line. The outline becomes nearly flat in the middle and incisal thirds. On the lingual, the height of contour is also in the cervical third, on the cingulum.

4. **MAXILLARY INCISOR ROOT FROM THE *PROXIMAL VIEWS***

The root of the **maxillary central incisor** is wide faciolingually at the cervix and tapers to a rounded apex. The lingual outline is nearly straight in the cervical third, then curves labially toward the tip in the middle and apical thirds. The labial outline is less convex (more nearly straight). In contrast, the root of the **maxillary lateral incisor** tapers more evenly throughout the root toward the blunt apex. This difference in root outline from the proximal view is evident in many incisors in Figure 4-5.

The *mesial* root surface of *all* maxillary incisors is likely be flat or have a depression, but the *distal* root surface is likely to be convex, without a longitudinal depression. The mesial longitudinal depression is in the middle third cervicoapically and slightly lingual to the center faciolingually. This mesial root depression is discernable in the shaded line drawings in Figure 4-5.

D.   MAXILLARY INCISORS FROM THE *INCISAL VIEW*

Refer to Figure 4-6 when studying the incisal view. To follow this description, a maxillary incisor should be held in such a position that the incisal edge is toward you, the labial surface is at the top, and you are looking *exactly along the root axis line*. You should see slightly more lingual surface than labial surface, because the incisal ridge is located somewhat labial to the root axis line (as in Fig. 4-6).

1. **MAXILLARY INCISOR CROWN PROPORTION FACIOLINGUALLY VERSUS MESIODISTALLY FROM THE *INCISAL VIEW***

The crown outline of the **maxillary central incisor** is noticeably wider mesiodistally than faciolingually [by an average of 1.5 mm] (Appendix 2h). The mesiodistal measurement of the **lateral incisor** crown is also greater than the labiolingual measurement but less so than on the central incisor [averaging only

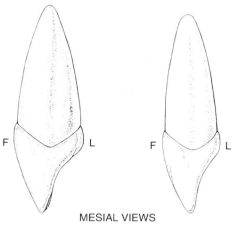

MESIAL VIEWS

Right maxillary
central incisor

Right maxillary
lateral incisor

FIGURE 4-5. Maxillary central and lateral incisors, *proximal views*, with traits that distinguish maxillary central from lateral incisors and traits that distinguish right and left sides.

Maxillary Incisors

Lefts

Rights

Centrals

Laterals

MESIAL SURFACES

DISTAL SURFACES

←——— Lingual   Facial———→

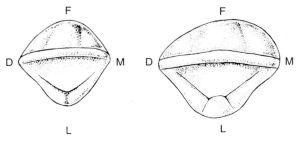

INCISAL VIEWS

Right maxillary
lateral incisor

Right maxillary
central incisor

FIGURE 4-6. Maxillary central and lateral incisors, *incisal views*, with traits that distinguish maxillary central from lateral incisors and traits that distinguish right and left sides.

TRAITS TO DISTINGUISH MAXILLARY CENTRAL FROM LATERAL INCISOR: INCISAL VIEW

CENTRAL INCISOR	LATERAL INCISOR
Crown noticeably wider M-D than F-L	Crown size M-D and F-L more similar
Crown outline roughly triangular	Crown outline more round or oval
Cingulum off center to distal	Cingulum centered
Incisal edge curves mesiodistally	Incisal edge straighter mesiodistally

TRAITS TO DIFFERENTIATE MAXILLARY RIGHT FROM LEFT INCISOR: INCISAL VIEW

CENTRAL INCISOR	LATERAL INCISOR
Cingulum more distal	Distal crown outline more rounded

0.4 mm greater]. On some lateral incisors, the two dimensions of the crown are almost the same size faciolingually as mesiodistally (Appendix 2h). Notice this difference in the teeth in Figure 4-6.

2.   **OUTLINE SHAPE OF MAXILLARY INCISOR CROWNS FROM THE *INCISAL VIEW***

The crown shape of the **maxillary central incisor** is roughly triangular, with a broadly curved labial outline forming the base that converges toward the cingulum. As was seen from the lingual view, the cingulum of the *maxillary central incisor* is slightly off-center to the distal, resulting in the mesial marginal ridge measuring longer than the distal marginal ridge (Appendix 2f).

The crown of the **lateral incisor** resembles the central incisor from this aspect, but its outline is more round or oval than triangular. The cingulum of the *lateral incisor* is nearly centered mesiodistally. These traits are evident in many teeth in Figure 4-6.

3. **INCISAL RIDGE CONTOUR OF MAXILLARY INCISORS FROM THE *INCISAL VIEW***

The incisal ridge or edge of the **maxillary central incisor** is 1.5–2 mm thick faciolingually and is slightly curved from mesial to distal, the convexity being on the labial side. It terminates mesially and distally at the widest portion of the crown. The position of the distoincisal angle is slightly more lingual than the position of the mesioincisal angle, which then gives the incisal edge its slight distolingual twist (Appendix 2g). The incisal ridge of the **lateral incisor** is straighter mesiodistally than on the central incisors.

4. **LABIAL CONTOUR OF MAXILLARY INCISORS FROM THE *INCISAL VIEW***

The labial outline of the **maxillary central incisor** crown usually appears broadly convex, but on some teeth, the center portion may be nearly flat. The labial outline of the **lateral incisor** is noticeably more convex than that of the central incisor. This characteristic difference is clearly seen in many teeth in Figure 4-6.

LEARNING EXERCISE

In determining a right from a left central incisor when it is not in the mouth (as on the bracket table with other incisors after multiple extractions), you need to distinguish the mesial from the distal surface. If you look at the facial surface of a tooth with its root aligned correctly for the correct arch and are able to identify the mesial or distal surface, you can place the tooth in its correct quadrant (right or left) and assign its Universal number. Evaluate the teeth in Figures 4-3 through 4-6, using the bottom chart in each figure to see how many "mesial vs. distal" traits can be used to differentiate the mesial from the distal surfaces, and therefore, right from left incisors. For example, look at the labial surface for the shape of the incisal angles (more rounded on distal), the position of the contact areas (more cervical on distal), the amount of cervical line curvature on the mesial and distal sides (more curved on mesial), as well as the flatter or concave mesial versus convex distal root surfaces. From the lingual view, look for the length of the marginal ridges (mesial is longer), and from the incisal view on the maxillary central, look for the distal location of the cingulum.

E. **VARIATIONS IN MAXILLARY INCISORS**

Racial differences in the maxillary incisor teeth have been reported in dental literature. For example, a high incidence of shovel-shaped incisors has been observed in Mongoloid peoples, including many groups of American Indians.[2,4,5,7] (Mongoloid pertains to a major racial division marked by a fold from the eyelid over the inner canthus, prominent cheekbones, straight black hair, small nose, broad face, yellowish complexion. Included are Mongols, Manchus, Chinese, Koreans, Eskimos, Japanese, Siamese, Burmese, Tibetans, and American Indians.) Caucasian and Black peoples are reported to have less frequent occurrences of this characteristic. Shovel-shape is the term commonly used to designate incisor teeth that have prominent marginal ridges and a deep fossa on their lingual surfaces (Fig. 4-1).

A study of the skulls of American Indians who lived in Arizona about 1100 AD has disclosed the occurrence of incisor teeth that have a mesial marginal ridge on the labial surface and a depression, or concavity, on the mesial part of the *labial* surface just distal to this ridge.[8] In these teeth, the distal part of the labial surface is rounded in an unusual manner. Such teeth have been referred to as "three-quarter double shovel-shaped," a descriptive, if ponderous, term. Labial "shoveling" has also been reported in some Eskimo peoples (see Figure 11.23).

FIGURE 4-7. Maxillary left central incisor with an unusual *labial ridge*.

A central incisor with a prominent labial ridge is seen in Figure 4-7. Other anomalies will be presented in chapter 11, such as palatal gingival grooves and peg-shaped lateral incisors.

SECTION III. Mandibular Incisor Type Traits: Similarities and Differences Useful to Distinguish Mandibular Central Incisors from Lateral Incisors (from All Views)

OBJECTIVES

This section is designed to prepare the learner to perform the following:
- Describe the type traits that can be used to distinguish the permanent mandibular central incisor from the mandibular lateral incisor.
- Describe and identify the labial, lingual, mesial, distal, and incisal surfaces for mandibular lateral incisors, and the facial, lingual and incisal surfaces for the symmetrical mandibular central incisor (where the mesial may be difficult to distinguish from the distal).
- Assign a Universal number to mandibular incisors present in a mouth (or on a model) with complete dentition. If possible, repeat this on a model with one or more mandibular incisors missing.
- Select and separate mandibular incisors from a selection of all teeth on a bench top.
- Holding a mandibular incisor, determine whether it is a central or a lateral and right or left. Then assign a Universal number to it.

A. MANDIBULAR INCISORS FROM THE *LABIAL VIEW*

Examine several extracted teeth and/or models as you read. Also refer to page 2 from the appendix and Figure 4-8 while you study the labial surface of mandibular incisors. Hold mandibular teeth with the root down and crown up, the position of the teeth in the mouth.

1. CROWN SHAPE OF MANDIBULAR INCISORS FROM THE *LABIAL VIEW*

Mamelons are usually present on newly emerged mandibular incisors (Fig. 4-1). Ordinarily, they are soon worn off by functional contacts against the maxillary incisors (attrition).

All mandibular incisor crowns are quite narrow relative to their crown length, but the **mandibular central incisor** crown is considerably narrower than the *maxillary* central incisor [on average only five-eighths, or 62%, as wide]. (Appendix 2p). Further, this tooth is so *symmetrical* that it is difficult to tell lefts from rights unless on casts or in the mouth. About the only difference to be found is the

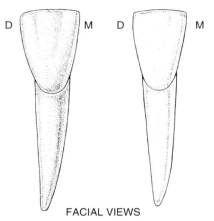

FACIAL VIEWS

Right mandibular lateral incisor

Right mandibular central incisor

FIGURE 4-8. Mandibular central and lateral incisors, *labial views*, with traits that distinguish mandibular central from lateral incisors and traits that distinguish right and left sides.

TRAITS TO DIFFERENTIATE MANDIBULAR CENTRAL FROM LATERAL INCISOR: LABIAL VIEW

CENTRAL INCISOR	LATERAL INCISOR
More symmetrical crown	Less symmetrical crown; tips to distal
No distal side bulge on crown	Distal side bulge on crown
Proximal contacts at same level M and D	Mesial proximal contact more incisal
Smaller than lateral in same mouth	Larger than central in same mouth

Facial

Centrals

Laterals

RIGHTS

LEFTS

◄——Distal——►

TRAITS TO DIFFERENTIATE MANDIBULAR RIGHT FROM LEFT INCISOR: LABIAL VIEW

CENTRAL INCISOR	LATERAL INCISOR
Very symmetrical: Can't tell right from left	Crown tips to distal
	Distal crown outline bulges more than M
	Distal proximal contact more cervical

greater mesial than distal curvature of the cervical line (visible only on extracted teeth). This trait would *not* be helpful in identifying one remaining central incisor after an orthodontist has realigned the teeth and closed the spaces on either side. The fairly straight mesial and distal crown outlines taper, becoming narrower toward the convex cervical line.

The crown of the **mandibular lateral incisor** resembles that of the mandibular central incisor, but it is not as bilaterally symmetrical. Its crown tilts distally on the root, giving the impression that the tooth has been bent at the cervix (Appendix 2l). This makes the curved distal outline of the crown (from proximal contact area to cervical line) shorter than the flatter mesial crown outline. Look at the incisors in Figure 4-8 and notice the asymmetry of most mandibular lateral incisors relative to the symmetry of the central incisors.

Unlike *maxillary* incisor crowns in the same mouth, where the central is larger than the lateral, the *mandibular lateral incisor* crown is a little larger in all dimensions than the mandibular central incisor in the same mouth, as seen when comparing many central and lateral incisors in Figure 4-8.

The labial surface of the *all mandibular incisors* are nearly smooth, but about half may have two shallow developmental depressions in the incisal third if you examine the surface closely. [Dr. Woelfel found these depressions on 48% of 793 centrals and on 51% of 787 lateral incisors.] The labial contour of all mandibular incisor crowns is convex mesiodistally in the cervical third (best viewed from the incisal) but nearly flat in the incisal third (feel it).

LEARNING EXERCISE

Look at your mouth in the mirror while you place your anterior teeth edge to edge and align the arch midlines over one another. Notice that the maxillary central incisor extends distal to the mandibular central incisor because it is the wider tooth by about 3.3 mm. Also notice that the mandibular central incisor appears smaller than the mandibular lateral incisor.

2. INCISAL PROXIMAL ANGLES OF MANDIBULAR INCISORS FROM THE *LABIAL VIEW*

The crown of the **mandibular central incisor** is nearly bilaterally symmetrical, so the mesioincisal and distoincisal angles are very similar: slightly rounded, forming nearly right angles (Appendix 2j). The distoincisal angle may barely be more rounded than the mesioincisal angle. The distoincisal angle of the **mandibular lateral incisor**, however, is noticeably more rounded than the mesioincisal angle (before attrition) (Appendix 2j). This helps to distinguish rights from lefts prior to attrition (wear).

3. PROXIMAL CONTACT AREAS OF MANDIBULAR INCISORS FROM THE *LABIAL VIEW*

The mesial and distal contact areas of the **mandibular central incisor** are at the same level: in the incisal third (Appendix 2i) almost level with the incisal edge. The mesial and distal contact areas of the **lateral incisor** are *not* at the same level (Appendix 2i). Although both the mesial and distal contacts are in the incisal third fairly near the incisal edge, the distal contact is noticeably cervical to the level of the mesial contact on lateral incisors.

4. ROOT-TO-CROWN PROPORTIONS OF MANDIBULAR INCISORS FROM THE *LABIAL VIEW*

Long but thin mesiodistally, mandibular incisor roots appear proportionally longer compared to their crown length than the maxillary incisors. Therefore, the root-to-crown ratio is larger for mandibular incisors.

5. ROOT SHAPE OF MANDIBULAR INCISORS FROM THE *LABIAL VIEW*

The roots of *all* mandibular incisors appear very narrow mesiodistally but wide faciolingually (ribbon-like) (compare proximal to labial surfaces in Appendix 2n) and taper uniformly on both sides from the cervical line to the apex. The apical end may curve slightly to the distal (seen in some incisors in Fig. 4-8).

B. MANDIBULAR INCISORS FROM THE *LINGUAL VIEW*

Refer to Figure 4-9 while studying the lingual surface of mandibular incisors.

1. LINGUAL ANATOMY (MARGINAL RIDGES, FOSSAE, AND CINGULUM) OF MANDIBULAR INCISORS FROM THE *LINGUAL VIEW*

The lingual fossae of *all* mandibular incisors are barely visible, smooth (without grooves, accessory ridges, or pits), and shallow, just slightly concave in the middle and incisal thirds (Appendix 2m). The adjacent marginal ridges, if distinguishable, are scarcely discernible, unlike with the maxillary incisors, where they are more likely to be quite prominent.

Mandibular Incisors (Lingual)

TRAITS TO DIFFERENTIATE MANDIBULAR CENTRAL FROM LATERAL INCISOR: LINGUAL VIEW

CENTRAL INCISOR	LATERAL INCISOR
Cingulum centered	Cingulum distal to center
Same length M and D marginal ridges	Longer mesial marginal ridge
Four outline characteristics from labial also apply to lingual view	

TRAITS TO DIFFERENTIATE MANDIBULAR RIGHT FROM LEFT INCISOR: LINGUAL VIEW

CENTRAL INCISOR	LATERAL INCISOR
Very symmetrical: Can't tell right from left	Same three traits as from labial
	Cingulum distal to center
	Shorter distal marginal ridge

FIGURE 4-9. Mandibular central and lateral incisors, *lingual views*, with traits that distinguish mandibular central from lateral incisors and traits that distinguish right and left sides.

2. **CINGULUM OF MANDIBULAR INCISORS FROM THE *LINGUAL VIEW***

As seen from this view, the cingulum of the **mandibular central incisor** is convex, small, and centered on the axis line of the root. The cingulum of the **lateral incisor** lies slightly distal to the axis line of the root (similar to the *maxillary* central incisor), making the mesial marginal ridge slightly longer than the distal marginal ridge.

3. **ROOT SHAPE OF MANDIBULAR INCISORS FROM THE *LINGUAL VIEW***

As with other incisor roots, the roots of *all* mandibular incisors are in general convex and slightly narrower on the lingual side than on the labial side. There are longitudinal depressions on *both* the mesial and distal sides of mandibular incisor roots (unlike the *maxillary* incisors, which normally only have mesial root depressions).

C. MANDIBULAR INCISORS FROM THE *PROXIMAL VIEWS*

Refer to Figure 4-10 while studying the proximal surfaces of the mandibular incisors.

1. **INCISAL EDGE ON MANDIBULAR INCISORS FROM THE *PROXIMAL VIEWS***

As on other mandibular anterior teeth, the incisal edges of *all* mandibular incisors are normally located on or lingual to the midroot axis (Appendix page 2). From the mesial side, the distolingual twist of the incisal ridge of the **mandibular lateral incisor** places the distal portion at the ridge even somewhat more lingual than on the mesial, unlike the mandibular central, which has no twist.

2. **CERVICAL LINE ON MANDIBULAR INCISORS FROM THE *PROXIMAL VIEWS***

The cervical line on the mesial of *all* mandibular incisors normally has a deep curvature of about 2 mm, extending incisally over one-fourth of the short crown length. As on other anterior teeth, the curvature on the distal is less [an average of 0.4 mm less on mandibular central incisors and 0.6 mm less on the mandibular lateral incisors for 234 teeth measured].

3. **HEIGHT (CREST) OF CONTOUR OF MANDIBULAR INCISORS FROM THE *PROXIMAL VIEWS***

Like the other anterior teeth, the heights of contour or greatest bulge on the *labial* surface of *all* mandibular incisors are in the cervical third, just incisal to the cervical line. The labial contour of the crown from the crest of contour to the incisal edge is so slightly curved that it often appears nearly flat, especially in the incisal half .

The *lingual* contours or outlines of *all* mandibular incisors are convex over the cingulum but concave in the middle third and straightening out in the incisal third (a shallow S outline), similar to all anterior teeth. The height of contour of the lingual surface is in the cervical third on the cingulum.

4. **ROOTS OF MANDIBULAR INCISORS FROM THE *PROXIMAL VIEWS***

The relatively large faciolingual dimension of the root at the cervix is very apparent from this view. The cervical portion of the roots on the mandibular incisors is 2 mm wider faciolingually than mesiodistally. The facial and lingual outlines of the roots of *all* mandibular incisors are nearly straight from the cervical line to the middle third; then the root tapers with its apex on the axis line (seen in mesial views of Appendix page 2).

The root contours of *all* mandibular incisors are noticeably flatter on their mesial and distal sides than the maxillary incisors (arch trait). In fact, there is usually a slight longitudinal depression on the middle third of the mesial *and* distal root surfaces, with the distal depression somewhat more distinct.

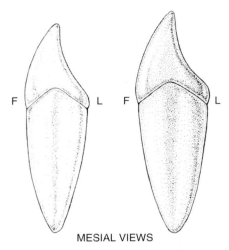

MESIAL VIEWS

Right mandibular central incisor

Right mandibular lateral incisor

FIGURE 4-10. Mandibular central and lateral incisors, *proximal views*, with traits that distinguish mandibular central from lateral incisors and traits that distinguish right and left sides.

Mandibular Incisors (Distal)

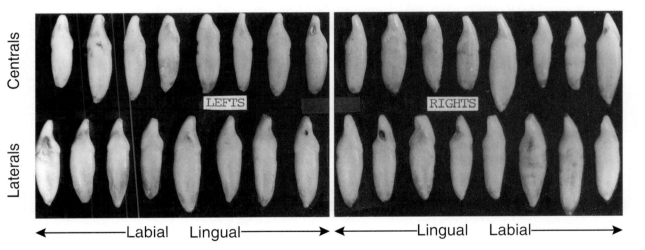

TRAITS TO DIFFERENTIATE MANDIBULAR CENTRAL FROM LATERAL INCISOR: PROXIMAL VIEWS

CENTRAL INCISOR	LATERAL INCISOR
This view is not good to differentiate central from lateral incisor.	

FIGURE 4-10. *Continues*

Mandibular Incisors (mesial)

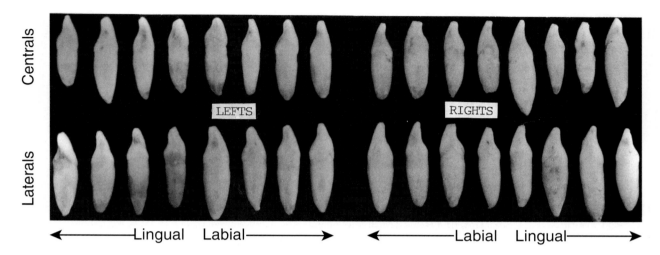

Centrals

Laterals

LEFTS RIGHTS

←—Lingual Labial—→ ←—Labial Lingual—→

TRAITS TO DIFFERENTIATE MANDIBULAR RIGHT FROM LEFT INCISOR: COMPARING PROXIMAL VIEWS

CENTRAL INCISOR	LATERAL INCISOR
D incisal ridge even with M incisal ridge	Distal incisal ridge may be more lingual
Mesial cervical line curve greater than distal on both central and lateral incisors	

FIGURE 4-10. *Continued*

D. MANDIBULAR INCISORS FROM THE *INCISAL VIEW*

To follow this description the tooth should be held in such a position that the incisal edge is toward the observer, the labial surface is at the top, and the observer is looking *exactly along the root axis line* as in Figure 4-11. You should see slightly more of the labial than the lingual surface, because the incisal ridge is just lingual to the root axis line.

1. CROWN PROPORTIONS OF MANDIBULAR INCISORS FROM THE *INCISAL VIEW*

The labiolingual measurements of *all* mandibular incisor crowns are greater than the mesiodistal measurement [by about 0.4 mm]. This is quite different from the measurements of the maxillary incisors, especially maxillary central incisors, which are considerably wider mesiodistally than faciolingually.

2. CROWN OUTLINE OF MANDIBULAR INCISORS FROM THE *INCISAL VIEW*

The **mandibular central incisor** is practically bilaterally symmetrical with little to differentiate the mesial half from the distal half. The greatest height of contour labially and lingually is centrally located. The **mandibular lateral incisor** is not bilaterally symmetrical, and this fact makes it easy to select rights from lefts and to determine centrals from laterals, especially from this view (Fig. 4-11).

3. INCISAL RIDGE CONTOUR (ALIGNMENT) OF MANDIBULAR INCISORS FROM THE *INCISAL VIEW*

The incisal ridge or edge of the **mandibular central incisor** is at right angles to the labiolingual root axis plane. It is nearly 2 mm thick and runs in a straight line mesiodistally toward the contact areas. It is lingual to the midroot axis. If you hold an extracted mandibular incisor with the root facing

INCISAL VIEWS

Right mandibular
central incisor

Right mandibular
lateral incisor

FIGURE 4-11. Mandibular central and lateral incisors, *incisal views*, with traits that distinguish mandibular central from lateral incisors and traits that distinguish right and left sides.

MANDIBULAR CENTRAL INCISORS (Incisal)

TRAITS TO DIFFERENTIATE MANDIBULAR CENTRAL FROM LATERAL INCISOR: INCISAL VIEW

CENTRAL INCISOR	LATERAL INCISOR
No distolingual twist of incisal edge	Distolingual twist of incisal edge
Cingulum is centered	Cingulum is off center to distal

Mandibular Lateral Incisors (Incisal)

TRAITS TO DIFFERENTIATE MANDIBULAR RIGHT FROM LEFT INCISOR: INCISAL VIEW

CENTRAL INCISOR	LATERAL INCISOR
Very symmetrical: Can't tell right from left	Distolingual twist of incisal edge
	Cingulum is off center to distal

directly away from your sight line, slightly more of the labial than lingual surface is visible because of the lingually positioned incisal ridge.

If you were to align a **mandibular lateral incisor** with its lingual *cingulum directly exactly downward* (represented roughly by the dotted vertical line with the arrow in Appendix 2k), the distal half of the incisal edge would be perceived as twisted lingually (called a distolingual twist). The twist of the incisal edge corresponds to the curvature of the mandibular dental arch; a tooth on the right side of the arch is twisted clockwise; one on the left is twisted counterclockwise. This twist is evident in most mandibular lateral incisors in Figure 4-11 and is an excellent way to distinguish mandibular central from lateral incisors and to distinguish the right from left mandibular lateral incisor.

4. CINGULUM OF MANDIBULAR INCISORS FROM THE *INCISAL VIEW*

If, instead of aligning the tooth with labiolingual root axis exactly vertical, you were to align the incisal edge of a lateral incisor exactly horizontal, the cingulum of the **mandibular lateral incisor** would be slightly off center to the distal (Appendix 2k). Recall that this was also seen on the maxillary central incisor. In comparison, the cingulum on the **mandibular central incisor** is centered, smooth, and makes a narrow convex outline.

5. LABIAL CONTOUR OF MANDIBULAR INCISORS FROM THE *INCISAL VIEW*

The labial surfaces of *all* mandibular incisors are only slightly convex in the incisal third labial to the incisal edge, but the outline in the cervical third is decidedly convex.

E. VARIATIONS IN MANDIBULAR INCISORS

There is more uniformity of shape in the mandibular incisor teeth than in other teeth. In some Mongoloid peoples, the cingulum of mandibular incisors is characteristically marked by a short deep groove running cervicoincisally. This groove is often a site of dental caries. In Chapter 11 on anomalies, you will see fused mandibular incisors, missing central incisors, and even a lateral incisor emerged distally to the canine.

LEARNING EXERCISE

Assign a Universal Number to a Hand-Held Incisor:

Suppose a patient just had all of his or her permanent teeth extracted. Imagine being asked to find tooth #8 from among a pile of 32 extracted teeth on the oral surgeon's tray because you wanted to evaluate a lesion on the root of that incisor. How might you go about it? Try the following steps:

- From a selection of all permanent teeth (extracted teeth or tooth models), select only the incisors (based on class traits).
- Determine whether each incisor is maxillary or mandibular. Review Table 4-2 if needed. You should never rely on only one characteristic difference between teeth to name them; rather, make a list of many traits that suggest that the tooth is a maxillary incisor, as opposed to only one trait that makes you think it belongs in the mandible. This way you can play detective and become an expert at recognition at the same time.
- If you determine that the tooth is maxillary, position the root up; if it is mandibular, position the root down.
- Next, using type traits, determine the type of incisor you are holding (central or lateral). Refer to the tables and teeth in Figures 4-3 through 4-6 and 4-8 through 4-11 as needed.
- Use characteristic traits for each surface to identify the facial surface. This will permit you to view the tooth as though you were looking into a patient's mouth.

continued

- Finally, determine which surface is the mesial. Refer to Figures 4-3 through 4-6 and 4-8 through 4-11 as needed. While viewing the incisor from the facial and picturing it within the appropriate arch (upper or lower) the mesial surface can be positioned toward the midline in only one quadrant, the right or left.
- Once you have determined the quadrant, assign the appropriate Universal number for the incisor in that quadrant. For example, the central incisor in the upper right quadrant is tooth # 8.

LEARNING QUESTIONS

Test your newly acquired knowledge by answering the following questions:

For each of the traits listed below, select the letter(s) of the permanent incisor(s) that normally exhibit(s) that trait. More than one answer may apply.

a. Maxillary central incisor
b. Maxillary lateral incisor
c. Mandibular central incisor
d. Mandibular lateral incisor

1. Mesiodistal dimension is larger than the labiolingual dimension.   a b c d
2. Incisal ridge exhibits a distolingual twist.   a b c d
3. Root is very narrow mesiodistally with mesial and distal root depressions.   a b c d
4. Incisal edge is positioned more to the lingual of the root axis line.   a b c d
5. The distal proximal height of contour is more cervical than the mesial height of contour.   a b c d
6. Has the widest (mesiodistally) incisor crown.   a b c d
7. Has the shortest root relative to its crown.   a b c d
8. Is the most symmetrical incisor.   a b c d
9. Has the largest curvature for the mesial cervical line.   a b c d
10. Has the narrowest incisor crown (mesiodistally).   a b c d

ANSWERS: 1-a, b; 2-a, d; 3-c, d; 4-c, d; 5-a, b, d; 6-a; 7-a; 8-c; 9-c; 10-c.

REFERENCES

1. Hanihara K. Racial characteristics in the dentition. J Dent Res 1967;46:923–926.
2. Carbonelli VM. Variations in the frequency of shovel-shaped incisors in different populations. In: Brothel DR, ed. Dental anthropology. London: Pergamon Press, 1963:211–234.
3. Brabant H. Comparison of the characteristics and anomalies of the deciduous and the permanent dentitions. J Dent Res 1967;48:897–902.
4. De Voto FCH. Shovel-shaped incisors in pre-Columbian Tastilian Indians. J Dent Res 1971; 50:168.
5. De Voto FCH, Arias NH, Ringuelet S, Palma NH. Shovel-shaped incisors in a northwestern Argentine population. J Dent Res 1968;47:820.
6. Taylor RMS. Variations in form of human teeth: I. An anthropologic and forensic study of maxillary incisors. J Dent Res 1969;48:5–16.
7. Dahlberg AA. The dentition of the American Indian. In: Laughlin WS, ed. The physical anthropology of the American Indian. New York: The Viking Fund, 1949.
8. Snyder RG. Mesial marginal ridging of incisor labial surfaces. J Dent Res 1960;39:361.

General Reference

Goose DH. Variability of form of maxillary permanent incisors. J Dent Res 1956;35:902.

Morphology of the Permanent Canine

Canines will be discussed in three sections, each with its own learning objectives:
I. General description of canines
    A. Functions
    B. General characteristics or class traits (similarities) of canines (both maxillary and mandibular)
II. Arch traits for canines: How to distinguish maxillary from mandibular canines (from each view)
    A. Canines from the labial view
    B. Canines from the lingual view
    C. Canines from the proximal views
    D. Canines from the incisal view
III. Variations in canine teeth

As in Chapter 4, "Appendix" followed by a number and letter (for example, "Appendix 3a") is used to denote reference to the page (number 3) and item (letter a) being referred to on that appendix page. The appendix pages are designed to be torn out to facilitate study and minimize page turns as you read the main text. This chapter will focus on Appendix pages 3 and 4.

SECTION I. General Description of Canines

OBJECTIVES

This section is designed to prepare the learner to perform the following:
- **Describe the functions of canines.**
- **List the class traits that apply to all canines. Include the incisor class traits that also apply to the canines.**
- **From a selection of all permanent teeth (or from drawings or photographs of all teeth from various views), select and separate out the canines.**

Use a cast of all permanent teeth and/or Figure 1.2 while studying about the position of the canines within the arch. There are four canines: one on either side in the maxillary arch (Universal numbers 6 and 11) and either side of the mandibular arch (numbers 22 and 27). They are longest of the permanent *teeth* [26.3 mm and 25.9 mm, respectively]. The canines are distal to the lateral incisors and are the third teeth from the midline. The mesial surface of the canine is in contact with the distal surface of the lateral incisor. The distal surface of each canine contacts the mesial surface of the first premolar.

The four canines are justifiably considered cornerstones of the arches, as they are located at the corners of the mouth or dental arches. They are often referred to as cuspids, eyeteeth, and fangs (nicknames and slang terminology). The use of such slang terminology should be discouraged. Frequently, the canines are the last teeth to be lost from dental disease (decay and/or periodontal problems). Have you known or seen an elderly person who is edentulous (toothless), except for one or more of the canines?

The name canine is of Greek origin and is found in the writings of Hippocrates and Aristotle of 2,350 years ago. Aristotle first described canine anatomy, stressing the intermediate nature of it between incisors and molars: it is sharp like an incisor and wide at the base like a molar. Celsus was the first writer to mention the roots of teeth, saying the canine was monoradicular.[1,2] The word cuspid in Spanish means "to spit." Therefore, the term cuspid would mean "spit tooth," a most unfair name for such an important tooth.

A. FUNCTIONS

In dogs, cats, and other animals with long, prominent canine teeth, the functions of these teeth are catching and tearing food and defense. As a matter of fact, *caninus* in Latin means "dog." Canines are essential to their survival. In human beings, these teeth usually function with the incisors (a) to support the lips and the facial muscles and (b) to cut, pierce, or shear food morsels. A steep overlap of the maxillary and mandibular canines, when present, serves as (c) a protective mechanism since the longer, opposing canines ride up over each other when the mandible moves to either side, causing all of the posterior teeth to separate (disclude). This canine guidance (also known as **canine protected occlusion**) relieves the premolars and molars from potentially damaging horizontal forces while chewing.

Canines, because of their large, long roots, are good anchor teeth (abutments) for a fixed dental bridge or removable partial denture attachments (clasps) when other teeth have been lost. As such, they often continue to function as a prime support for the replacement teeth for many years.

B. GENERAL CHARACTERISTICS OR CLASS TRAITS (SIMILARITIES) OF CANINES (BOTH MAXILLARY AND MANDIBULAR)

Using the maxillary right canine as a representative example for all canines, refer to the Appendix, page 3, while studying the traits of all canines.

1. SIZE OF CANINES

The canines are the longest *teeth* in the mouth. They have particularly long roots [average: 16.2 mm] and thick roots (faciolingually) that help to anchor them securely in the alveolar process. Table 5-1 provides all canine dimensions.

2. INCISAL RIDGES AND CUSP TIPS OF CANINES

The incisal ridges of canine, rather than being nearly straight horizontally like the incisors, are divided into two inclines called the **mesial** and **distal cusp ridges** (or cusp slopes or cusp arms). Subsequently, canine crowns from the facial view resemble a five-sided pentagon (Appendix 3a). The mesial cusp ridge is shorter than the distal cusp ridge (Appendix 3b). In older individuals, the lengths of the cusp ridges are often altered by wear (attrition). Canine teeth do not ordinarily have mamelons, but may have a notch on either cusp ridge, as seen clearly in Figure 5-1.

Table 5-1

SIZE OF CANINES (MEASURED BY DR. WOELFEL AND HIS DENTAL HYGIENE STUDENTS, 1974–1979)

DIMENSION MEASURED	321 MAXILLARY CANINES		316 MANDIBULAR CANINES	
	Average (mm)	Range (mm)	Average (mm)	Range (mm)
Crown length	10.6	8.2–13.6	11.0	6.8–16.4
Root length	16.5	10.8–28.5	15.9	9.5–22.2
Overall length	26.4	20.0–38.4	25.9	16.1–34.5
Crown width M-D	7.6	6.3–9.5	6.8	5.7–8.6
Root width (cervix)	5.6	3.6–7.3	5.2	4.1–6.4
Faciolingual crown size	8.1	6.7–10.7	7.7	6.4–9.5
Faciolingual root (cervix)	7.6	6.1–10.4	7.5	5.8–9.4
Mesial cervical curve	2.1	0.3–4.0	2.4	0.2–4.8
Distal cervical curve	1.4	0.2–3.5	1.6	0.2–3.5

FIGURE 5-1. *Labial view* of a maxillary right canine with a prominent labial ridge and notches on mesial and distal cusp ridges.

3. LABIAL CONTOUR OF CANINES

The labial surface of a canine is prominently convex with a vertical **labial ridge** (Appendix 3c). Canines are the only teeth with a *labial* ridge although premolars have a similar looking ridge called a *buccal* ridge.

4. CROWN PROPORTIONS OF CANINES

The measurement of the crown is greater labiolingually than it is mesiodistally [on maxillary canines by 0.5 mm and on mandibular canines by 0.9 mm; averages from 637 teeth] (Appendix 3d). The root cervix measurements are even more oblong faciolingually [greater faciolingually by 2.0 mm on maxillary canines and 2.3 mm on mandibular canines]. (Compare the facial and mesial views in Appendix 3i.)

5. CANINE TRAITS THAT ARE SIMILAR TO INCISOR TRAITS

Similar to most incisors (EXCEPT the mandibular central, where contacts are at the same level), the distal contact area is more cervical in position than the mesial contact area (Appendix 3g), and the crown outline is more convex on the distal than on the mesial surface (Appendix 3f). From the *proximal views*, canine crowns are wedge shaped (Appendix 3o). The height of contour on the facial surface is in the cervical third, and on the lingual surface is on the cingulum, which makes up the cervical third of the crown length (Appendix 3p). The remaining outline of the lingual surface (lingual ridge) is slightly concave in the middle third and is straight or slightly convex in the incisal third. Combined, the lingual outline is S-shaped, as on all other anterior teeth (Appendix 3q). Further similarities with incisors include the following: crowns taper, narrowing from the contact areas toward the cervix (Appendix 3e); cervical lines curve more on the mesial than on the distal surface (compare mesial and distal views in Appendix 3n); and marginal ridges (as well as crowns) taper lingually from the contact areas toward the cingulum (Appendix 3-l); so the crown is narrower on the lingual half than on the facial half. Facial outlines are less convex than lingual outlines (Appendix 3s), and the incisal edges extend from mesial to distal contact areas (Appendix 3r). Further, roots taper, narrowing on the lingual half, and narrowing from the cervix toward the apex (Appendix 3h), with the root tip or apex often bending to the distal (Appendix 3j). Roots are also longer than crowns (Appendix 3k).

The location of incisal edge tooth wear on canines is similar to wear on incisors. Facets on the **mandibular** canine cusp tip and cusp ridge normally form more on the labial border, not the lingual border of the cusp ridge as occurs on the **maxillary** canine. *If* you find wear facets on the lingual surface of a mandibular canine, or on the labial surface of a maxillary canine, it is probably because the teeth were not aligned with the normal overlapping of anterior teeth described in Chapter 3. Refer back to Figure 4-2 for an illustration of this concept on incisors.

SECTION II. Arch Traits for Canines: How to Distinguish Maxillary from Mandibular Canines (from Each View)

Unlike incisors where there are two types, a central and a lateral, there is only one type of canine. Therefore, type traits do not apply to canines, but arch traits are useful to distinguish maxillary from mandibular canines.

OBJECTIVES

This section is designed to prepare the learner to perform the following:

- Describe the arch traits that can be used to distinguish the permanent maxillary canines from mandibular canines.
- Describe and identify the labial, lingual, mesial, distal, and incisal surfaces for all canines.
- Assign a Universal number to canines present in a mouth with a complete permanent dentition, (or on a model or in an illustration), based on its shape as well as its position in the quadrant.
- Holding a canine, determine whether it is a maxillary or mandibular, and whether it belongs on the right or left side. Then picture it within the appropriate quadrant and assign a universal number to it.

A.   CANINES FROM THE *LABIAL VIEW*

Examine several extracted canines and/or models as you study this section. Hold maxillary canines with crowns down and mandibular canines with crowns up, as you examine them. This is the way they are oriented in the mouth. Also, while reading this section, tear out and refer to the Appendix study page 4 on canines.

1.   CANINE MORPHOLOGY FROM THE *LABIAL VIEW*

Along with the tooth models and the Appendix pages, refer to Figure 5-2 for viewing similarities and the range of differences of canines from the labial view.

The facial side of any canine crown is formed from three labial lobes like the incisors. (The cingulum on the lingual side of the crown is from the fourth lobe.) The middle lobe on the facial forms the *labial ridge* (Appendix 3c), which can be quite prominent on the **maxillary canine**. The labial ridge runs cervicoincisally near the center of the crown in the middle and incisal thirds. Shallow depressions lie mesial and distal to the labial ridge.

The labial surface of **mandibular canines** is more smooth and convex. A labial ridge is often present but not as pronounced as on the maxillary canines. In the incisal third, the labial crown surface is convex but slightly flattened mesial to the labial ridge and even a little more flattened distal to the ridge. (Feel it.)

2.   CANINE SHAPE AND SIZE FROM THE *LABIAL VIEW*

The outline of the *mesial* half of the **maxillary canine** crown is broadly convex in the middle third, becoming nearly flat in the cervical third (Appendix 4b). The outline of the *distal* portion of this crown forms a shallow S shape, being convex in the middle third and slightly concave in the cervical third.

The **mandibular canine** crown appears longer and narrower than the crown of the maxillary canine (Appendix 4a). [The mandibular canine is actually 0.4 mm longer and 0.8 mm narrower; averages from 637 teeth.] The *mesial* outline of the mandibular crown is almost flat to slightly convex, *nearly in line* with the mesial side of the root, and not projecting beyond it (Appendix 4b). This conspicuous feature is quite evident in most mandibular canines in Figure 5-2, but is not seen on maxillary canines. In other words, the mesial side of the mandibular canine crown does not bulge or project beyond the root outline. The *distal* side of the crown may be slightly concave in the cervical third; it is convex in the incisal two-thirds. There is noticeably more of the crown distal to the root axis line than mesial to it. This often makes the lower canine crown appear to be tilted or bent distally when the root is held in a vertical position.

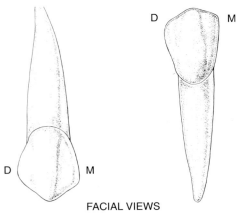

FACIAL VIEWS

Right maxillary canine   Right mandibular canine

FIGURE 5-2. *Labial views of canines* with traits to distinguish maxillary from mandibular canines and traits to distinguish rights from lefts.

Canines(Labial)

Rights   Lefts

Maxillary

Mandibular

← Distal →

TRAITS TO DISTINGUISH MAXILLARY FROM MANDIBULAR CANINE: LABIAL VIEW

MAXILLARY CANINE	MANDIBULAR CANINE
Cusp angle sharper, more acute (105°)	Cusp angle more blunt (120°)
	Mesial cusp ridge almost horizontal
M,D contacts more cervical	M,D proximal contacts more incisal
Crown wider M-D	Crown narrower M-D
Mesial cusp ridge shorter than distal	Mesial cusp ridge *much* shorter than distal
Mesial of crown bulges beyond root outline	Mesial crown-to-root outline continuous
More pronounced labial ridge	Less pronounced labial ridge
More pointed root tip	Blunter root tip

TRAITS TO DIFFERENTIATE RIGHT FROM LEFT CANINES: LABIAL VIEW

MAXILLARY CANINE	MANDIBULAR CANINE
Mesial crown outline less curved than D	Mesial crown outline flatter than distal
Mesial crown outline bulges beyond root	Mesial crown outline is in line with root
	Mesial cusp ridge more horizontal

Distal crown outline curves more than mesial crown outline
Distal contact more cervical than mesial contact
Mesial cusp ridge shorter than distal

3. **CANINE CUSP TIP AND INCISAL RIDGES FROM THE *LABIAL VIEW***

Recall that the mesial ridges are normally shorter than the distal ridges for *all* canines. The cusp ridges and the cusp of the **maxillary canine** make up nearly one-third of the cervicoincisal length of the crown, because the angle formed by the cusp ridges is relatively sharp, slightly more than a right angle (105°) (Appendix 4c). Compare this to the cusp tip of the **mandibular canine**, where cusp ridges form a less sharp, more obtuse (blunt) angle (120°) (Appendix 4c). The *mesial* cusp ridge of the mandibular canine is also almost horizontal compared to its longer distal cusp ridge, which slopes more steeply in an apical direction. Shorter, more horizontal mesial cusp ridges are seen clearly on most mandibular canines in Figure 5-2. Wear on the incisal edge may alter the length of the cusp slopes, sometimes even completely obliterating the cusp.

4. **CANINE CONTACT AREAS FROM THE *LABIAL VIEW***

The *mesial* contact area of the **maxillary canine** is located at the junction of the incisal and middle thirds. The *distal* contact area of the maxillary canine, like all anterior teeth, is in a more cervical location on the distal side than on the mesial side. It is located in the middle third, just cervical to the junction of the incisal and middle thirds (recall Appendix 3g). This is the only canine proximal contact area (mesial or distal) located in the middle third.

The *mesial* contact area of the **mandibular canine** is in a more incisal position than on the maxillary canine due to its nearly horizontal mesial cusp ridge. It is in the incisal third just cervical to the mesioincisal angle. The *distal* contact area is, as expected, more cervical than the mesial, at the junction of the middle and incisal thirds.

5. **CANINE TOOTH PROPORTIONS FROM THE *LABIAL VIEW***

The **maxillary canine** crown is nearly as long as the maxillary central incisor, but the root is much longer [3.5 mm longer than the average on 719 teeth] making this, on average, the *longest tooth* in the mouth (Appendix 3k). The **mandibular canine** is considerably larger than either of the mandibular incisors, particularly in length [by 4.1 mm] and mesiodistal width [1.3 mm].

6. **CANINE ROOT CONTOUR FROM THE *LABIAL VIEW***

The labial surface of a canine root is normally convex. The root of the **maxillary canine** is long, slender, and conical. The apical third is narrow mesiodistally and the apex may be pointed or sharp. The apical third of the root often bends distally. [On 100 maxillary canines examined by Dr. Woelfel, 58 bent distally, 24 were straight, and 18 had the apical end of their roots bending slightly toward the mesial.] Three maxillary canine roots can be seen bending mesially in Figure 5-2.

The **mandibular canine** root tapers apically to a somewhat more blunt apex. The apical end of the root is more often straight rather than curving toward the mesial or distal sides. [On 100 mandibular canines inspected by Dr. Woelfel, 45 had absolutely straight roots, 29 had the apical third bending mesially, and 26 bent slightly toward the distal.] Therefore, on mandibular canines, the root curvature should not be used to differentiate rights and lefts. Mandibular canine roots are shorter than the roots of maxillary canines [0.6 mm shorter on 637 teeth].

B. CANINES FROM THE *LINGUAL VIEW*

Refer to Figure 5-3 while studying similarities and differences of canines from the lingual view.

1. **CANINE LINGUAL RIDGES AND FOSSAE FROM THE *LINGUAL VIEW***

The **maxillary canine** has a prominent lingual ridge running cervicoincisally from the cusp to the cingulum (Appendix 4d). The mesial and distal lingual fossae lie on either side of the lingual ridge and are usually shallow. Sometimes the lingual surface of the maxillary canine is naturally smooth or worn smooth from attrition so that the lingual ridge and the two fossae on either side of it are not easily discernible. By examining a number of specimens you will find some with considerable wear or attrition on the lingual surface, sometimes entirely obliterating the lingual ridge.

TRAITS TO DISTINGUISH MAXILLARY FROM MANDIBULAR CANINE: LINGUAL VIEW

MAXILLARY CANINE	MANDIBULAR CANINE
More prominent anatomy on lingual:	Smoother lingual surface:
Lingual marginal ridges pronounced	Lingual marginal ridges less pronounced
Prominent lingual ridge and fossae	Less prominent ridge and fossae
Most prominent lingual ridge (46%)	Most prominent distal ridge (63%)
Cingulum centered	Cingulum centered or to distal

Also, six outline traits from facial view also apply to lingual view.

TRAITS TO DIFFERENTIATE RIGHT FROM LEFT CANINES: LINGUAL VIEW

MAXILLARY CANINE	MANDIBULAR CANINE

Cingulum distal to center
Outline traits that are seen from facial view also are seen from lingual view
Mesial marginal ridge longer than distal marginal ridge

FIGURE 5-3. *Lingual views of canines* with traits to distinguish maxillary from mandibular canines and traits to distinguish rights from lefts.

The lingual surface of the **mandibular canine** is not subject to lingual wear as on the maxillary canine but, even without wear, the ridge and fossae are normally less prominent.

2. **CANINE CINGULUM FROM THE *LINGUAL VIEW***

The **maxillary canine** cingulum is large. Its incisal border is sometimes pointed in the center, resembling a small cusp or tubercle (seen clearly in the far right maxillary canine in Fig. 5-3). The cingulum and the tip of the cusp are usually centered mesiodistally (seen best from the incisal view in Appendix 4e). The cingulum of the **mandibular canine** is low, less bulky, and less prominent than on maxillary canines. Unlike maxillary canines, the cingulum lies just distal to the midroot axis line. This distal location of the cingulum becomes most apparent when you are viewing the tooth with neither the mesial nor distal corners of the incisal ridge twisted toward you (apparent from the incisal view in Appendix 4e).

3. CANINE MARGINAL RIDGES FROM THE *LINGUAL VIEW*

The elevated mesial and distal marginal ridges of the **maxillary canines** are usually of moderate size, and the *lingual ridge* is often most prominent. The distal marginal ridge is slightly more elevated than the mesial marginal ridge (prior to attrition). [Dr. Woelfel's dental hygiene students inspected 455 maxillary canines on dental stone casts. The lingual ridge was found to be the most elevated of the three lingual ridges 46% of the time, the distal ridge was most elevated 36% of the time, and the mesial marginal ridge was most elevated only 18% of the time.] The mesial marginal ridge (extending from the proximal contact area to the cingulum) is longer than the distal marginal ridge because of the shorter mesial cusp slope and the more incisally located mesial contact area.

The marginal ridges of **mandibular canines** are not prominent, and much of the lingual surface appears smooth when compared to that of the maxillary canines (arch trait). The somewhat inconspicuous mesial marginal ridge may be longer and straighter than the shorter, more elevated, and curved distal marginal ridge. The *distal marginal ridge* is usually slightly more prominent or elevated than either the lingual ridge or the mesial marginal ridge. [Of 244 mandibular canines on dental stone casts inspected by dental hygiene students, the distal marginal ridge was the most prominent of the three lingual ridges on 63% of the teeth and the mesial marginal ridge was the most prominent on only 18%. The lingual ridge was most prominent only on 19% of these unworn lingual surfaces.]

4. CANINE ROOTS FROM THE *LINGUAL VIEW*

All canine roots are usually convex on the lingual and are narrower on the lingual side than on the labial side. Therefore, it is often possible to see both mesial and distal sides of the root and one or both of the proximal longitudinal root depressions from this view.

C. CANINES FROM THE *PROXIMAL VIEWS*

Refer to Figure 5-4 while studying the similarities and differences of canines from the mesial or distal views.

1. CANINE OUTLINE FROM THE *PROXIMAL VIEWS*

The wedge-shaped **maxillary canine** crown from this view has a bulky cusp because of the prominent labial and lingual ridges. The **mandibular canine** crown is also wedge shaped but thinner in the incisal portion than the crown of the maxillary canine because of a less bulky lingual ridge. Observe this difference in cusp thickness in the canines in Figure 5-4.

2. INCISAL RIDGE AND CUSP TIP OF CANINES FROM THE *PROXIMAL VIEWS*

The incisal ridge and cusp tip of the **maxillary canine** is usually located *labial* to the midroot axis line. The incisal ridge and cusp tip of the **mandibular canine** are most often located slightly *lingual* to the root axis line, but it may be centered over it (Appendix 4h). This is a good distinguishing trait between mandibular and maxillary canines. Observe this difference in cusp tip location (more labial on the maxillary canine and more lingual on mandibular canines) in a majority of canines in Figure 5-4. Further, the distoincisal angle of the mandibular canine is slightly more lingual in position than the cusp tip because of the distolingual twist of the crown so that much of the lingual surface is visible from the mesial aspect, similar to the mandibular lateral incisors (seen from the incisal view on Appendix 4f).

3. CANINE HEIGHT OF CONTOUR FROM THE *PROXIMAL VIEWS*

As with all teeth, the *labial* height of contour of the **maxillary canine** is in the cervical third of the crown, but it may not be as close to the cervical line as the corresponding curvature on the incisor

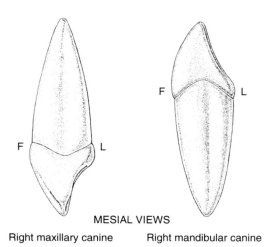

MESIAL VIEWS

Right maxillary canine   Right mandibular canine

FIGURE 5-4. *Proximal views of canines* with traits to distinguish maxillary from mandibular canines, and traits to distinguish rights from lefts.

Canines (Proximal)

Lefts   Rights

Maxillary

Mandibular

MESIAL SURFACES   DISTAL SURFACES

⟵ Lingual   Labial ⟶

TRAITS TO DISTINGUISH MAXILLARY FROM MANDIBULAR CANINE: PROXIMAL VIEW

MAXILLARY CANINE	MANDIBULAR CANINE
Cingulum more prominent	Cingulum less prominent
Cusp tip labial to root axis line	Cusp tip lingual to root axis line
Labial height of contour less cervical	Labial height of contour closer to cervical line
Labial height of contour more pronounced	Labial height of contour less pronounced
Incisal wear is more lingual, even in fossa	Incisal wear more labial
Cusp tip appears thicker F-L	Cusp tip appears less thick F-L

TRAITS TO DIFFERENTIATE RIGHT FROM LEFT CANINES: COMPARING *PROXIMAL VIEWS*

MAXILLARY CANINE	MANDIBULAR CANINE

Cervical line curves more on the mesial than distal surface.
Distal root depression is more distinct than mesial.

teeth or on the mandibular canine. The labial surface is much more convex than on the incisors (feel it and compare the curvatures of the incisors and the canines).

The height of contour of the *labial* surface of the **mandibular canine** crown is closer to the cervical line than on a maxillary canine. There is an almost continuous crown-root outline on mandibular canines with minimal facial or lingual crown bulge when viewed from the proximal aspects. This lack of discernable cervical crown bulge beyond the root facially and lingually is clearly evident in many mandibular canines in Figure 5-4. This feature can be helpful when distinguishing mandibular from maxillary canines.

As with all anterior teeth, the *lingual* heights of contour of *all canines* are usually in the cervical third, on the cingulum.

4. CANINE CERVICAL LINE FROM THE *PROXIMAL VIEWS*

The cervical lines of *all canines* from the proximal views usually curve incisally quite a bit (over 2 mm on maxillary canines). As on incisors, the curvature is greater on the mesial surface than on the distal surface, but it is less on the canines than on the incisors. [Of the 321 **maxillary canines** measured by Dr. Woelfel's dental hygiene students, the *mesial* cervical curvature averaged 2.1 mm, with a range from 0.3–4.0 mm; the *distal* curvature averaged 1.4 mm with a range of 0.2–3.5 mm. Such wide variability is not unusual.]

The **mandibular canine** cervical line appears to curve more incisally than on maxillary canines. The fact that the mandibular canine crown is narrower faciolingually than the maxillary canine [by 0.4 mm] and has a greater mesial cervical line curve [by 0.3 mm] accentuates the apparent greater depth of the curve [averages from 637 canines]. However, one of the mandibular canines had a mesial cervical curvature of 4.8 mm, whereas another one's curve was almost flat [at 0.2 mm]. So, once again, the tremendous variation between the same kind of teeth is evident. As with most other teeth, the cervical line curves less on the distal surface than on the mesial surface [by 0.8 mm; of the 316 mandibular canines measured, the *mesial* curvature averaged 2.4 mm; the *distal* curvature averaged 1.6 mm].

5. CANINE ROOT FROM THE *PROXIMAL VIEWS*

The labial outlines of the roots of *all canines* are often *slightly* convex with the lingual outline more convex, although this varies. *All canine* roots usually have vertical longitudinal (cervicoapical) depressions on the mesial *and* distal surfaces, and the distal depression is usually more distinct (deeper) especially on the lowers. [Mesial: On 100 *maxillary* canines examined by Dr. Woelfel, 70 had a longitudinal depression on the *mesial* root surface (six fairly deep), 23 were flat, and only 8 had convex mesial middle third root surfaces with no depression. On 100 *mandibular* canines examined by Dr. Woelfel, 88 had a longitudinal *mesial* root depression (28 were fairly deep), 8 were flat, and 4 were considered to be convex. Distal: On 100 *maxillary* canines examined by Dr. Woelfel, 90 had a longitudinal depression on the *distal* surface (20 were rather deep), and only 10 had no distal root depression. Of 100 *mandibular* canines examined by Dr. Woelfel, 97 had a longitudinal depression on the *distal* surface (40 were fairly deep), and only 3 had flat distal root surfaces. None of the distal root surfaces were judged to be convex on the middle third of the root.]

D. CANINES FROM THE *INCISAL VIEW*

Refer to Figure 5-5 for a comparison of similarities and differences of canines from the incisal view. To follow this description, the tooth should be held so that the incisal edge (cusp tip) is toward the observer, the labial surface is at the top, and the observer is looking *exactly down the midroot axis line*. You should see more of the lingual surface of the maxillary canine, because the cusp tip and the cusp ridges are labial to the midroot axis line, and you may see more of the labial surface of mandibular canines because the cusp ridges are lingual to, or centered on, the midroot axis line, as seen on most canines in Figure 5-5.

1. CANINE CROWN PROPORTIONS FROM THE *INCISAL VIEW*

The **maxillary canine** crown outline is not symmetrical. The labiolingual dimension of the crown is slightly greater than mesiodistally [by 0.5 mm] (recall Appendix 3d). This is similar to the *mandibu-

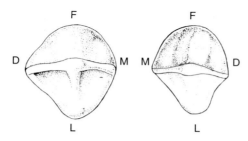

INCISAL VIEWS

Right maxillary canine   Right mandibular canine

FIGURE 5-5. *Incisal views of canines* with traits to distinguish maxillary from mandibular canines, and traits to distinguish rights from lefts.

CANINES (Incisal)
Facial Surfaces

Lingual Surfaces

TRAITS TO DISTINGUISH MAXILLARY FROM MANDIBULAR CANINE: *INCISAL VIEW*

MAXILLARY CANINE	MANDIBULAR CANINE
More asymmetrical crown outline	More symmetrical crown outline
Slightly greater F-L than M-D	Much greater F-L compared to M-D
Distal half of crown pinched in F-L	Distal crown pinch F-L not as evident
Cingulum centered	Cingulum to distal (or centered)
Incisal edge more horizontal M-D	Incisal edge with DL twist
Facets on lingual-incisal or lingual surface	Facets on labial-incisal of cusp ridge
Contour traits noted from lingual view are also seen from incisal view	

TRAITS TO DIFFERENTIATE RIGHT FROM LEFT CANINES: *INCISAL VIEW*

MAXILLARY CANINE	MANDIBULAR CANINE
More faciolingual bulk in mesial half	Cingulum often to distal
	Incisal ridge more lingual on distal half
Distal half of crown pinched faciolingually	Distal half of crown may be pinched F-L
Contour traits seen from lingual are also viewed from incisal.	

lar anteriors but uncharacteristic of the *maxillary incisors*. The labiolingual dimension of the **mandibular canine** crown is noticeably greater than the mesiodistal measurement [by an average of 0.9 mm on 316 teeth]. This characteristic oblong faciolingual outline is seen on many mandibular canines in Figure 5-5.

2. **CANINE INCISAL EDGE (CUSP TIP) CONTOUR FROM THE *INCISAL VIEW***

The incisal edge (made up of the cusp tip and thick cusp ridges) of the **maxillary canine** is located slightly labial to the labiolingual center of the root, and this edge is aligned almost horizontally (Appendix 4f).

The cusp tip of the **mandibular canine** is near the center labiolingually, or it may be lingual to the center. When the tooth is held with the faciolingual axis of the cervix of the root exactly vertical, the distal cusp ridge is directed slightly lingually from the cusp tip, placing the distoincisal angle in a position somewhat lingual to the position of the cusp tip (Appendix 4f). This lingual placement of the distoincisal angle gives the incisal part of the crown a slight distolingual twist like the mandibular lateral incisor. From this view, the *distolingual twist* of the crown would match closely the curvature of the dental arch.

3. **CANINE CINGULUM AND MARGINAL RIDGES FROM THE *INCISAL VIEW***

The **maxillary canine** cingulum is large and is located in the center mesiodistally (Appendix 4e). On the lingual outline of the **mandibular canine**, the height (crest) of contour of the cingulum is centered or slightly distal to the centerline (Appendix 4e). The mesial marginal ridge (extending from the contact area to the cingulum) appears longer than the distal marginal ridge because of the slight distal placement of the cingulum, and the lingual positioning of the distal cusp ridge placing it closer to the cingulum. This may be better appreciated from the lingual view.

4. **CANINE LABIAL CONTOUR FROM THE *INCISAL VIEW***

The labial outline of the **maxillary canine** is convex, more than either maxillary incisor, since the labial ridge is often quite prominent. The *mesial* half of the labial outline is quite convex, whereas the *distal* half of the labial outline is frequently somewhat concave, giving this portion of the crown the appearance that it has been pinched in on the facial (Appendix 4g). This observation is most helpful and is a reliable guide in determining right from left maxillary canines and is seen on many upper canines in the top row in Figure 5-5.

The outline of the **mandibular canine** crown is more symmetrical than a maxillary canine. However, the labial crown outline mesial to the centerline is noticeably more convex, whereas the labial outline distal to the center is more flat, or even slightly concave.

5. **CANINE LINGUAL CONTOUR FROM THE *INCISAL VIEW***

The lingual ridge of the **maxillary canine** divides the lingual surface in half with a shallow fossa on each side. This ridge and fossae are less evident in the **mandibular canine**.

LEARNING EXERCISE

Assign a Universal number to a hand-held tooth:
A patient just had all of his permanent teeth extracted. Imagine being asked to find tooth #6 from among a pile of 32 extracted teeth on the oral surgeon's tray because you want to evaluate a lesion on the root of that canine. How might you go about it? Try the following steps:
- From a number of extracted teeth or tooth models, select the canines based on class traits.
- Determine whether the canine is maxillary or mandibular. You should never rely on only one

characteristic difference between teeth to name them; rather, make a list of many traits that suggest the tooth is a maxillary canine as opposed to only one trait that makes you think it belongs in the mandible. This way you can play detective and become an expert at recognition at the same time. Refer to the arch traits in Figures 5-2 through 5-5 as needed.

- If you determine that the tooth is maxillary, position the root up; if it is mandibular, position the root down.
- With the tooth aligned correctly, use characteristic traits for each surface to identify the facial surface. This will permit you to view the tooth as though you were looking into a patient's mouth.
- Finally, determine which surface is the mesial. (Refer to the right/left traits in Figs. 5-2 through 5-5 as needed.) While viewing the tooth from the facial, and picturing it within the appropriate arch (upper or lower), the mesial surface can be positioned toward the midline in only one quadrant, the right or left.
- Once you have determined the quadrant, assign the appropriate Universal Number for the canine in that quadrant. For example, the canine in the upper right quadrant is tooth #6.

SECTION III. Variations in Canine Teeth

Probably the most conspicuous variation in canine teeth is found in the mandibular canine. For example, although it is rare to find a maxillary canine tooth with the root divided, this division is known to occur. The division results in labial and lingual roots, and may be split only in the apical third or it may extend into the cervical third of the root (Fig. 5-6).

FIGURE 5-6. Two mandibular canines with split (furcated) root with facial and lingual root tips.

Observe the enormous variation in size and shape among several maxillary and mandibular canines in Figure 5-7. Referring to the measurements of 637 canines in Table 5-1 under the range column: maxillary canine crowns from shortest to longest varied by 5.4 mm, root length differed by 17.7 mm, and overall length differed by 18.4 mm. In the 1962 issue of the *Journal of the North Carolina Dental Society* (46:10), there was a report of an extraction, without incident, of a maxillary left canine 47 mm long. On mandibular canines, crown length, root length, and overall length ranges varied by 9.6, 12.7, and 18.4 mm, respectively. Can you imagine one mandibular canine with a crown 9.6 mm longer than another one? The shortest mandibular canine (cusp tip to root apex) was only 16.1 mm long. Two of the mandibular canine crowns in Figure 5-7 are that short. See if you can spot these teeth. A maxillary canine with an unusual notch on its mesial cusp slope is seen in Figure 5-8.

Other anomalies will be noted in subsequent chapters. These will include a maxillary canine with a palatal gingival groove on the lingual side of a maxillary canine crown and root (in Chapter 8) and a very unusual maxillary canine with a shovel-shaped lingual surface (in Chapter 7). Perhaps the most unique canines of all occur on the male Babirusa (type of wild boar) seen in Figure 5-9. His two enormous maxillary canines curve backward, piercing the upper lip and bony snout on each side. Then they curve in a large arc upward, backward, and finally down toward the forehead. These unusual maxillary canines serve only to protect the boar's eyes and upper face. The Babirusa's mandibular canines are also very large, tusk-like, and curve up and back, possibly serving to protect the side of his face and for fighting or piercing food when his jaw is opened widely.

FIGURE 5-7. Canines of differing size showing tremendous variation.

FIGURE 5-8. Maxillary right canine with a deep notch in the mesial cusp ridge.

FIGURE 5-9. A male Babirusa (type of wild boar) with extremely unique canines that actually pierce the upper lip and bony snout on each side.

LEARNING QUESTIONS

For each trait described below, indicate the letter of the best response from the five selections provided. Each trait has only one best answer.

a. Maxillary central incisor
b. Maxillary canine
c. Mandibular canine
d. All of the above
e. None of the above
1. This tooth exhibits less cervical line curvature on the distal aspect than on the mesial aspect.   a b c d e

LEARNING QUESTIONS, cont.

2. The cingulum is centered mesiodistally.   a b c d e
3. There is an almost continuous crown-root outline
    on the mesial surface of this tooth.   a b c d e
4. The mesial contact area is located more incisally .
    than the distal contact area on the same tooth   a b c d e
5. The cusp tip is positioned lingual to the midroot
    axis line from the proximal view.   a b c d e
6. Mamelons could be observed on this tooth.   a b c d e
7. On which tooth is the cusp angle most acute?   a b c d e
8. The mesiodistal width of this tooth is greater than
    its labiolingual width.   a b c d e
9. The mesial and distal marginal ridges are positioned
    more vertically than horizontally on the lingual surface.   a b c d e
10. The tooth (teeth) develop(s) from four lobes.   a b c d e
11. The tooth (teeth) develop(s) from three lobes.   a b c d e

ANSWERS 1–d; 2–b; 3–c; 4–d; 5–c; 6–a; 7–b; 8–a; 9–d; 10–d; 11–e.

REFERENCES

1. Cootjans G. The cuspid in Greaco-Latin literature. Rev Belge Med Dent 1971;26(3):387–392.
2. Year Book of Dentistry. Chicago: Year Book Medical Publishers, 1973:354.

General References

Taylor RMS. Variations in form of human teeth: II. An anthropologic and forensic study of maxillary canines. J Dent Res 1969;48:173–182.

6 Morphology of Premolars

The morphology of premolars will be presented in three sections, each with its own learning objectives:

I. Overview of premolars
   A. General description of premolars
   B. Functions of premolars
   C. Class traits of premolars
   D. Arch traits that differentiate maxillary from mandibular premolars
II. Type traits that differentiate *maxillary* first from maxillary second premolars
   A. Type traits of maxillary premolars from the *buccal view*
   B. Type traits of maxillary premolars from the *lingual view*
   C. Type traits of maxillary premolars from the *proximal views*
   D. Type traits of maxillary premolars from the *occlusal view*
III. Type traits that differentiate *mandibular* first from second premolars
   A. Type traits of mandibular premolars from the *buccal view*
   B. Type traits of mandibular premolars from the *lingual view*
   C. Type traits of mandibular premolars from the *proximal views*
   D. Type traits of mandibular premolars from the *occlusal view*

SECTION I. Overview of Premolars

OBJECTIVES

This section is designed to prepare the learner to perform the following:
- Describe the functions of premolars.
- List class traits common to all premolars.
- List arch traits that can be used to distinguish maxillary from mandibular premolars.
- From a selection of all teeth, select and separate out the premolars.
- Divide a selection of all premolars into maxillary and mandibular.

Using the maxillary right second premolar as a representative example for all premolars, refer to the Appendix, page 5, while reading Section I of this chapter. Throughout this chapter, "Appendix" followed by a number and letter (Appendix 5a) is used to denote reference to the page (number 5) and item (letter a) being referred to on that appendix page. The appendix pages are designed to be torn out to facilitate study and minimize page turns.

A. GENERAL DESCRIPTION OF PREMOLARS

The term premolar is used to designate any tooth in the permanent (secondary) dentition of mammals that replaces a primary molar. There are eight premolars: four in the maxillary arch and four in the mandibular arch. They are the fourth and fifth teeth from the midline in each quadrant. The maxillary premolars can be identified by the universal numbering system as teeth numbers 5 and 12 (maxillary right and left *first* premolars, respectively) and numbers 4 and 13 (maxillary right and left *second* premolars, respectively). The mandibular right and left *first* premolars are numbers 28 and 21, respectively, with the mandibular right and left *second* premolars numbered 29 and 20, respectively.

The mesial surfaces of first premolars contact the distal surfaces of adjacent canines, whereas distal surfaces contact the mesial surfaces of adjacent second premolars. The distal sides of second premolars are in contact with the mesial sides of adjacent first molars.

B. FUNCTIONS OF PREMOLARS

The premolars (upper and lower) function with the molars (a) in the mastication of food and (b) in maintaining the vertical dimension of the face. The first premolars (c) assist the canines in shearing or cutting food morsels, and all premolars (d) support the corners of the mouth and cheeks to keep them from sagging. This is more discernible in older people. Patients who unfortunately have lost all of their molars can still masticate or chew quite well if they still have four to eight occluding premolars. However, it is very noticeable when a person smiles and is missing one or more maxillary premolars.

C. CLASS TRAITS OF PREMOLARS

1. CLASS TRAITS SIMILAR TO ANTERIOR TEETH

Consider first the similarities between premolars and anterior teeth by examining models of the entire maxillary and mandibular arches as you read the following.

Number of Developmental Lobes: Like anterior teeth, the facial (or buccal) surfaces of all premolars develop from three *facial* lobes, usually evidenced by two shallow, vertical depressions separating a center ridge on the facial surface of the crown from mesial and distal portions (Appendix 5a). This centered buccal ridge is more conspicuous on first than second premolars, and is more pronounced on maxillary than mandibular premolars. (The prominent buccal ridge on the maxillary first premolar is similar to the pronounced labial ridge on the maxillary canine.) Also, the lingual surfaces of most premolars (like anterior teeth) develop from one *lingual* lobe. In premolars, this lobe forms one lingual cusp; in anterior teeth, it forms the cingulum (recall Fig. 3-23). An EXCEPTION occurs in a common variation of the mandibular second premolar, the three-cusp type, which develops from three facial and *two* (not one) *lingual* lobes, forming two lingual cusps. Due to this variation of the mandibular second premolar with three cusps, the term bicuspid (referring to *two* cusps) is hardly appropriate for this group of teeth.

Crowns Taper Toward the Cervical: From the facial, crowns are narrower in the cervical third than occlusally (Appendix 5m). This is because the widest *proximal* heights (crests) of contour (or contact areas) are located in the occlusal to middle thirds on posterior teeth (similar to the location on anterior teeth in the incisal to middle thirds).

Cervical Lines: Similar to all anterior teeth, cervical lines, when viewed from the proximal, curve toward the biting surfaces (occlusal or incisal) (Appendix 5o) and, when viewed from the facial or lingual, are curved toward the apex (Appendix 5n). Also, the amount of curvature is slightly greater on the mesial than on the distal surface.

Root Shape: Like anterior teeth, facial and lingual root surfaces are convex, and roots taper apically (Appendix 5q). Also, the root tapers toward the lingual resulting in a narrower lingual side of the root mesiodistally. The apical third is usually bent distally (Appendix 5p).

2. CLASS TRAITS THAT DIFFER FROM ANTERIOR TEETH

Tooth Surface Terminology: Compared to the anterior teeth, the facial surfaces of the posterior teeth are called *buccal* (resting against the cheeks) instead of *labial*, and posterior teeth have *occlusal* surfaces instead of *incisal* edges. Occlusal surfaces have cusps, ridges, and grooves on the occlusal surface that are usually oriented in a horizontal plane.

Occlusal Cusps versus Incisal Edges: Unlike anterior teeth with incisal edges or ridges and a cingulum, premolars have one buccal (or facial) cusp, and most have one lingual cusp (Appendix 5b). The EXCEPTION is the mandibular second premolar, which often has two lingual cusps [54% of the time].

Marginal Ridges: The marginal ridges of premolars are oriented in a horizontal plane versus a more lingually sloping plane in the anterior teeth (Appendix 5c). However, the mesial marginal ridge of the mandibular first premolar is an EXCEPTION since it is aligned almost halfway between horizontal and vertical.

Table 6-1

A. SIZE OF MAXILLARY PREMOLARS (MILLIMETERS) (MEASURED BY DR. WOELFEL AND HIS DENTAL HYGIENE STUDENTS, 1974–1979)

DIMENSION MEASURED	234 FIRST PREMOLARS		224 SECOND PREMOLARS	
	Average	Range	Average	Range
Crown length	8.6	7.1–11.1	7.7	5.2–10.5
Root length	13.4	8.3–19.0	14.0	8.0–20.6
Overall length	21.5	15.5–28.9	21.2	15.2–28.4
Crown width M-D	7.1	5.5–9.4	6.6	5.5–8.9
Root width (cervix)	4.8	3.6–8.5	4.7	4.0–5.8
Faciolingual crown size	9.2	6.6–11.2	9.0	6.9–11.6
Faciolingual root (cervix)	8.2	5.0–9.4	8.1	5.8–10.5
Mesial cervical curve	1.1	0.0–1.7	0.9	0.4–1.9
Distal cervical curve	0.7	0.0–1.7	0.6	0.0–1.4

B. SIZE OF MANDIBULAR PREMOLARS (MILLIMETERS) (MEASURED BY DR. WOELFEL AND HIS DENTAL HYGIENE STUDENTS, 1974–1979)

DIMENSION MEASURED	238 FIRST PREMOLARS		227 SECOND PREMOLARS	
	Average	Range	Average	Range
Crown length	8.8	5.9–10.9	8.2	6.7–10.2
Root length	14.4	9.7–20.2	14.7	9.2–21.2
Overall length	22.4	17.0–28.5	22.1	16.8–28.1
Crown width M-D	7.0	5.9–8.8	7.1	5.2–9.5
Root width (cervix)	4.8	3.9–7.3	5.0	4.0–6.8
Faciolingual crown size	7.7	6.2–10.5	8.2	7.0–10.5
Faciolingual root (cervix)	7.0	5.5–8.5	7.3	6.1–8.4
Mesial cervical curve	0.9	0.0–2.0	0.8	0.0–2.0
Distal cervical curve	0.6	0.0–1.6	0.5	0.0–1.3

Crown Length: Premolar crowns are shorter than *anterior* tooth crowns [maxillary premolar crowns are 0.8–3.5 mm shorter and mandibular premolars are 0.3-2.5 mm shorter]. Maxillary premolar roots are about the same length as maxillary incisor roots [within 1 mm], but are shorter than the roots of maxillary canines [by 2.5–3.1 mm for 1,472 teeth]. Mandibular premolar roots are longer than mandibular incisor roots [by 1-1.9 mm] but are shorter than the mandibular canine root [by 1.3 mm.] (Complete data can be found in Table 6-1A and B)

Height (Crest) of Contour: From both mesial and distal aspects, the *facial* heights of contour of premolar crowns are in the cervical third, like on anterior teeth. However, the heights of contour are more occlusal in position than the corresponding crests of curvature on the anterior teeth (Appendix 5d). In other words, the greatest facial bulge is farther from the cervix on premolars. An EXCEPTION is the buccal height of contour of the mandibular first premolar, which may be located as far cervically as on anterior teeth. The location of the *lingual* height of contour for premolars is also farther from the cervix relative to anterior teeth. Lingually, it is located in the *middle third* occlusocervically compared to the cervical third as on anterior teeth.

Contact Areas: The proximal contact areas are more cervically located and broader than on anterior teeth.

3. OTHER CLASS TRAITS CHARACTERISTIC OF ALL PREMOLARS

Evaluate the similarities of all premolars while comparing models or extracted specimens of all four types of premolars from the views indicated. Also, use the study pages from the Appendix to identify the class traits. It is important to note that although general characteristics are described in this book, there is considerable variation from these descriptions in nature.[1–3] Please remember when studying the *maxillary* premolars to hold them with their facial side toward you, crown down and roots upward. With *mandibular* premolars, have the crowns upward and the roots below. In this manner, the teeth will be oriented as they were in the mouth.

a. Class Traits of All Premolars from the *Buccal View*

Crown Outline Shape: The crown from the buccal view is broadest at the level of the contact areas and more narrow at the cervix: shaped roughly like a five-sided pentagon, similar to the canine crown shape (Appendix 5g). The mesial and distal outlines of the crown are nearly straight or slightly convex from contact areas to the cervical line.

Convex Contact Areas: Both mesial and distal sides of the crown are convex around the contact areas, similar to canines. *Mesial* proximal contacts are near the junction of the occlusal and middle thirds, and the *distal* contacts are normally slightly more cervical, in the middle third (Appendix 5e), EXCEPT on mandibular first premolars where, mesial contacts are usually more cervical than the distal contacts.

Cusp Ridge Size: As with canines, when viewed from the facial, the tip of the facial cusp is often slightly mesial to the vertical root axis line of the tooth (Appendix 5h), with the *mesial* cusp ridge of the buccal cusp shorter than the *distal* ridge (Appendix 5i). The EXCEPTION to this general rule is the maxillary first premolar where the buccal cusp tip is located slightly to the distal of the root axis line and the mesial cusp ridge is *longer*.

b. Class Traits of All Premolars from the *Lingual View*

Crown Shape (Outline): The crown is narrower on the lingual side than on the buccal side, EXCEPT some three-cusp mandibular second premolars that may be wider on the lingual half. The lingual surface is convex.

c. Class Traits of All Premolars from the *Proximal Views*

Marginal Ridges: The *mesial* marginal ridge is more occlusally positioned than the *distal* marginal ridge, so if you first look at the mesial side and then the distal side of this tooth, you should be able to see less of the triangular ridges from the mesial view (Appendix 5j). An EXCEPTION is the mandibular first premolar, where the *distal* marginal ridge is in a more occlusal position than the *mesial* marginal ridge.

d. Class Traits of All Premolars from the *Occlusal View*

Tooth Proportions: All premolars are wider faciolingually than mesiodistally (Appendix 5k). [Measuring 923 premolars, their crowns were wider faciolingually by 1.2 mm and roots by 2.8 mm.]

Cusp Ridges and Marginal Ridges Bound the Occlusal Table: Like canine cusps, both the buccal and lingual premolar cusps have mesial and distal cusp ridges. On premolars these merge laterally with the marginal ridges to surround the portion of the tooth known as the **occlusal table** (Appendix 5l).

Triangular Ridges Form Transverse Ridges: The triangular ridges of the buccal and lingual cusps slope toward the occlusal sulcus and converge at the central groove (see Fig. 6-5). On premolars with only two cusps, the two triangular ridges (one buccal and one lingual) join together to form a transverse ridge, which can be best observed from the occlusal aspect. An EXCEPTION: The three triangular ridges on the three-cusped mandibular second premolar do *not* meet, so do *not* form a transverse ridge (seen later in Fig. 6-15).

Grooves and Fossae: A groove (or grooves) runs mesiodistally across the occlusal surface on premolars. (EXCEPTION: The mandibular first premolar has a pronounced triangular ridge, often without a groove running mesiodistally across it.) The groove (or grooves), when present, ends mesially in the mesial fossa and distally in the distal fossa. These fossae are bounded on one side by the buccal and lingual triangular ridges and on the other side by a marginal ridge.

Proximal Contacts Viewed from the *Occlusal View*: Proximal contacts from the occlusal view are either on or slightly buccal to the faciolingual midline of the crown (Appendix 5f).

D. ARCH TRAITS THAT DIFFERENTIATE MAXILLARY FROM MANDIBULAR PREMOLARS

Refer to Appendix page 6 and while reading about differences between maxillary and mandibular premolars.

Relative Shape and Size: The maxillary first and second premolars appear more alike than the mandibular premolars (yet the *maxillary first* premolar crown is larger than the second in all dimensions).

Lingual Crown Tilt in Mandibular Premolars: From either proximal aspect, the **mandibular** premolar crowns appear to be *tilted* lingually relative to the roots (the first premolar noticeably more than the second). This lingual tilting of the crown is characteristic for all mandibular posterior teeth and enables their buccal cusps to fit and function both beneath and lingual to the **maxillary** buccal cusps, which are aligned more directly over their roots. This difference is easy to recognize when comparing the proximal views of maxillary and mandibular premolars in Appendix 6j and 6a.

Cusp Size and Location: The buccal cusp is larger than the lingual cusp (or cusps) on all premolars, but this is much more evident on **mandibular** premolars (compare Appendix 6c and 6p). *Lingual* cusp tips are positioned off center *to the mesial* most often on maxillary premolars and may be centered or positioned to the mesial on mandibular first and second (two-cusp) premolars (seen from lingual views in Appendix 6i and 6q).

Distal Crown Tilt on Mandibular Premolars: From the buccal and lingual aspects, many mandibular premolar crowns, especially mandibular first premolars, appear to be tilted somewhat distally at the cervix. This distal tilting is characteristic of all *mandibular posterior* teeth (including the three molars) and the mandibular canines.

Buccal Ridge Prominence: The buccal ridge is more prominent on the maxillary first premolar than on the mandibular first premolar.

Crown Proportions: From the occlusal view, **maxillary** premolars are more *oblong* or rectangular (considerably wider faciolingually than mesiodistally), whereas **mandibular** premolars are more *square* (closer to equal dimension faciolingually as mesiodistally). (This difference is apparent when comparing premolar dimensions in Appendix 6d).

Now is a good time to review the major differences between maxillary and mandibular premolars in Table 6-2.

Table 6-2

MAJOR ARCH TRAITS THAT DISTINGUISH MAXILLARY FROM MANDIBULAR PREMOLARS

MAXILLARY PREMOLARS	MANDIBULAR PREMOLARS
BUCCAL VIEW	
Buccal ridge is more prominent	Buccal ridge is less prominent
No distal crown tilt relative to root	Crown exhibits slight distal tilt on root
LINGUAL VIEW	
Lingual cusps relatively longer than mandibular lingual cusps	Lingual cusps relatively shorter than maxillary lingual cusps
Tip of lingual cusp toward mesial	Lingual cusp tip centered or 2 L cusps
PROXIMAL VIEWS	
Crown aligned over root	Crown tilts to lingual relative to root
Lingual cusp is just slightly shorter than buccal	Lingual cusp is much shorter than buccal
OCCLUSAL VIEW	
Crown shape oval	Crown shape closer to square
Crown considerably wider FL than MD	Crown less oblong FL

SECTION II. Type Traits That Differentiate Maxillary First from Maxillary Second Premolars

OBJECTIVES

This section prepares the reader to perform the following:

- Describe the type traits that can be used to distinguish the permanent maxillary *first* premolar from the maxillary *second* premolar.
- Describe and identify the labial, lingual, mesial, distal, and occlusal surfaces for all maxillary premolars.
- Assign a universal number to maxillary premolars present in a mouth (or on a model) with complete dentition. If possible, repeat this on a model with one or more maxillary premolars missing.
- Holding a maxillary premolar, determine whether it is a *first* or a *second* and *right* or *left*. Then assign a universal number to it.

A. TYPE TRAITS OF MAXILLARY PREMOLARS FROM THE *BUCCAL VIEW*

From the buccal view, compare the maxillary first and second premolars in Figure 6-1. Compare tooth models and/or extracted maxillary premolars as you read the following characteristics, holding the crowns down, roots up, just as they are oriented in the mouth.

1. RELATIVE SIZE OF MAXILLARY PREMOLAR CROWNS FROM THE *BUCCAL VIEW*

The *crown* of the *maxillary first premolar* is larger than the maxillary second premolar [wider by 0.5 mm and longer by 0.9 mm], and the root is longer overall [by 1.3 mm; measurements on 458 teeth]. The **shoulders** (junction of cusp slopes and proximal surfaces) seem more broad, bulging, and angular (especially on the mesial) on the first premolar than on the more gently convex second premolar.

The mesial and distal sides of the crown, from the contact areas to the cervical line, converge more noticeably on the maxillary first premolar than second premolar. This makes the cervical portion of the crown of the second premolar appear relatively wider. Observe the more prominent mesial shoulders and increased crown taper on many maxillary first premolars in Figure 6-1.

2. LOCATION OF CONTACTS FOR MAXILLARY PREMOLARS FROM THE *BUCCAL VIEW*

For *both* types of maxillary premolars, mesial contacts are usually in the middle third, near the junction of the occlusal and middle thirds. Distal contacts are slightly more cervical, still in the middle third (recall Appendix 5e).

3. LOCATION OF BUCCAL CUSP TIP OF MAXILLARY PREMOLARS FROM THE *BUCCAL VIEW*

The *maxillary first premolar* has its buccal cusp tip placed slightly to the *distal* of the vertical midroot axis line with a longer mesial cusp ridge, as compared to the distal cusp ridge (Appendix 6e and most maxillary first premolars in Fig. 6-1). This is an EXCEPTION to all other premolars and canines, which have their buccal cusp tip placed more to the mesial or centered with their mesial slope shorter than their distal.

4. SHAPE OF THE BUCCAL CUSP OF MAXILLARY PREMOLARS FROM THE *BUCCAL VIEW*

The buccal cusp of the **maxillary first premolar** is relatively long and pointed or sharp (Appendix 6f), resembling a maxillary canine, with the mesial and distal slopes meeting at almost a right angle (100–110°), compared to the **second premolar**, which is less pointed and more obtuse (125–130°), as seen on most second premolars in Figure 6-1.

D   M   D   M

25%   2%   2%   52%

Right maxillary second premolar   Right maxillary first premolar

FIGURE 6-1. *Buccal views of maxillary premolars* with type traits to distinguish maxillary first from second premolars and traits to distinguish rights from lefts. Percentages give the frequency of notches on each cusp ridge.

Maxillary Premolars (Buccal)

Rights   Lefts

Firsts

Seconds

← Distal →

TRAITS TO DISTINGUISH MAXILLARY FIRST FROM SECOND PREMOLAR: BUCCAL VIEWS

MAXILLARY FIRST PREMOLAR	MAXILLARY SECOND PREMOLAR
Mesial buccal ridge depression [52%]	Distal buccal ridge depression [25%]
Sharper buccal cusp angle (105°)	More blunt buccal cusp angle (125°)
Bulging shoulders and angular outline	Narrow, more rounded shoulders
Tapers more from contacts cervically	Less taper from contacts cervically
Mesial cusp arm longest	Distal cusp arm longest
Prominent buccal ridge	Less prominent buccal ridge

TRAITS TO DIFFERENTIATE MAXILLARY RIGHT FROM LEFT PREMOLARS: BUCCAL VIEWS

MAXILLARY FIRST PREMOLAR	MAXILLARY SECOND PREMOLAR
Longer mesial cusp ridge	Shorter mesial cusp ridge
Depression mesial to buccal ridge [52%]	Depression distal to buccal ridge [25%]

Root often, but not always, curves to distal for both

5. **BUCCAL RIDGE AND DEPRESSIONS OF MAXILLARY PREMOLARS FROM THE *BUCCAL VIEW***

The buccal ridge is prominent on the **maxillary first premolar** (Appendix 6g). A shallow vertical depression mesial to the buccal ridge in the occlusal third of the crown was found about half of the time in the first premolars [52% of 452], but rarely on the distal [2%]. The buccal ridge is less prominent on the *maxillary* **second premolar**, and depressions were found only 27% of the time on second premolars [506 teeth].

6. **ROOT OF MAXILLARY PREMOLARS FROM THE *BUCCAL VIEW***

Most of the time, the **maxillary first premolar** has a divided root with buccal and lingual portions or roots coming off a common trunk in the apical third (seen best from the proximal view in Appendix 6h, but both root tips may also be seen from the buccal view). [On 200 teeth, 61% had two roots, 38% had one root, and 1% had three roots.] The buccal and lingual roots are usually relatively straight except for a frequent distal curve of the buccal root near the apex. Sometimes you can see the tip of the lingual root when it is straighter or bends in a different direction than the buccal root. This is evident in several maxillary first premolars in Figure 6-1.

The single root of the **second premolar** is longer on the average than on the first premolar [by 0.6 mm] and is nearly twice as long as the crown. The root to crown ratio is 1.8:1, which is the highest for any maxillary tooth.

The apical end of the root of *all* premolars frequently bends distally [58% of 343 second premolars and 66% of 426 first premolars], but these roots may also be straight or bend mesially.

B. **TYPE TRAITS OF MAXILLARY PREMOLARS FROM THE *LINGUAL VIEW***

Compare the lingual view of maxillary first and second premolars in Figure 6-2.

1. **RELATIVE CUSP SIZE OF MAXILLARY PREMOLARS FROM THE *LINGUAL VIEW***

The lingual cusp is shorter than the buccal cusp, considerably more so on the maxillary first premolar. This trait is seen in almost all first premolars in Figure 6-2 and is evident on the lingual views of maxillary premolars in Appendix page 6. [Maxillary *first* premolar lingual cusps were 1.3 mm shorter on the average, ranging from 0.3 to 3.3 mm shorter on 317 teeth; *second* premolar lingual cusps averaged only 0.4 mm shorter on 300 teeth.] The crown is a little narrower on the lingual side than on the buccal side, more obviously so on the first premolar than on the second premolar.

2. **CUSP RIDGES OF MAXILLARY PREMOLARS FROM THE *LINGUAL VIEW***

The mesial and distal ridges of the lingual cusp of the **maxillary first premolars** meet at the cusp tip at a somewhat rounded angle, but the angle is still sharp or steep compared to the molar cusps. The tip of the lingual cusp of the **second premolar** is relatively sharper.

3. **MARGINAL RIDGES OF MAXILLARY PREMOLARS FROM THE *LINGUAL VIEW***

From the lingual view, differences in marginal ridge heights are apparent on hand-held teeth when rotating the tooth just enough one way to see the mesial ridge height, then just enough in the opposite direction to compare the distal ridge height. The *distal* marginal ridges of *both* types of maxillary premolars are more cervical in position than the mesial marginal ridge (recall Appendix 5j). (This relative positioning is true of all posterior teeth, with the EXCEPTION of the *mandibular* first premolar, where the distal marginal ridge is the more occlusal one.)

4. **LINGUAL CUSP POSITION FOR MAXILLARY PREMOLARS FROM THE *LINGUAL VIEW***

The tips of the unworn lingual cusps of *both* maxillary premolars are consistently positioned to the *mesial* of the midroot axis line (Appendix 6i). This trait is an excellent way to tell rights from lefts, especially for the maxillary second premolar which is, in most other ways, nearly symmetrical.

MAXILLARY PREMOLARS (Lingual)

FIGURE 6-2. *Lingual views of maxillary premolars* with type traits to distinguish maxillary first from second premolars and traits to distinguish rights from lefts.

TRAITS TO DISTINGUISH MAXILLARY FIRST FROM SECOND PREMOLAR: LINGUAL VIEWS

MAXILLARY FIRST PREMOLAR	MAXILLARY SECOND PREMOLAR
Lingual cusp shorter: see both cusps	B and L cusps same length and width
Crown narrower on lingual	Less taper toward lingual
Outline traits visible from buccal view are also visible from lingual view	

TRAITS TO DIFFERENTIATE MAXILLARY RIGHT FROM LEFT PREMOLARS: LINGUAL VIEWS

MAXILLARY FIRST PREMOLAR	MAXILLARY SECOND PREMOLAR
Lingual cusp tip is bent toward the mesial for both	
Length of buccal cusp ridges: M longest on 1st and D longest on 2nd	

5. **ROOTS OF MAXILLARY PREMOLARS FROM THE *LINGUAL VIEW***

The lingual root of a two-rooted maxillary *first premolar* is usually shorter than the buccal root [0.8 mm for 93 teeth]. The apical end of the lingual root of the teeth may bend toward either the mesial or the distal. *Both* first and second premolar roots taper to the lingual.

C. **TYPE TRAITS OF MAXILLARY PREMOLARS FROM THE *PROXIMAL VIEWS***

Compare the proximal views of maxillary first and second premolars in Figure 6-3.

1. **CROWN SHAPE AND MORPHOLOGY OF MAXILLARY PREMOLARS FROM THE *PROXIMAL VIEWS***

All maxillary premolars are shaped like a trapezoid from the proximal view (Appendix 6b). *Maxillary first premolars* have a prominent mesial concavity cervical to the contact area; *second premolars* do not

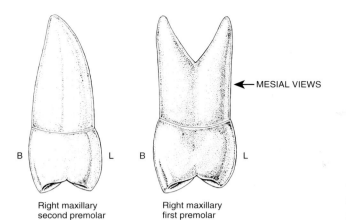

← MESIAL VIEWS

Right maxillary second premolar | Right maxillary first premolar

FIGURE 6-3. *Proximal views of maxillary premolars* with type traits to distinguish maxillary first from second premolars and traits to distinguish rights from lefts.

Maxillary Left Premolars
Mesial Surfaces

Firsts

Seconds

←——— Lingual   Buccal ———→

Maxillary Right Premolars
Distal Surfaces

←——— Lingual Buccal ———→

Firsts

←——— Buccal Lingual ———→

Seconds

TRAITS TO DISTINGUISH MAXILLARY FIRST FROM SECOND PREMOLAR:
COMPARE PROXIMAL VIEWS

MAXILLARY FIRST PREMOLAR	MAXILLARY SECOND PREMOLAR
Buccal cusp longer than lingual [1.3 mm]	Buccal and lingual cusps same length
Cusp tips closer together	Cusp tips farther apart
Mesial crown *and* root depression	Mesial root but *not* crown depression
Mesial root depression deeper than D	Distal root depression deeper than M
Divide or two roots [62%]	Single root
Mesial marginal ridge groove [97%]	Less likely mesial marginal ridge [37%]

TRAITS TO DIFFERENTIATE MAXILLARY RIGHT FROM LEFT PREMOLARS:
PROXIMAL VIEWS

MAXILLARY FIRST PREMOLAR	MAXILLARY SECOND PREMOLAR
Mesial crown depression	No mesial crown depression
Mesial root depression at cervix	Flat/convex mesial root surface at cervix
Deeper mesial than distal root depression	Deeper distal than mesial root depression
Mesial marginal ridge groove [97%]	Mesial marginal ridge groove [only 37%]
Greater mesial than distal cervical line curvature for both	
Distal marginal ridge is more cervical than mesial for both	

(Appendix 6j). This unique *mesial crown concavity* is perhaps the most consistent and obvious trait of the maxillary first premolar crown that can be used to distinguish it from a maxillary second premolar, and can be used to confirm the mesial surface on the maxillary first premolar.

2. **RELATIVE CUSP HEIGHT OF MAXILLARY PREMOLARS FROM THE *PROXIMAL VIEWS***

From this view, as from the lingual, the buccal cusp is noticeably longer than the lingual cusp on **maxillary first premolars**, compared to the **second premolar**, which has two cusps of nearly equal length (Appendix 6c). Observe this difference when comparing first and second premolars in Figure 6-3. From this view, it is a challenge telling buccal from lingual on the mandibular second premolar since the cusp heights are so similar.

3. **HEIGHT (CREST) OF CONTOUR OF MAXILLARY PREMOLARS FROM THE *PROXIMAL VIEWS***

Like most posterior teeth, the *buccal* height of contour of maxillary premolars is in the cervical third. Specifically, it is near the junction of the middle and cervical third. Lingually it is more occlusal, in the middle third (near the center of the crown). This trait helps distinguish the buccal from lingual surfaces on the majority of maxillary premolars from the proximal views in Figure 6-3.

4. **DISTANCE BETWEEN CUSPS ON MAXILLARY PREMOLARS FROM THE *PROXIMAL VIEWS***

The average distance between the buccal and lingual cusp tips of maxillary first and second premolars is 5.9 mm and 5.7 mm, respectively [or 65 to 67% of the faciolingual dimension for 243 teeth]. However, both cusp tips are located over and *well within the boundary of the root contour*, an important relationship imparting good functional support for a large chewing area.

5. **MARGINAL RIDGE GROOVES OF MAXILLARY PREMOLARS FROM THE *PROXIMAL VIEWS***

The *mesial* marginal ridge of **maxillary first premolars** is almost always crossed by a developmental groove called a marginal ridge groove [on 97% of 600 maxillary first premolars]. This marginal ridge groove serves as a spillway for food during mastication (best seen from the occlusal view in Appendix 6k). The *distal* marginal ridge groove occurs less frequently [39% of 600 teeth]. Short mesial *and* distal marginal ridge grooves were even less likely to be found crossing the ridges of **second premolars** [only present on 37% of 641 mesial marginal ridges and 30% of distal marginal ridges of maxillary second premolars].

6. **CERVICAL LINES OF MAXILLARY PREMOLARS WHEN COMPARING THE *PROXIMAL VIEWS***

The cervical line on the *mesial* of the **maxillary first premolar** curves occlusally in a broad but shallow arc [averaging only 1.1 mm high on 234 teeth]. As expected, the mesial curvature was slightly greater than on the distal side of these teeth [by 0.4 mm]. The cervical line on the *lingual* surface is in a more occlusal position than on the buccal border. This accentuates the appearance that the lingual cusp is definitely shorter than the buccal cusp. The cervical line curvature on the mesial of the **second premolar** is also greater than on the distal [by 0.3 mm].

7. **ROOTS AND ROOT DEPRESSIONS OF MAXILLARY PREMOLARS FROM THE *PROXIMAL VIEWS***

The roots of the maxillary premolars, when viewed from the mesial or distal aspect, often have root depressions of varying depths. Knowledge of the frequency with which these depressions occur, as well as the relative location and depth of these depressions, can be helpful clinically when evaluating root surfaces for the presence of calcified depositions that contribute to periodontal disease and when identifying areas of decay on the roots.

The **maxillary first premolar**, as stated previously, is the only premolar with an obvious concavity or depression on the mesial surface of the *crown*, and this depression continues onto the *root* [100% of teeth studied]. This important type trait is seen clearly on the mesial views of all maxillary premolars in Figure 6-3. Recall that this tooth usually has two roots [61% of 100 teeth] with the lingual root slightly shorter [by 0.8 mm] than the buccal root. A bifurcation occurs in the apical third of the root.

Even when there is only one root, there is a *mesial* root depression. There is also a *distal* root depression found on both double and single rooted teeth [100% of 100 teeth]. This depression is located on the middle third of the undivided portion of the root. Near the cervix, however, the distal side of the root is usually convex or flat with little or *no* depression. The *mesial* side longitudinal root depression is deeper than on the distal side.

The **maxillary second premolar** usually has one root, but like the maxillary first premolar, it also has root depressions on both sides. The longitudinal depression on the *mesial* root surface [78% of 100 teeth] does *not* extend onto the crown. The longitudinal depression on the *distal* root surface is located in the middle third of the root, and is usually *deeper than on the mesial root surface*. This feature is the opposite from the maxillary first premolar, which usually has the deepest mid-root depression on the mesial.

D. TYPE TRAITS OF MAXILLARY PREMOLARS FROM THE *OCCLUSAL VIEW*

Compare occlusal views of maxillary first and second premolars in Figure 6-4. To follow this description, the teeth or tooth models you are using should be held as those displayed in Figure 6-4, so that the buccal surface is at the top and you are sighting down along the vertical midroot axis.

1. RELATIVE SIZE OF MAXILLARY PREMOLARS FROM THE *OCCLUSAL VIEW*

In the same mouth, the *maxillary first premolar* was judged to be larger than the second premolar in 55% of the specimens examined and smaller than the second premolar in only 18% [1392 comparisons were done on dental stone casts].

2. GROOVES AND FOSSAE OF MAXILLARY PREMOLARS FROM THE *OCCLUSAL VIEW*

Characteristically, central developmental grooves run mesiodistally across the center of *both* maxillary premolars with a pit at both ends. The length of the central groove of the **maxillary first premolar** is more than one-third the mesiodistal width of the occlusal surface [average length was 2.7 mm of 408 teeth]. The groove of the **second premolar** averaged 2.1 mm, shorter than on first premolars [by 0.6 mm based on 818 teeth] (Appendix 6l). This longer central groove is one of the distinguishing characteristics of the maxillary first premolar, compared to the central groove length of the second premolar, and is quite obvious when comparing the maxillary premolars in Figure 6-4.

Because the central groove is longer on the *maxillary first premolar*, the mesial and distal pits are relatively closer to the marginal ridges than on maxillary second premolars. In other words, the pits are farther apart on maxillary first premolars.

There are fewer supplemental grooves on **maxillary first premolars** than on maxillary second premolars. On **second premolars**, there are usually supplementary grooves radiating buccally and lingually from the pit at the depth of each triangular fossa.

As was seen from the mesial view of the **maxillary first premolar**, a mesial marginal ridge groove almost always crosses the mesial marginal ridge and connects with the central groove in the mesial triangular fossa (Fig. 6-5). The mesial marginal groove is one of the distinguishing characteristics of the maxillary first premolar, where it occurs with much greater frequency [97% of 600 first premolars] than on **second premolars** [only 37%]. Distal marginal grooves were also less common [30-39% of second and first premolars, respectively].

The distal triangular fossae are usually larger than the mesial fossae on *both* types of maxillary premolars. [The distal triangular fossa was larger on 55% of the 184 maxillary *first* premolars and 53% of 209 maxillary *second* premolars. The mesial triangular fossa was considered to be largest on 27% of first premolars and 17% of second premolars.]

3. RELATIVE PROPORTIONS OF MAXILLARY PREMOLARS FROM THE *OCCLUSAL VIEW*

The oblong (somewhat rectangular) outline of the maxillary premolar crown is greater buccolingually than mesiodistally [by 2.1 mm on 234 maxillary first premolars, and by 2.4 mm on second premolars]. This is obvious in all maxillary premolars in Figure 6-4.

Right maxillary second premolar

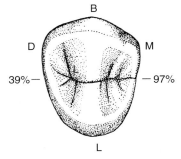

Right maxillary first premolar

FIGURE 6-4. *Occlusal views of maxillary premolars* with type traits to distinguish maxillary first from second premolars and traits to distinguish rights from lefts. Percentages give the frequency of marginal ridge grooves on each marginal ridge.

Maxillary Premolars (Occlusal)

TRAITS TO DISTINGUISH MAXILLARY FIRST FROM SECOND PREMOLAR: OCCLUSAL VIEWS

MAXILLARY FIRST PREMOLAR	MAXILLARY SECOND PREMOLAR
Crown asymmetrical, more hexagonal	Crown symmetrical and more oval
Mesial side concave or flat	Mesial side more convex
Proximal surfaces converge lingually	Little tapering toward lingual
Longer central groove	Shorter central groove
Triangular fossae closer to marginal ridge	Triangular fossae closer to tooth center
Mesial marginal ridge groove [97%]	Less common mesial marginal ridge
More prominent buccal ridge	Less prominent buccal ridge
Fewer supplemental grooves	More supplemental grooves

TRAITS TO DIFFERENTIATE MAXILLARY RIGHT FROM LEFT PREMOLARS: OCCLUSAL VIEWS

MAXILLARY FIRST PREMOLAR	MAXILLARY SECOND PREMOLAR
Distal contact is more buccal	Mesial contact is more buccal
Mesial marginal ridge groove [97%]	M marginal ridge groove less
Mesial crown outline is concave or flat	Mesial crown outline is convex
MB corner is a right angle	MB corner is obtuse angle.
Lingual cusp tipped toward mesial for both	
Distal marginal ridge longer than mesial for both	

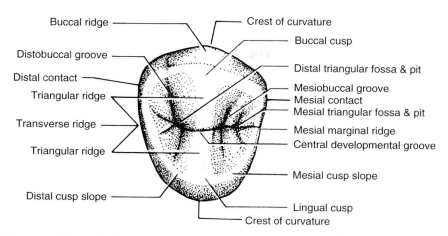

Buccal ridge
Crest of curvature
Buccal cusp
Distobuccal groove
Distal triangular fossa & pit
Distal contact
Mesiobuccal groove
Triangular ridge
Mesial contact
Mesial triangular fossa & pit
Transverse ridge
Mesial marginal ridge
Triangular ridge
Central developmental groove
Mesial cusp slope
Distal cusp slope
Lingual cusp
Crest of curvature

FIGURE 6-5. Maxillary right first premolar; occlusal surface, with normal landmarks. Notice the proximal contact locations.

4. OUTLINE OF MAXILLARY PREMOLARS FROM THE *OCCLUSAL VIEW*

On *both* types of maxillary premolars, the lingual side of the tooth is narrower than the buccal side, more so on first premolars.

From the occlusal aspect, the outline of the buccal surface of the **maxillary first premolar** is a rounded and inverted V-shape because of the prominent buccal ridge (less prominent on the second premolar as seen in Fig. 6-4). This is the only part of the occlusal outline that looks symmetrical. The lingual three-fourths of the tooth seems to be bent slightly mesially. This *asymmetrical occlusal outline* is a distinguishing feature of maxillary first premolars and is not found on most second premolars (compare outline shapes in Appendix 6m). The mesiobuccal cusp ridge joins the mesial marginal ridge at an almost right angle (not so on second premolars). The *mesial* outline of the *maxillary first premolar* and the *mesial* marginal ridge form a nearly straight or concave (bent inward) outline buccolingually. This mesial marginal ridge is shorter buccolingually than the more convex distal marginal ridge (note this characteristic on the occlusal surfaces of most maxillary first premolars in Fig. 6-4).

Seen from the occlusal aspect, the **second premolar** is typically much more symmetrical than the first premolar. Its occlusal outline is less angular than that of the first premolar, and it has an oblong or oval shape. This smoother, more symmetrical outline is obvious on the maxillary second premolars in Figure 6-4.

5. CONTACT AREAS AND HEIGHTS OF CONTOUR OF MAXILLARY PREMOLARS FROM THE *OCCLUSAL VIEW*

Mesial contacts for *both* types of maxillary premolars are near or at the junction of the buccal and middle thirds (slightly more buccal on first premolars) (Fig. 6-5). Recall that one-third of the tooth from this aspect means one-third of the total buccolingual measurements of the crown, rather than one-third of the occlusal surface measurement. *Distal* contacts are in the middle third on **maxillary second premolars**, located more lingually than mesial contacts. Just the opposite is true on **first premolars** with their asymmetry, where the distal contact is more buccal than the mesial contact (Fig. 6-5). Picture this asymmetry when viewing the outline presented in Appendix 6m for the maxillary first premolar.

The *lingual* height of contour is usually *mesial* to the center line of the tooth for *both* first and second premolars, with the tip of the *lingual cusp always mesial to the center* of the tooth.

LEARNING EXERCISE

Review the summary tables of type traits that differentiate the maxillary first from second premolars and maxillary right from left premolars in Figures 6-1 through 6-4.

SECTION III. Type Traits That Differentiate Mandibular First from Mandibular Second Premolars

OBJECTIVES

The section prepares the reader to perform the following:
- Describe the type traits that can be used to distinguish the permanent mandibular first premolar from the mandibular second premolar.
- Describe and identify the labial, lingual, mesial, distal, and occlusal surfaces for all mandibular premolars on a photograph, model, or extracted tooth.
- Assign a Universal number to mandibular premolars present in a mouth (or on a model) with complete dentition. If possible, repeat this on a model with one or more mandibular premolars missing.
- Holding a mandibular premolar, determine whether it is a first or a second and right or left. Then assign a Universal number to it.

For this section, compare mandibular first and second premolars on Appendix page 6. To appreciate differences in mandibular first and second premolars, it is first important to know that there are two common types of mandibular second premolars.3 They are a two-cusp type with one buccal and one lingual cusp and a three-cusp type with one buccal and two lingual cusps (seen from the occlusal views in Fig. 6-10). The frequency of these two types on 808 dental hygiene students from Ohio is given in Table 6-3.

LEARNING EXERCISE

Look in your own mouth and determine which of these categories matches your mandibular second premolars. The three-cusp type occurs with only slightly greater frequency than the two-cusp type [54.2% of 532 teeth for three cusps type versus 43.0% for the two-cusp type.]

The morphologic details of mandibular premolars are difficult to describe because of the great amount of variation. To list all of the frequent variations would lead to confusion rather than to clarification. Bear in mind while studying these teeth that one description will not exactly fit every tooth.[1-3] Most descriptions in this book are for unworn teeth. Most extracted tooth specimens will have signs of attrition, and some will show evidence of tooth decay (caries).

Examine several extracted mandibular premolars or models as you read. Hold them with the crowns up and the roots down.

TABLE 6-3

OCCURRENCE OF LINGUAL CUSPS ON MANDIBULAR SECOND PREMOLARS (808 FEMALES, 1,532 TEETH)

NUMBER AND FREQUENCY	PERCENTAGE	COMMENT
2 lingual cusps on both sides	44.2%	Almost half
1 lingual cusp on both sides	34.2%	One-third
2 lingual cusps on one side	18.2%	One-fifth
3 lingual cusps on both sides	1.7% }	1 in 29
3 lingual cusps on one side	1.7% }	
Overall frequency	{ 3-cusp type 54.2% 2-cusp type 43.0% 4-cusp type 2.8% }	1,532 teeth
Same type on both sides	80.1% }	702 comparisons
Different type on each side	19.9% }	

A. TYPE TRAITS OF MANDIBULAR PREMOLARS FROM THE BUCCAL VIEW

Refer to views from the buccal of mandibular first and second premolars in Figure 6-6.

1. RELATIVE CROWN SHAPE AND SIZE OF MANDIBULAR PREMOLARS FROM THE *BUCCAL VIEW*

As with all premolars and canines, the premolar crown shape from the facial view is roughly a five-sided pentagon. From this view, *both* types of mandibular premolars appear nearly symmetrical except for the shorter mesial than distal cusp ridge, and the greater distal bulge of the crown. Some teeth have a slight distal tilt of the crown on the root.

The crown of the **mandibular first premolar** bears some resemblance from this aspect to the second premolar, but there are differences that make first premolars distinguishable. In general, the first premolar is slightly longer overall than the second with a longer crown [by 0.6 mm] and a shorter root [by 0.3 mm average for 465 teeth]. Just like maxillary premolars, the mandibular *first* premolar has a sharper buccal cusp [110°] than on the *second*. The buccal cusp of the mandibular first premolar crown appears longer, is centered over the root, and resembles a maxillary canine from this aspect.

The crown of the **mandibular second premolar** also has a pentagon shape, but appears closer to square than the first premolar because it is shorter overall, wider in the cervical third, and its buccal cusp is less pointed than on the mandibular first premolar, with cusp slopes meeting at an angle of about 130°. (Appendix 6n). The shape of the buccal surface of the second premolar is similar on both *two-cusp* and *three-cusp* types.

Shallow *notches* are commonplace on both cusp ridges on unworn premolars. These notches serve as spillways for food during mastication (sometimes called Thomas notches, named after Peter K. Thomas, who recommended carving them in all occlusal restorations and crowns because spillways for food are so important).

The most common occurrence and frequency of such notches and of depressions in the occlusal third of the buccal surface on the cusp ridges is evident in Figure 6-7. On the **mandibular first premolar**, the shorter *mesial* cusp ridge of the buccal cusp is more likely to have a notch [65% of 1,348 teeth] than the longer distal cusp ridge [46% of 1,348 teeth]. On the **second premolar**, the frequency of notches is reversed. Its crown is more likely to have a notch on the *distal* cusp ridge [66% of 1,522 teeth] than on the mesial cusp ridge [43% of 1,522 teeth].

2. MORPHOLOGY OF MANDIBULAR PREMOLARS FROM THE *BUCCAL VIEW*

The buccal ridge and adjacent depressions of *both* types of mandibular premolars are less discernible than on the maxillary premolars. However, when vertical depressions on either side of the indistinct buccal ridge are present on the mandibular *first* premolar, the *mesial* crown depression is more likely to be deeper, whereas on the mandibular *second* premolar, the *distal* crown depression is more likely to be deeper. [Eighty percent of 285 mandibular *first* premolars had a smooth buccal surface in the occlusal third without depressions; 17% had a deeper depression on the *mesial* side of the buccal ridge, and only 3% had a deeper distal depression; 74% of mandibular *second* premolars had no discernible depressions, 25% had a deeper *distal* than mesial depression, and only 1% had a deeper mesial depression.] The location of these deeper depressions (mesial or distal) is consistent with the location of cusp ridge notches.

3. CERVICAL LINES OF MANDIBULAR PREMOLARS FROM THE *BUCCAL VIEW*

The cervical line of the first premolar on the buccal surface curves more mesiodistally than on second premolars.

4. CONTACT AREAS OF MANDIBULAR PREMOLARS FROM THE *BUCCAL VIEW*

Because of the greater length of the buccal cusp, the contact areas on the **mandibular first premolar** are located more cervically from the cusp tip than they are on mandibular second premolars. On **mandibular second premolars**, both contact areas are positioned closer to the cusp tip or are in a more occlusal position than on the mandibular first premolars because the second's cusp ridges join at a less steep angle.

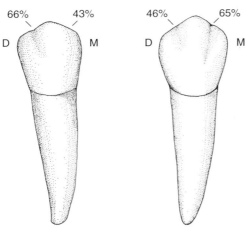

66%   43%   46%   65%

D   M   D   M

Right mandibular   Right mandibular
second premolar   first premolar

FIGURE 6-6. *Buccal views of mandibular premolars* with type traits to distinguish mandibular first from second premolars and traits to distinguish rights from lefts. Percentages give the frequency of notches on each cusp ridge.

Mandibular Premolars (Buccal)

Rights   Lefts

Firsts

Seconds

←—— Distal ——→

TYPE TRAITS TO DISTINGUISH MANDIBULAR FIRST FROM SECOND PREMOLARS: *BUCCAL VIEWS*

MANDIBULAR FIRST PREMOLAR	MANDIBULAR SECOND PREMOLAR
Longer crown	Shorter wider crown
More crown taper from contact to cervix	Crown relatively wider at cervix
More pointed cusp (110°)	Less pointed cusp (130°)
More prominent buccal ridge	Less prominent buccal ridge
Shorter root with pointed apex	Longer root with blunt apex

TRAITS TO DIFFERENTIATE MANDIBULAR RIGHT FROM LEFT PREMOLARS: *BUCCAL VIEWS*

MANDIBULAR FIRST PREMOLAR	MANDIBULAR SECOND PREMOLAR
M cusp ridge notch more common [65%]	D cusp ridge notch more common [66%]
Lower mesial than distal contact	Lower distal than mesial contact
Mesial cusp ridge is shorter than distal on both mandibular premolars	

FIGURE 6-7. Mandibular first and second premolars depicting the most common type of *notch* on the buccal cusp ridges with a shallow depression beneath it on the buccal surface (see arrows). Depressions were found in these locations on 17% of first premolars and 25% of second premolars.

Mesial contacts of *both* types of mandibular premolars are near the junction of the occlusal and middle thirds (slightly more occlusal on second premolars). The *distal* contact of the **mandibular second premolar** follows the general rule: Distal contact is slightly *cervical* to the mesial contact area (Appendix 6o). The distal contact area of the **mandibular first premolar** is an EXCEPTION to most other teeth; here the distal contact is slightly more *occlusal* in position than the mesial contact area (Appendix 6o). (The mandibular first premolar is one of only two teeth which have a more occlusally [incisally] located distal than mesial contact; the other tooth is the primary maxillary canine).

5. **ROOTS OF MANDIBULAR PREMOLARS FROM THE *BUCCAL VIEW***

The roots of mandibular premolars taper gradually to the apex. The roots are noticeably more blunt on mandibular second premolars than on first premolars. As with most roots, there is a tendency for the apical third of the root to bend distally [on 58% of 424 teeth mandibular first premolars, and 62% of 343 teeth mandibular second premolars. The tendency for a mesial bend was 23% and 17% on first and second premolars, respectively.]

The root of the *mandibular second premolar* appears thicker [0.2 mm wider mesiodistally] and is longer than the root of the first premolar. The root of the mandibular second premolar is nearly twice as long as the crown, with a root-to-crown ratio of 1.80:1.

B. **TYPE TRAITS OF MANDIBULAR PREMOLARS FROM THE *LINGUAL VIEW***

For the lingual aspect, refer to lingual views of mandibular first and second premolars in Figure 6-8.

1. **CROWN SHAPE OF MANDIBULAR PREMOLARS FROM THE *LINGUAL VIEW***

On **mandibular first premolars**, as on most teeth, the crown is much narrower on the lingual side than on the buccal side. This can also be seen on **second premolars** with *one* lingual cusp. However, the width of the lingual side of the second premolar with *two* lingual cusps is usually as wide or wider mesiodistally than the buccal side. ONLY this tooth and some maxillary first molars have their crowns wider on the lingual side than on the buccal side.

2. **LINGUAL CUSP AND GROOVES OF MANDIBULAR PREMOLARS FROM THE *LINGUAL VIEW***

The lingual cusp of the **mandibular first premolar** is quite small and is often pointed at the tip. It is nonfunctional, and could be considered a transition between the canine cingulum and prominent lingual cusp or cusps of the second premolar (best appreciated from the proximal views in Fig. 6-9). Much of the occlusal surface of this tooth can be seen from the lingual aspect because of the most obvious shortness of the lingual cusp. [Of 321 first premolars measured, the lingual cusp averaged 3.6 mm shorter than the buccal cusp (range from 1.7 to 5.5 mm shorter).] This tooth may have almost no lingual cusp or as many as four lingual cusplets.

On **mandibular second premolars** with *one lingual cusp*, the single lingual cusp is smaller than the buccal cusp, but it is larger (longer and wider) than the lingual cusp of the first premolar. This single

MANDIBULAR PREMOLARS (Lingual)

LEFTS — RIGHTS

FIRSTS

SECONDS

← DISTAL →

TYPE TRAITS TO DISTINGUISH MANDIBULAR FIRST FROM SECOND PREMOLARS: LINGUAL VIEWS

MANDIBULAR FIRST PREMOLAR	MANDIBULAR SECOND PREMOLAR
Crown much narrower on lingual	Crown quite wide on lingual
Lingual cusp very short, narrow	If one lingual cusp, not as short as 1st
One nonfunctional lingual cusp	Many have two functional L cusps
Mesial marginal ridge with ML groove	Lingual groove between two L cusps
Mesial marginal ridge lower than D	Distal marginal ridge lower than M
Buccal outline traits also apply since lingual cusps are short	

TRAITS TO DIFFERENTIATE MANDIBULAR RIGHT FROM LEFT PREMOLARS: LINGUAL VIEWS

MANDIBULAR FIRST PREMOLAR	MANDIBULAR SECOND PREMOLAR
Mesial marginal ridge lower than distal	Distal marginal ridge lower than mesial
Mesiolingual groove present [67%]	If 3-cusp type, mesiolingual cusp larger
More occlusal visible on mesial	More occlusal visible on distal
Buccal outline traits also apply from this view	

FIGURE 6-8. *Lingual views of mandibular premolars* with type traits to distinguish mandibular first from second premolars and traits to distinguish rights from lefts.

lingual cusp is either just mesial to (often) or on the center line of the root (Appendix 6q). The mesial and distal ridges of the lingual cusp merge into the mesial and distal marginal ridges.

In the *two lingual cusp* variation, there is one large buccal and two smaller lingual cusps. The mesiolingual cusp is almost always larger and longer than the distolingual cusp [90% of 818 teeth; the two lingual cusps were rarely equal in size, only on 3%, and the distolingual cusp is rarely larger, only 7%].

3. MARGINAL RIDGES OF MANDIBULAR PREMOLARS FROM THE *LINGUAL VIEW*

From the lingual view, differences in marginal ridge heights are apparent on hand held teeth when rotating the tooth first enough in one direction to see the mesial marginal ridge height, then enough in the opposite direction to compare the distal ridge height. As with most other posterior teeth, the *distal* marginal ridges of the **mandibular second premolars** are slightly more cervically located than the mesial marginal ridges (evident on all mandibular second premolars in Fig. 6-8). An EXCEPTION to all other adult teeth is the **mandibular first premolar**, the only adult tooth where the *mesial* marginal ridge is more cervically located than the distal marginal ridge (evident in Fig. 6-8 for many mandibular first premolars).

4. GROOVES ON MANDIBULAR PREMOLARS FROM THE *LINGUAL VIEW*

On **mandibular second premolars** with *two lingual cusps* [present 54% of the time], a *lingual groove* passes between the mesiolingual and distolingual cusps and extends slightly onto the lingual surface of the crown (seen in Fig. 6-15). On **mandibular first premolars**, there is frequently a *mesiolingual groove* separating the mesial marginal ridge from the mesial slope of the small lingual cusp (Appendix 6r) [present in 67% of 609 first premolars]. Rarely, a similar groove might be present between the distal marginal ridge and the distal slope of the lingual cusp [8% of these 609 first premolars].

5. ROOTS OF MANDIBULAR PREMOLARS FROM THE *LINGUAL VIEW*

The roots of second mandibular premolars are tapered and only slightly longer than the roots of first premolars [0.3 mm longer on average for 465 teeth].

C. TYPE TRAITS OF MANDIBULAR PREMOLARS FROM THE *PROXIMAL VIEWS*

When studying the proximal views of mandibular first and second premolars, refer to Figure 6-9.

1. CROWN SHAPE OF MANDIBULAR PREMOLARS FROM THE *PROXIMAL VIEWS*

As on all mandibular posterior teeth, the crown of the **mandibular first premolar** tilts noticeably toward the lingual surface at the cervix (much more than any other premolar). This tilt places the tip of the buccal cusp almost over the midroot axis line (obvious on all mandibular first premolars in Fig. 6-9). As was also seen from the lingual aspect, the lingual cusp of the mandibular first premolar is considerably shorter than the buccal cusp by more than one-third of the total crown length [3.6 mm average for 321 teeth]. By virtue of being so short and narrow mesiodistally, it is a *nonfunctioning* cusp (Appendix 6p). The tip of the short lingual cusp results in the cusp tip location usually being in line vertically with the lingual outline of the cervical portion of the root.

The **mandibular second premolar** crown (both types) also tips lingually, but not as much as the mandibular first premolar. The tip of the buccal cusp of the *mandibular second premolar* is usually located on a line that would divide the crown vertically between the buccal and middle thirds. As with the first premolar, the tip of the lingual cusp (or of the mesiolingual cusp) of this second premolar is usually about on a line with the lingual surface of the root.

The lingual cusps (or mesiolingual cusps for three-cusp types) of *second premolars* are closer in length to the buccal cusp than on first premolars [average of only 1.8 mm shorter than the buccal cusp; range 0.1–3.8 mm for 317 teeth]. From the mesial view, the mesiolingual cusp conceals the shorter distolingual cusp, while looking from the distal, both lingual cusp tips are usually visible (as seen on several mandibular second premolars viewed from the distal in Fig. 6-9).

2. MARGINAL RIDGES OF MANDIBULAR PREMOLARS FROM THE *PROXIMAL VIEWS*

The *mesial* marginal ridge of the **mandibular first premolar** slopes cervically from the buccal toward the center of the occlusal surface at nearly a 45° angle and is nearly parallel to the triangular ridge of the buccal cusp (Appendix 6s, and mesial views of the mandibular first premolars in Fig. 6-9). The *distal* marginal ridge of the *mandibular first premolar* is in a more horizontal position compared to the *mesial marginal* ridge, and is longer from buccal to lingual than the mesial marginal ridge. The difference in

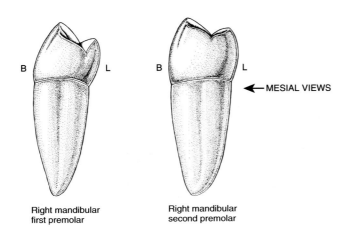

B   L   B   L

← MESIAL VIEWS

Right mandibular
first premolar

Right mandibular
second premolar

FIGURE 6-9. *Proximal views of mandibular premolars* with type traits to distinguish mandibular first from second premolars and traits to distinguish rights from lefts.

Mandibular Right Premolars (Proximal)

MESIAL SURFACES   DISTAL SURFACES

Firsts

Seconds

←——— Buccal Lingual ———→   ←——— Lingual Buccal ———→

TYPE TRAITS TO DISTINGUISH MANDIBULAR FIRST FROM SECOND PREMOLARS: PROXIMAL VIEWS

MANDIBULAR FIRST PREMOLAR	MANDIBULAR SECOND PREMOLAR
Severe lingual crown tip	Less lingual crown tip
L cusp much shorter than B cusp	L cusp slightly shorter than B cusp
M marginal ridge parallel to B cusp ridge	M marginal ridge higher and horizontal
Can see much of occlusal from mesial	Cannot see much of occlusal from M
Mesiolingual groove on most [67%]; No lingual groove	Lingual groove on 3-cusp type No mesiolingual groove
Root may be divided in apical third	Root not divided
Mesial root depression [45%]	Mesial root flat or convex [81%]

TRAITS TO DIFFERENTIATE MANDIBULAR RIGHT FROM LEFT PREMOLARS: PROXIMAL VIEWS

MANDIBULAR FIRST PREMOLAR	MANDIBULAR SECOND PREMOLAR
Mesial marginal ridge is lower than distal	Distal marginal ridge is lower than M
Deeper distal root depression [69%]	No mesial root depression [81%] but distal
More occlusal is visible from mesial	More occlusal is visible from distal
Mesial marginal ridge parallel to buccal triangle ridge	Mesiolingual cusp larger [90%] on 3-cusp

marginal ridge angle is most helpful in differentiating rights from lefts (by identifying the sloping mesial surface). Also, the *triangular* ridge of the *lingual* cusp is short and is in a nearly horizontal plane.

The horizontal *mesial* marginal ridge of the **second premolar** is occlusally located hiding much of the occlusal surface when viewed from the mesial (Fig. 6-9). The *distal* marginal ridge is concave, somewhat longer buccolingually, and definitely in a more cervical position than the mesial marginal ridge (compare mesial and distal views in Fig. 6-9).

3. MESIAL MARGINAL RIDGE GROOVES AND MESIOLINGUAL GROOVES ON MANDIBULAR PREMOLARS FROM THE *PROXIMAL VIEWS*

When present [67% of the teeth studied], the *mesiolingual grooves* on **mandibular first premolars** lie between the mesial marginal ridge and the mesial slope of the lingual cusp in the lingual third of the tooth (Appendix 6r). There is seldom a groove between the *distal* marginal ridge and the distal slope of the lingual cusp [8% of 609 mandibular first premolars]. Mesiolingual grooves are *not* present on **mandibular second premolars,** and the *mesial* marginal ridges of these teeth are *not* frequently crossed by a marginal ridge groove [only 21 of 100 teeth]. Only rarely is the *distal* marginal ridge crossed by a marginal ridge groove [4 of 100 teeth].

4. HEIGHT (CREST) OF CONTOUR OF MANDIBULAR PREMOLARS FROM THE *PROXIMAL VIEWS*

In general, the height of contour of *both* types of mandibular premolar crowns on the *buccal* surface is in the cervical third. On the **mandibular first premolar,** the *buccal* height of contour of the crown is just occlusal to the cervical line, like the mandibular canine next to it (Fig. 6-9). The buccal height of contour on **second premolars** is near the junction of the cervical and middle thirds. The *buccal* crown outline of the second premolar is flatter or less convex than on the first mandibular premolar from the height of contour to the cusp tip.

For *all* mandibular premolars, the height of contour of the *lingual* surface of the crown is in the middle third, about in the center of the total crown length. On the mandibular first premolar, this is not far from the tip of the lingual cusp (clearly seen on mandibular first premolars in Fig. 6-9). Because of the extreme lingual tilting of the crown, the lingual surfaces of *all* mandibular premolar crowns extend lingually beyond the lingual surface of the root.

5. CERVICAL LINES OF MANDIBULAR PREMOLARS FROM THE *PROXIMAL VIEWS*

Similar to other teeth, the occlusal curve of the cervical line on the proximal surfaces of premolars is greater on the mesial surface than on the distal. [The *mesial* cervical line of the mandibular *first* premolar curves an average of 0.9 mm for 238 teeth versus 0.6 mm on the *distal*; *mesial* of *second* mandibular premolar curves occlusally an average of 0.8 mm for 227 teeth versus 0.5 mm (almost flat) on the *distal*.] It is also located more occlusally on the lingual than on the buccal [by as much as 2 mm on first premolars]. This makes the crowns appear to be quite short on the lingual side.

6. ROOTS OF MANDIBULAR PREMOLARS FROM THE *PROXIMAL VIEWS*

Both types of mandibular premolar roots taper apically, with the least taper in the cervical third. Rarely, an anomaly occurs where a mandibular premolar has a furcated root (i.e., the apical part of the root is divided into a buccal and lingual portion [seen in the chapter on anomalies]).

7. ROOT DEPRESSIONS OF MANDIBULAR PREMOLARS FROM THE *PROXIMAL VIEWS*

Mandibular first premolars have a shallow longitudinal depression in the apical and middle thirds of the *mesial* root surface about half of the time [45 of 100 teeth], but are even more likely to have a longitudinal depression on the *distal* surface [86 of 100 teeth], which is deeper than on the mesial [69% of the time]. Comparison depths of the depressions on mesial and distal root surfaces of this tooth are not a positive basis on which to determine rights from lefts.

Most **mandibular second premolars** [81%] have *no* depression on the mesial root surface, but are likely to have a longitudinal depression in the middle third of the *distal* root surface [73% of 100 teeth].

D.   TYPE TRAITS OF *MANDIBULAR PREMOLARS FROM THE* OCCLUSAL VIEW

For the occlusal view of mandibular first and second premolars, refer to Figure 6-10. To follow this description, the teeth or tooth models should be held with the occlusal surface toward the observer, the buccal surface up, and the observer looking exactly along the vertical midroot axis.

1.   OUTLINE SHAPE OF MANDIBULAR PREMOLARS FROM THE *OCCLUSAL VIEW*

There is much variation in the occlusal morphology of the **mandibular first premolar**.[2] The outline of the crown is *not* symmetrical (more bulk in the distal half) as seen in practically all mandibular first premolars in Figure 6-10. It often looks as though the mesial side of the crown has been *pushed inward on the mesiolingual corner* (toward the distal) (Appendix 6u). This results in a somewhat diamond-shaped outline (also Appendix 6u).

The distal marginal ridge is often nearly at right angles to the distal cusp ridge of the buccal cusp, whereas the mesial marginal ridge meets the mesiobuccal cusp ridge at a more acute angle on the first premolars. The cusp ridges of the buccal cusp are in a nearly straight line mesiodistally. The contact areas, as seen from the occlusal view, are at the point of broadest mesiodistal dimension just lingual to the line of the buccal cusp ridges and cusp tip.

Sometimes the mesial and distal marginal ridges may converge symmetrically to the lingual in such a way that the occlusal table (surface) is nearly an equilateral triangle with the base made up of the buccal cusp ridges, and the apex is the lingual cusp tip. On this symmetrical type of mandibular first premolar, it is more difficult to determine right from left by looking at the occlusal design.

On **mandibular first premolars**, the buccal ridge is not prominent, and the buccal crest of contour is slightly mesial to center. The crest of contour of the lingual surface is often distal to the center line of the tooth. Much of the buccal surface is visible from this view since the tip of the buccal cusp is slightly buccal to tooth center from this view (clearly seen in almost all mandibular first premolars in Fig. 6-10).

On the **two-cusp mandibular second premolars**, the crown is round or oval shaped, but with a relatively square occlusal table. The crown outline tapers to the lingual so the crown is more broadly rounded on the lingual side than on the buccal side.

On the **three-cusp second premolars**, the occlusal surface is more nearly square than is the occlusal surface of the two-cusp type because the crown is wider with two cusps on the lingual side. When the lingual cusps are large, the occlusal surface is broader on the lingual side than on the buccal side (seen on a number of three cusp premolars in Figs. 6-10 and 6-11). This is quite different than the two-cusp mandibular premolars (Fig. 6-12). Three-cusp premolar teeth often have greater faciolingual bulk in the distal than mesial half of the crown (tapering from distal to mesial), which is an EXCEPTION to the normal taper to the distal. [This was true on 56% of 229 specimens examined, but more than one-third (38%) tapered the more conventional way (mesial to distal), like two-thirds of the two-cusp type.] Examples of these types of crown taper are seen on mandibular second premolars in Figure 6-11. The mesiolingual cusp is most often larger than the distolingual cusp [90% of 818 teeth]. This difference in size may be little or great.

2.   OCCLUSAL MORPHOLOGY OF THE MANDIBULAR PREMOLARS FROM THE *OCCLUSAL VIEW*

a.   Ridges and Fossae and Grooves of the *Mandibular First Premolars* from the *Occlusal View*

Due to the much larger buccal than lingual cusp on the *mandibular first premolars*, the triangular ridge of the buccal cusp is long and slopes lingually from the cusp tip to where it joins the very short triangular ridge of the lingual cusp. Most often the two triangular ridges unite smoothly near the center of the occlusal surface and form an uninterrupted pronounced *transverse ridge* that completely separates the mesial and distal circular fossae.

On the *mandibular first premolar*, there is a mesial fossa and a distal fossa; both are called *circular*, not triangular; the mesial fossa is more linear buccolingually. Each fossa has a pit. These deep pits are susceptible to decay (caries) and are therefore often restored with gold, amalgam, or, more often, with a tooth-colored composite resin (Fig. 6-13. The distal fossa is usually larger or deeper [largest of 82 of 100 teeth examined, with the mesial fossa largest on only 8 teeth].

Rarely, the pronounced transverse ridge of the *mandibular first premolar* is crossed near the center of the occlusal surface by a shallow central groove, which extends from the mesial to the distal fossa. Commonly, there are *mesial* and *distal* developmental grooves running in a nearly buccolingual direction, flaring buccally from the mesial and distal fossae (Fig. 6-14). The mesial

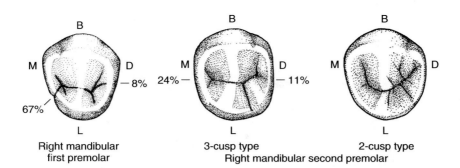

Right mandibular
first premolar

3-cusp type
Right mandibular second premolar

2-cusp type

Mandibular Premolars (Occlusal)

TYPE TRAITS TO DISTINGUISH MANDIBULAR FIRST FROM SECOND PREMOLARS:
OCCLUSAL VIEWS

MANDIBULAR FIRST PREMOLAR	MANDIBULAR SECOND PREMOLAR
Nonsymmetrical crown outline	Outline nearly square
Small nonfunctional occlusal table	Larger, functional occlusal table
Converges toward lingual, esp. on mesial	Crown may be wider on lingual
Mesiolingual groove common [67%]	Lingual groove on 3-cusp type
Two circular fossae (mesial and distal)	Two circular fossae on 2-cusp type
Definite transverse ridge	3-cusp type has no transverse ridge
Mesial and distal grooves and pits	"Y" groove pattern on 3-cusp type

TRAITS TO DIFFERENTIATE MANDIBULAR RIGHT FROM LEFT PREMOLARS:
OCCLUSAL VIEWS

MANDIBULAR FIRST PREMOLAR	MANDIBULAR SECOND PREMOLAR
Asymmetrical crown outline: convex on distal; ML "corner" flat (chopped off)	Wider FL on distal than mesial
ML groove common [67%]	L groove on 3-cusp type with ML cusp
	Lingual cusp mesial or centered (3-cusp)
Distal fossa larger than mesial fossa	Distal fossa larger (2-cusp type);
	Distal fossa smallest (3-cusp type)
Shorter mesiobuccal cusp ridge on both	

FIGURE 6-10. *Occlusal views of mandibular premolars* with type traits to distinguish mandibular first from second premolars and traits to distinguish rights from lefts. Percentages give the frequency of marginal ridge grooves on each marginal ridge.

FIGURE 6-11. *Mandibular second premolar* (three-cusp type) and *first molar* (four-cusp type), which are both *wider lingually than buccally*. Note that the distolingual cusp on the second premolar is wider than the mesiolingual cusp (found on only 7%) and that the second premolar is larger than the first premolar (a common occurrence unlike the maxillary premolars). Also observe the pronounced mesiolingual groove on the first premolar.

FIGURE 6-12. Closeup view of a *mandibular left second premolar* (*two-cusp type*): buccal above and mesial at right. The single lingual cusp is slightly mesial to the center line. The central groove is U-shaped.

FIGURE 6-13. Two left and one smaller right *mandibular first premolars* that have *amalgam restorations* in the mesial and distal fossae. These restorations are sometimes nicknamed "snake eyes."

groove is continuous with the mesiolingual groove (when present). The grooves on the first premolars are fewer in number but may be deeper than those on the second premolars.

b. **Ridges, Fossae, and Grooves of the *Two-Cusp Mandibular Second Premolars* from the *Occlusal View***

Mandibular second premolars (two-cusp type), as on maxillary second premolars, have more numerous supplemental grooves on their occlusal surfaces than do first premolars.[4] On the *two-cusp* type mandibular second premolar, the lingual cusp is smaller than the buccal cusp. There is a large triangular ridge on the buccal cusp and a correspondingly smaller one on the lingual cusp that join to form a transverse ridge (unlike the three-cusp type). There is a curved *central developmental groove* but no lingual groove on the two-cusp type of second mandibular premolar. The central groove extends mesiodistally across the occlusal surface. Sometimes this groove is short and nearly straight; sometimes it is U-shaped or like a crescent, with the open end directed buccally (Fig. 6-12). It may be interrupted near its center by a union of the buccal and lingual triangular ridges as they form the transverse ridge. The central groove ends in the *circular* mesial and circular distal fossae, where it often joins a mesiobuccal and distobuccal groove. The distal fossa is generally larger than the mesial fossa.

c. **Ridges, Fossae, and Grooves of the *Three-Cusp Mandibular Second Premolar***

On the *three-cusp* type of *mandibular second premolar*, there are three triangular ridges: one each on the two lingual cusps and one on the buccal cusp. These three ridges converge toward the central fossa (Fig. 6-15), but there is no transverse ridge. This tooth has mesial and distal fossae like all other premolars, but it is the ONLY PREMOLAR to also have a *central fossa*. The large central fossa is located quite distal to the center of the occlusal surface and in the middle buccolingually. Comparing size and depth of the mesial triangular fossa and central fossa, the central fossa was usually largest [on 65% of 200 teeth; the mesial fossa was largest on only 25% of the teeth].

The *three-cusp* type of *mandibular second premolar* does *not*, by definition, have a central groove. Rather, what appears similar to a central groove is actually the joining of a mesial and distal groove. The longer *mesial* groove extends from a small mesial *triangular* fossa to the central fossa. The shorter *distal* groove continues from the central fossa to the minute distal *triangular* fossa (Fig. 6-15). The distal triangular fossa is so small it appears to be in the outer edge of the

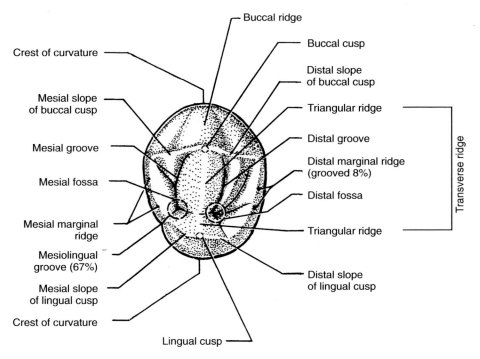

FIGURE 6-14. Occlusal surface of a *mandibular right first premolar* with normal landmarks.

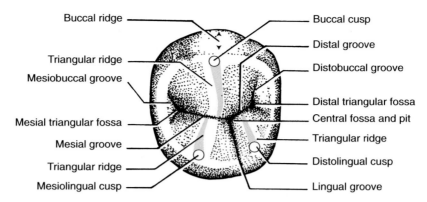

Buccal ridge — — Buccal cusp

— Distal groove

Triangular ridge —

Mesiobuccal groove — — Distobuccal groove

— Distal triangular fossa

Mesial triangular fossa — — Central fossa and pit

Mesial groove — — Triangular ridge

Triangular ridge — — Distolingual cusp

Mesiolingual cusp — — Lingual groove

FIGURE 6-15. *Mandibular right second premolar (three-cusp type).* Occlusal surface with normal landmarks.

central fossa. A *lingual groove* (also UNIQUE to this three-cusp mandibular second premolar) begins in the central fossa at the junction of the mesial and distal grooves, and extends lingually between the mesiolingual and distolingual cusps and onto the lingual surface. The junction of three grooves forms a Y-shaped occlusal groove pattern found only on this tooth (Fig. 6-15).

d. Marginal Ridge Grooves of Mandibular Premolars from the *Occlusal View*

On both the *two-cusp* and *three-cusp* second premolar types, grooves crossing the marginal ridges are not commonplace. [On the mesial marginal ridge, 24% of 200 teeth, compared to distal marginal ridge grooves on only 11%.] The first premolar is much more likely to have a mesiolingual groove.

LEARNING EXERCISE

1. First, review all arch traits that differentiate the maxillary from the mandibular premolars in Table 6-3. Then, review the summary tables of type traits that differentiate the first from second premolars, and the right from left premolars.

2. **Assign a Universal number to a hand-held premolar:**

Suppose a patient just had all of his/her permanent teeth extracted and you were asked to find tooth #4 from among a pile of 32 extracted teeth on the oral surgeon's tray because you wanted to evaluate a lesion on the root of that premolar that had been seen on the radiograph. How might you go about it? Try the following steps:

*   From a selection of all permanent teeth (extracted teeth or tooth models), select only the premolars (based on class traits).

*   Determine whether each premolar is maxillary or mandibular. *You should never rely on only one characteristic difference* between teeth to name them; rather, make a list of many traits that suggest the tooth is a maxillary premolar, as opposed to only one trait that makes you think it belongs in the mandible. This way you can play detective and become an expert at recognition at the same time.

*   If you determine that the tooth is maxillary, position the root up; if it is mandibular, position the root down.

*   Next, using type traits, determine the type of premolar you are holding (first or second).

*   Use characteristic traits for each surface to identify the buccal surface. This will permit you to view the tooth as though you were looking into a patient's mouth.

*   Finally, determine which surface is the mesial. While viewing the incisor from the facial, and picturing it within the appropriate arch (upper or lower), the mesial surface can be positioned toward the midline in only one quadrant, the right or left.

- Once you have determined the quadrant, assign the appropriate universal number for the premolar in that quadrant. For example, the second premolar in the upper right quadrant is tooth # 4.

3. A. Name the ridges on this mandibular second premolar, two-cusp type in Figure 6-16A.

   B. Name the ridges on this mandibular second premolar, three-cusp type in Figure 6-16B.

4. What problem do you see in Figure 6-17

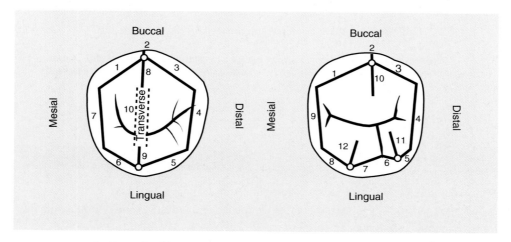

A. Name the ridges   B. Name the ridges

Ridges	Name		Ridges	Name
1.	___		1.	___
2.	___		2.	___
3.	___		3.	___
4.	___		4.	___
5.	___		5.	___
6.	___		6.	___
7.	___		7.	___
8.	___		8.	___
9.	___		9.	___
10.	___		10.	___
			11.	___
			12.	___

ANSWERS

A. Ridges for two-cusp type: 1. mesial cusp ridge of buccal cusp; 2. buccal ridge; 3. distal cusp ridge of buccal cusp; 4. distal marginal ridge; 5. distal cusp ridge of lingual cusp; 6. mesial cusp ridge of lingual cusp; 7. mesial marginal ridge; 8. triangular ridge of buccal cusp; 9. triangular ridge of lingual cusp; 10. transverse ridge.

B. Ridges for three-cusp type: 1. mesial cusp ridge of buccal cusp; 2. buccal ridge; 3. distal cusp ridge of buccal cusp; 4. distal marginal ridge; 5. distal cusp ridge of distolingual cusp; 6. mesial cusp ridge of distolingual cusp; 7. distal cusp ridge of mesiolingual cusp; 8. mesial cusp ridge of mesiolingual cusp; 9. mesial marginal ridge; 10. triangular ridge of buccal cusp; 11. triangular ridge of distolingual cusp; 12. triangular ridge of mesiolingual cusp.

FIGURE 6-16. A. Mandibular second premolar, two-cusp type. B. Mandibular second premolar, three-cusp type.

FIGURE 6-17. What is wrong with the teeth in this photograph?

ANSWER: The maxillary second premolar is rotated so its lingual surface is facing in a buccal direction. You can tell this by the taper of the tooth (which should be from buccal to lingual).

LEARNING QUESTIONS

Maxillary and Mandibular First and Second Premolars:
For each of the following traits or statements, circle the letter or letters of the premolars (if any) that apply. More than one answer may be correct.

a. Maxillary first premolar
b. Maxillary second premolar
c. Mandibular first premolar
d. Mandibular second premolar (2-cusp type)
e. Mandibular second premolar (3-cusp type)

1. Mesial ridge of the buccal cusp is longer than the distal cusp ridge.	a b c d e
2. Has a nonfunctioning lingual cusp.	a b c d e
3. Two premolars that most frequently have a groove crossing the mesial marginal ridge or one groove just lingual to it.	a b c d e
4. Has a depression in the cervical one-third of the mesial side of the *crown* and root	a b c d e
5. Maxillary premolar that has the longer sharper buccal cusp	a b c d e
6. Largest maxillary premolar	a b c d e
7. Mandibular premolar with the longest and sharpest buccal cusp	a b c d e
8. Maxillary premolar that is most symmetrical (occlusal view)	a b c d e
9. Two premolars without a central groove.	a b c d e
10. Crowns tipped lingually with respect to the root axis line (proximal view)	a b c d e
11. From buccal view, crown is tipped distally from the root axis	a b c d e
12. Mesial marginal ridge is more cervically located than its distal marginal ridge	a b c d e
13. Has no transverse ridge	a b c d e
14. Has the longer central groove	a b c d e
15. Has two major cusps almost the same size and length	a b c d e
16. Has a central fossa	a b c d e
17. Premolars with two circular fossae	a b c d e

18. Premolars with only two triangular fossae   a b c d e
19. Has a central fossa and two triangular fossae   a b c d e
20. Has a lingual groove   a b c d e

Answers: 1–a; 2–c; 3–a,c; 4–a; 5–a; 6–a; 7–c; 8–b; 9–c,e; 10–c,d,e; 11–c,d,e; 12–c; 13 e; 14–a; 15–b; 16–e; 17–c,d; 18–a,b; 19–e; 20–e.

REFERENCES

1. Morris DH. Maxillary premolar variations among Papago Indians. J Dent Res 1967;46:736–738.
2. Kraus BS, Furr ML. Lower first premolars. Part I. A definition and classification of discrete morphologic traits. J Dent Res 1953;32:554.
3. Ludwig FJ. The mandibular second premolar: morphologic variations and inheritance. J Dent Res 1957;36:263–273.
4. Brand RW, Isselhard DE. Anatomy of Orofacial Structures. St. Louis: C.V. Mosby, 1998.
5. Takeda Y. A rare occurrence of a three-root mandibular premolar. Ann Dent 1988;44:43–44.
6. Osborn JR, ed. Dental Anatomy and Embryology. Oxford: Blackwell Scientific Publications, 1981:133.
7. Palmer RS. Elephants. In: World Book Encyclopedia, Vol. 6. 1979:178c.
8. Brant D. Beaver. In: World Book Encyclopedia, Vol. 2. 1979:147.
9. Zoo Books: Elephants. Wildlife Education Ltd. San Diego: Frye & Smith, 1980:14.

General References

Grundler H. The Study of Tooth Shapes: A Systematic Procedure. (Weber L, trans.) Berlin: Buch-und Zeitschriften-Verlag "Die Quintessenz," 1976.

Oregon State System of Higher Education. Dental Anatomy: A Self-Instructional Program. 9th ed. East Norwalk: Appleton-Century-Crofts, 1982.

Renner RP. An Introduction to Dental Anatomy and Esthetics. Chicago: Quintessence Publishing, 1985.

7 Morphology of Permanent Molars

The morphology of molars is presented in four sections, each with its own learning objectives.

I. Overview of molars
  A. General description
  B. Functions of molars
  C. Class traits of all molars
  D. Arch traits that differentiate maxillary from mandibular molars

II. Type traits that differentiate mandibular second molars from mandibular first molars
  A. Type traits of mandibular molars from the buccal view
  B. Type traits of mandibular molars from the lingual view
  C. Type traits of mandibular molars from the proximal views
  D. Type traits of mandibular molars from the occlusal view

III. Type traits that differentiate maxillary second molars from maxillary first molars
  A. Type traits of the maxillary first and second molars from the buccal view
  B. Type traits of maxillary molars from the lingual view
  C. Class traits of first and second maxillary molars from the proximal views
  D. Class traits of maxillary molars from the occlusal view

IV. Maxillary and mandibular third molar type traits
  A. Type traits of all third molars (different from first and second molars)
  B. Size and shape of third molars
  C. Similarities and differences of third molars crowns compared with first and second molars in the same arch
  D. Similarities and differences of third molars roots compared with first and second molars in the same arch

Using the mandibular right second molar as a representative example for all molars, refer to the Appendix, page 7 while reading Section I of this chapter. Throughout this chapter, "Appendix" followed by a number and letter (e.g., Appendix 7a) is used within the text to denote reference to the page (number 7) and item (letter a) being referred to on that appendix page. The appendix pages are designed to be torn out to facilitate study and minimize page turns. Other appendix pages will be referred to throughout this chapter.

SECTION I. Overview of Molars

OBJECTIVES

This section is designed to prepare the learner to perform the following:

- Describe the functions of molars.
- List class traits common to all molars.
- List arch traits that can be used to distinguish maxillary from mandibular molars.
- From a selection of all teeth, select and separate out the molars.
- Divide a selection of all molars into maxillary and mandibular.

A. GENERAL DESCRIPTION

There are 12 permanent molars—six maxillary and six mandibular. The six permanent molars in each arch are the first, second, and third molars on either side of the arch. They are the sixth, seventh, and eighth teeth from the midline. Using the Universal Numbering System, the maxillary molars are numbers 1, 2, and 3 for the right third, second, and first molars, and numbers 14, 15, and 16 for the left first, second, and third molars, respectively. The mandibular molars are numbers 17, 18, and 19 for the left third, second, and first molar, and numbers 30, 31, and 32 for the right first, second, and third molars, respectively.

In the adult dentition, the first molars are distal to second premolars. The permanent first molars are located near the center of each arch, anteroposteriorly. This is one reason that their loss is so devastating to arch continuity (allowing movement and tipping of the teeth on either side). They are the largest and strongest teeth in each arch. The second molars are distal to the first molars, and the third molars are distal to the second molars. Said another way, in the adult dentition the mesial surface of the first molar contacts the distal surface of the second premolar. The mesial surface of the second molar contacts the distal of the first molar, and the mesial surface of the third molar contacts the distal of the second molar.

The third molar is the last tooth in the arch, and its distal surface is not in contact with any other tooth. Unfortunately, this tooth's nickname is "wisdom tooth." It also has unfairly been given a bad reputation for having soft enamel, not serving any function, readily decaying, causing crowding of the anterior teeth, and other dental problems. The reason for this bad reputation is probably its posterior location that makes it difficult to keep clean. Frequently, one or more of the third molars are congenitally missing (never develop); this occurs in nearly 20% of the population.

The combined mesiodistal width of the three mandibular molars on one side make up over half (51%) of the mesiodistal dimension of their quadrant. The maxillary molars constitute 44% of their quadrant's mesiodistal dimension, still a significant portion.

B. FUNCTIONS OF MOLARS

The permanent molars, like the premolars, (a) play a major role in the mastication of food (chewing and grinding to pulverize) and (b) are most important in maintaining the vertical dimension of the face (preventing a closing of the bite or vertical dimension, a protruding chin, and a prematurely aged appearance). They are also (c) important in maintaining continuity within the dental arches, thus keeping other teeth in proper alignment. You have probably seen someone who has lost all 12 molars (six upper and six lower) and has sunken cheeks. The molars, therefore, have (d) at least a minor role in esthetics or keeping the cheeks normally full or supported, as well as keeping the chin a proper distance from the nose.

The loss of a first molar is really noticed and missed by most people when it has been extracted. More than 80 mm^2 of efficient chewing surface is gone; the tongue feels the huge space between the remaining teeth; and during mastication of coarse or brittle foods, the attached gingiva in the region of the missing molar often becomes abraded and uncomfortable. Loss of six or more molars would also predispose problems in the temporomandibular joints.

C. CLASS TRAITS OF ALL MOLARS

Refer to Appendix page 7 while reading about the following class traits of all molars.

1. CROWN SIZE FOR ALL MOLARS

Molars have an occlusal (chewing) surface with three to five cusps. Molars are larger than the other teeth in their respective arches. (Refer to Tables 7-1 and 7-2 for the average and range in size of maxillary and mandibular molars in all dimensions.) They have broader occlusal surfaces than other posterior teeth (i.e., the premolars) both faciolingually and mesiodistally [averaging 2.2 mm and 3.0 mm, respectively, in maxillary molars and 2.1 mm and 3.2 mm, respectively, in mandibular molars]. However, molar crowns are shorter cervico-occlusally than all other crowns. The crowns of *both* the mandibular and maxillary molars are wider mesiodistally than long cervico-occlusally (Appendix 7a).

2. TAPER FROM BUCCAL TO LINGUAL FOR ALL MOLARS

From the occlusal view, molar crowns taper (get narrower) from the buccal to the lingual (that is, the mesiodistal width on the buccal half is wider than on the lingual half; see Appendix 7b), EXCEPT

Table 7-1

SIZE OF MAXILLARY MOLARS (MILLIMETERS) (MEASURED BY DR. WOELFEL AND HIS DENTAL HYGIENE STUDENTS, 1974–1979)

Dimension Measured	308 FIRST MOLARS		309 SECOND MOLARS		303 THIRD MOLARS	
	Average	Range	Average	Range	Average	Range
Crown length*	7.5	6.3–9.6	7.6	6.1–9.4	7.2	5.7–9.0
Root length						
Mesiobuccal*	12.9	8.5–18.8	12.9	9.0–18.2	10.8	7.1–5.5
Distobuccal	12.2	8.9–15.5	12.1	9.0–16.3	10.1	6.9–14.5
Lingual	13.7	10.6–17.5	13.5	9.8–18.8	11.2	7.4–15.8
Overall length*	20.1	17.0–27.4	20.0	16.0–26.2	17.5	14.0–22.5
Crown width (M-D)	10.4	8.8–13.3	9.8	8.5–11.7	9.2	7.0–11.1
Root width (cervix)	7.9	6.4–10.9	7.6	6.2–8.4	7.2	5.3–9.4
Faciolingual crown size	11.5	9.8–14.1	11.4	9.9–14.3	11.1	8.9–13.2
Faciolingual root (cervix)	10.7	7.4–14.0	10.7	8.9–12.7	10.4	7.5–12.5
Mesial cervical curvature	0.7	0.0–2.1	0.6	0.0–2.2	0.5	0.0–2.0
Distal cervical curvature	0.3	0.0–1.4	0.2	0.0–1.0	0.2	0.0–1.7

* Overall length from mesiobuccal root apex to tip of mesiobuccal cusp. Root length is from cervical line to root apex. Crown length is from cervical line to tip of mesiobuccal cusp (slanted).

Table 7-2

SIZE OF MANDIBULAR MOLARS (MILLIMETERS) (MEASURED BY DR. WOELFEL AND HIS DENTAL HYGIENE STUDENTS, 1974–1979)

Dimension Measured	281 FIRST MOLARS		296 SECOND MOLARS		262 THIRD MOLARS	
	Average	Range	Average	Range	Average	Range
Crown length*	7.7	6.1–9.6	7.7	6.1–9.8	7.5	6.1–9.2
Root length						
Mesial*	14.0	10.6–20.0	13.9	9.3–18.3	11.8	7.3–14.6
Distal	13.0	8.1–17.7	13.0	8.5–18.3	10.8	5.2–14.0
Overall length*	20.9	17.0–27.7	20.6	15.0–25.5	18.2	14.8–22.0
Crown width (M-D)	11.4	9.8–14.5	10.8	9.6–13.0	11.3	8.5–14.2
Root width (cervix)	9.2	7.7–12.4	9.1	7.4–10.6	9.2	6.4–10.7
Faciolingual crown size	10.2	8.9–13.7	9.9	7.6–11.8	10.1	8.2–13.2
Faciolingual root (cervix)	9.0	7.3–11.6	8.8	7.1–10.9	8.9	7.0–11.5
Mesical cervical curvature	0.5	0.0–1.6	0.5	0.0–1.4	0.4	0.0–1.4
Distal cervical curvature	0.2	0.0–1.2	0.2	0.0–1.2	0.2	0.0–1.0

* Overall length from mesial root apex to tip of mesiobuccal cusp. Root length is from cervical line to root apex. Crown length is from cervical line to tip of mesiobuccal cusp.

some maxillary first molars with large distolingual cusps, where crowns actually taper from lingual toward the buccal.

3. TAPER TO THE DISTAL FOR ALL MOLARS

For both arches, molar crowns from the occlusal view tend to taper distally, so that the distal side is narrower buccolingually than the mesial side (Appendix 7c). Also, from the buccal (or lingual) views, all molar occlusal surfaces slope toward the cervix from mesial to distal (Appendix 7d). This, along with the more cervical placement of the distal marginal ridge, makes more of the occlusal surface visible from the distal aspect than from the mesial aspect (compare mesial to distal views in Appendix page 7).

4. HEIGHT (CREST) OF CONTOUR FOR ALL MOLARS

As with premolars, the height of contour on the buccal of molars viewed from the proximal is in the cervical third; on the lingual, it is in the middle third (Appendix 7e).

5. CONTACT AREAS FOR ALL MOLARS

The contact areas of all molars from the buccal (or lingual) views are at or near the junction of the occlusal and middle thirds mesially and are more cervical on the distal, near the middle of the tooth (Appendix 7f).

D. ARCH TRAITS THAT DIFFERENTIATE MAXILLARY FROM MANDIBULAR MOLARS

Compare extracted maxillary and mandibular molars and/or tooth models while reading about these differentiating arch traits. Also refer to study page 8 in the Appendix.

1. CROWN OUTLINE TO DISTINGUISH MAXILLARY FROM MANDIBULAR MOLARS

From the occlusal view, the crowns of **mandibular molars** are oblong: they are characteristically much wider mesiodistally than faciolingually (by 1.2 mm on 839 teeth). This is just the opposite of the **maxillary molars**, which have their greater dimension faciolingually (by 1.2 mm on 920 teeth). From the occlusal view, *maxillary* molars have a more square or twisted parallelogram shape; *mandibular* molars have a rectangular or even a pentagon crown shape. Compare the outline shapes in Appendix 8a, and 8k.

2. NUMBER AND RELATIVE SIZE OF CUSPS

Mandibular molar crowns have four major cusps, two buccal and two lingual, often with a fifth minor one (the minor cusp is distal and found on the first, and sometimes the third, molar). The two lingual cusps are of nearly equal size (much different from the maxillary molars). The crowns of **maxillary molars** have three larger cusps (mesiobuccal, distobuccal, and mesiolingual) with a fourth cusp of lesser size (distolingual). The longest and largest mesiolingual cusp is connected by an *oblique ridge* to the distobuccal cusp (unique to maxillary molars) (Appendix 8d). A fifth minor cusp (of Carabelli) is often found on the lingual surface of the mesiolingual cusp of maxillary first molars (Appendix 8i).

3. LINGUAL AND DISTAL TILT THAT DISTINGUISHES MAXILLARY FROM MANDIBULAR MOLARS

When examined from the mesial or distal views, **mandibular molar** crowns appear to be tilted lingually (true for all mandibular posterior teeth), whereas the crowns of **maxillary molars** are centered over their roots (Appendix 8b). *Mandibular* molar crowns also tip distally relative to the long axis of the root (due in part to the increased taper from the distal contact to the cervical line (Appendix 8g).

4. ROOTS TO DISTINGUISH MAXILLARY FROM MANDIBULAR MOLARS

Perhaps the most obvious trait to differentiate *extracted* maxillary from mandibular molars is the number of roots. **Maxillary molars** have *three* roots of generous size that are nearly twice as long as the crown: mesiobuccal, distobuccal, and lingual (palatal). The lingual root is usually the longest; the distobuccal root the shortest. The roots converge into a broad cervical root trunk. **Mandibular molars** have only *two* roots: a mesial root and a slightly shorter distal root [mesial roots averaged 1 mm longer than the distal roots for 839 mandibular molars]. The root furcation on lower molars is usually close to the cervical line (especially on first molars), making the root trunk shorter than on the maxillary molars (see Appendix 8c). Table 7-3 includes a summary of arch traits that can be used to differentiate maxillary from mandibular molars.

Table 7-3

ARCH TRAITS TO DISTINGUISH MANDIBULAR FROM MAXILLARY MOLARS

MAXILLARY MOLARS	MANDIBULAR MOLARS
BUCCAL VIEW	

Two buccal cusps:
   Mesiobuccal and distobuccal
   ML cusp tip visible from buccal
	Two or three buccal cusps:
	   M-B, D-B, and distal
	   Both lingual cusp tips visible from buccal

One buccal groove	Two buccal grooves on first molars [81%]
Three roots (2 buccal and 1 lingual)	Two roots (1 mesial and 1 distal)
Root trunk longer	Root trunk shorter
Crown centered over root	Crown tipped distally on root
LINGUAL VIEW	
Lingual groove off center	Lingual groove centered
M-L cusp much larger than D-L cusp	M-L and D-L cusps size and height more equal
Cervix of crown tapers more to lingual	Cervix of crown tapers less to lingual
Cusp of Carabelli or groove on 70% of first molars	No Carabelli cusp
PROXIMAL VIEWS	
Crown more centered over root	Crown tipped more lingually over root

DL cusp on second molars [62%] or no
   DL cusp [38%]
	Distal cusp (3rd B cusp) seen from distal on
	   first molars [81%]

OCCLUSAL VIEW	
Crowns wider faciolingually than M-D	Crowns wider mesiodistally than F-L
Oblique ridge present from M-L to D-B;	No oblique ridge
One transverse ridge MB to ML	Two transverse ridges MB-ML and DB-DL

Parallelogram (or square) shape crown:
   Three-cusp seconds are heart shaped
	Pentagon or rectangular shape crown:
	   Second molars are rectangular

Four fossae: including large central and cigar-shaped distal	Three fossae: central fossa is large
Central groove not across oblique ridge	Central pit with Y or + groove pattern

First molars have four cusps plus
   Carabelli cusp/groove [70%]
	Five cusps on first [81%]: (distal cusp is fifth
	   cusp)

First molars wider on lingual than buccal	First molars wider on buccal than lingual
Second molars have four cusps [62%] or three cusps (heart shaped) [38%]	Second molars have four cusps:
M-L cusp much larger than D-L	M-L cusp slightly larger than D-L

SECTION II. Type Traits That Differentiate Mandibular Second Molars from Mandibular First Molars

OBJECTIVES

The section prepares the reader to perform the following:

- Describe the type traits that can be used to distinguish the permanent mandibular *first* molar from the mandibular *second* molar.
- Describe and identify the buccal, lingual, mesial, distal, and occlusal surfaces for all mandibular molars.
- Assign a universal number to mandibular molars present in a mouth (or on a model) with complete dentition. If possible, repeat this on a model with one or more mandibular molars missing.
- Holding a mandibular molar, determine whether it is a *first* or a *second* and *right* or *left*. Then assign a Universal number to it.

Mandibular first and second molars have specific traits that can be used to distinguish one from the other. The third molars vary considerably, often resembling a first or a second molar while still having their own unique traits that will be discussed later in Section IV. For this section, hold a mandibular first and second molar in front of you (with crowns up, roots down) and refer to Appendix page 8 while making the following comparisons.

A. TYPE TRAITS OF MANDIBULAR MOLARS FROM THE *BUCCAL VIEW*

Refer to Figure 7-1 for similarities and differences of mandibular first and second molars.

1. CROWN PROPORTIONS FROM THE *BUCCAL VIEW*

For *both* types of mandibular molars, the crowns are wider mesiodistally than high cervico-occlusally, but more so on the larger first molars [3.7 mm larger on first molars versus 3.1 mm for second molars].

2. RELATIVE NUMBER AND SIZE OF MANDIBULAR MOLAR CUSPS (AND GROOVES THAT SEPARATE THEM) FROM THE *BUCCAL VIEW*

The crown of the **mandibular first molar** is usually larger than the crown of the second molar in the same mouth. [In one study, second *mandibular* molars were larger than first molars in 10% of Ohio Caucasians and in 19% of Pima Indians.[23] In contrast, Dr. Woelfel examined more than 600 sets of complete dentition casts of young dental hygienists' mouths and found only a few where *mandibular* second molars were slightly larger than the first molars. There were a few more in which the mandibular third molar crowns were as large as the first molars and larger than the mandibular second molars.]

The *mandibular first molar* has the largest mesiodistal dimension (11.4 mm) of any tooth [includes measurements of 2392 maxillary and 2180 mandibular teeth].

The mandibular first molar usually has *five* cusps: three buccal [81% of the time] and two lingual. They are, in order from longest to shortest: mesiolingual, distolingual, mesiobuccal, distobuccal, plus the smallest distal cusp. The mesiobuccal cusp is the largest, widest, and highest cusp *on the buccal* side. [The mesiobuccal cusp was widest in 61%, compared to only 17% for the distobuccal cusp, for 1367 *mandibular first molars*.] The *distobuccal* cusp is slightly smaller, shorter, and may be sharper than the *mesiobuccal* cusp. [After examination of 430 teeth, it was considered to be sharper than the mesiobuccal cusp 55% of the time, compared to only 17% for the mesiobuccal cusp. The rest were equally sharp.] The minor *distal* cusp, present about 81% of the time, is located on the distobuccal angle of the crown. It is the smallest of the five cusps. [In Mongoloid peoples this cusp is often positioned lingually. It may also be split into two parts by a fissure.[1]]

Right mandibular second molar   Right mandibular first molar

Mandibular Molars (Buccal)

Rights   Lefts

Firsts

Seconds

⟵——— Distal ———⟶

TRAITS TO DISTINGUISH MANDIBULAR FIRST MOLARS FROM SECOND MOLARS: BUCCAL VIEW

MANDIBULAR FIRST MOLAR	MANDIBULAR SECOND MOLAR
Three buccal cusps [81%]: MB, DB, and Distal	Two buccal cusps: MB and DB
Two buccal grooves	One buccal groove
Crowns tipped less distally on root	Crowns tipped distally on root
Wider root spread, shorter trunk	Less root spread, longer trunk
Roots more curved	Straighter, less curved roots

TRAITS TO DISTINGUISH MANDIBULAR RIGHT FROM LEFT MOLARS: BUCCAL VIEW

MANDIBULAR FIRST MOLAR	MANDIBULAR SECOND MOLAR
Distal cusp is smallest buccal cusp	Distobuccal cusp is smaller than MB

Crown tapers and is shorter toward distal.
Distal contact more cervical than mesial contact.
Crown appears to tilt distally on its root.
Mesiobuccal root is longer than distobuccal root.

FIGURE 7-1. *Buccal views* of **mandibular molars** with traits to distinguish mandibular first from second molars, and traits to distinguish rights from lefts.

The *mesiolingual* cusp of the *mandibular first molar*, which is the highest or longest of all the cusps of the mandibular first molar, is just visible behind the mesiobuccal cusp even from the buccal view. The *distolingual* cusp is visible behind the distobuccal cusp and is usually the second highest cusp when the tooth is oriented vertically. This is clearly seen in the first molars in Figure 7-1. Even though the lingual cusps are higher than buccal cusps when viewing extracted teeth with the root axis held vertically, the lingual cusp tips are at a lower level than the buccal cusps *in the mouth* due to the lingual tilt of the root axis in the mandible (helping to create the curve of Wilson shown in Fig. 10.7c).

When there are three buccal cusps on the *mandibular first molar*, there are two buccal grooves: the longer mesiobuccal and shorter distobuccal. The *mesiobuccal groove* on the buccal surface separates the mesiobuccal cusp from the distobuccal cusp. There may be a deep pit at the cervical end of the mesiobuccal groove. This pit is sometimes a site of caries. (This pit is common in the teeth of Mongoloid persons.) Six of the *mandibular first molars* in Figure 7-1 have pits at the end of the mesiobuccal groove, and a seventh has an amalgam restoration. The *distobuccal groove* separates the distobuccal cusp from the distal cusp. It is shorter than the mesiobuccal groove [70% of the time on 720 molars] and is *not* frequently pitted. One of the *mandibular first molars* in Figure 7-1 has this pit; can you find it?

The **mandibular second molar** has *four* cusps: two buccal and two lingual. These cusps, in order from longest to shortest, are the mesiolingual, distolingual, mesiobuccal, and distobuccal, the same order as for the four major cusps of the mandibular first molar. As on the first molar, the mesiobuccal cusp is usually wider mesiodistally than the distobuccal cusp. [The mesiobuccal cusp was considered widest on 66%, compared to only 19% with a wider distobuccal cusp, for 1,514 mandibular second molars examined on dental stone casts.] As on the first molar, the lingual cusp tips are visible from the buccal side. The tips of the slightly longer mesiolingual and distolingual cusps are seen behind the mesiobuccal and distobuccal cusps (Fig. 7-1).

Mandibular second molars have only one *buccal* groove, separating the mesiobuccal and the distobuccal cusps. The buccal groove may end on the middle of the buccal surface in a pit (seen in two of the 10 second molars in Fig. 7-1). There is *no* distobuccal groove as on the first molar.

3. PROXIMAL CONTACTS OF MANDIBULAR MOLARS FROM THE *BUCCAL VIEW*

Both types of mandibular molars (in fact, all molars) have their *mesial* contact located more occlusally than the distal, at the junction of middle and occlusal thirds of the crown. The *distal* contact is located more cervically, in the middle third (near the middle of the tooth cervico-occlusally). This difference in proximal contact height can be seen in most mandibular molars in Figure 7-1.

4. CERVICAL LINES OF MANDIBULAR MOLARS FROM THE *BUCCAL VIEW*

The cervical lines of both mandibular first and second molars are often nearly straight across the *buccal* surface. On *mandibular first molars*, there is often a ridge of cementum crossing the space in the root bifurcation in a mesiodistal direction,[6] but sometimes there is a point of enamel that dips down nearly into the root bifurcation (seen later in Fig. 8-15B) [This point of enamel is reported to occur in 90% of Mongoloid peoples studied.] Sometimes there is dipping down of enamel on both the buccal and the lingual surfaces, and these extensions may meet in the root bifurcation[1,2] (Fig. 7-1, leftmost mandibular second molar). Such enamel extensions may cause periodontal problems because of the deep gingival sulcus in these regions.

5. TAPER OF MANDIBULAR MOLARS FROM THE *BUCCAL VIEW*

There is proportionally more tapering of the crown from the contact areas to the cervical line on *mandibular first molars* than on *second* molars because of the bulge of the distal cusp (Appendix 8g). The crown of the second molar appears to be wider at the cervix than the first molar because of the absence of a distal cusp (less taper toward the cervix below the contact points). The *mesial* sides of mandibular molar crowns are nearly straight, or slightly concave, from the cervical line to the convex contact area (Fig. 7-1). The *distal* sides are straight, or slightly convex, from the cervical line to the contact areas.

Also, the occlusal surface of *both* types of mandibular molars slopes cervically from mesial to distal because the crown is tipped distally on its two roots (somewhat less so on first molars, again due partly to the shortest distal cusp).

6. VARIATIONS IN MANDIBULAR MOLAR CROWNS FROM THE *BUCCAL VIEW*

The distal cusp of *mandibular first molars* is absent about a fifth of the time (Fig. 7-2). [Among 874 dental hygiene students at the Ohio State University College of Dentistry (1971–1983), dental stone casts revealed that 81% of 1,327 first molars without restorations had five cusps and 19% had only four cusps. Seventy-seven percent of the females had five-cusp first molars on both sides, 16% had four-cusp first molars on both sides, and 3% had one four-cusp and one five-cusp mandibular first molar]. Consequently, *not all four-cusp molars are second molars. Almost one-fifth may be mandibular first molars.*

The mandibular first molar sometimes has an extra cusp on the buccal surface of the mesiobuccal cusp, about in the middle third of the crown. Studies have shown this to occur frequently in the Pima Indians of Arizona[3, 14] and in Indian (Asian) populations.[4,5] An extra cusp in the same location has also been found on second and, most frequently, on third molars (see Fig. 7-3).

7. ROOTS OF MANDIBULAR MOLARS FROM THE *BUCCAL VIEW*

Both mandibular first and second molars have *two* roots, one slightly longer mesial root and one distal root. [The mesial root averaged only 1 mm longer than the distal root on 281 *first* molars, and 0.9 mm longer on 296 *second* molars.] Both roots are nearly twice as long as the crown [root to crown ratio for first molars is 1.83:1, the highest of any tooth].

The root bifurcation of the **mandibular first molar** is near the cervical line with a depression existing between the bifurcation and cervical line, and its root trunk is relatively short (shorter than on second molars). The roots of the mandibular first molar are widely separated, more so than on the second where they are more parallel (Appendix 8f). Greater root divergence can be seen in most *mandibular first molars* in Figure 7-1.

The *mesial* root of the mandibular first molar bows out mesially, such that the mesial side of this root may extend mesial to the mesial surface of the first molar crown, but the apical half curves distally. The curvature and direction of the roots is enough that the apex of the mesial root may be in line with the mesiobuccal groove of the crown, and the apex of the distal root often lies distal to the distal surface of the crown. (See the drawing of the mandibular first molar in the upper portion of Figure 7-1 and compare it to the other first molars on that page.) From the buccal aspect, it is possible to see the distal surface of the mesial root because of the way it is twisted on the trunk. The *distal* root is straighter than the mesial root and may have a more pointed apex.

FIGURE 7-2. A mandibular first molar with *only four cusps* (whereas most have five cusps). Buccal view (below) and occlusal view (above).

FIGURE 7-3. Four-cusp mandibular right third molar, buccal surface. Note the bulbous crown and the extra cusplet on the buccal surface of the mesiobuccal cusp. This extra cusp or cusplet is *not* called a Carabelli cusp.

The roots of **mandibular second molars** are less widely separated or more parallel. The root trunk is slightly longer. There is a depression on the root trunk from the cervical line to the root bifurcation (Fig. 7-1). Both roots taper apically and are more pointed than the roots of the first molar. Often the apices of both roots are directed toward the centerline of the tooth similar in shape to the handle of pliers (2 of the 10 mandibular molars in Fig. 7-1; see if you can find them), or both roots may curve distally.

8. VARIATIONS IN MANDIBULAR MOLAR ROOTS FROM THE *BUCCAL VIEW*

Observe the wide variation from the normal in the roots with extreme distal root curvature seen in Figure 7-4, lower row. This condition is called **flexion** [FLEK shen].

Occasionally, the mesial root is divided into a mesiobuccal and a mesiolingual root, making three roots on the mandibular first molar. It is reported that this condition is found in 10–20% of the mandibular first permanent molars in Eskimos.[7]

In Mongoloid peoples, there is usually a longer root trunk.[1] In Mongoloid peoples, 10% of the *mandibular first molars* have an additional distolingual root, and sometimes the mesial root is bifurcated, resulting in a four-rooted first molar.[8] It is reported that in both deciduous and permanent dentitions, three-rooted mandibular molars occur frequently in Mongoloid (Chinese) peoples, but rarely in European groups.[1,9] A small, third root can be seen in Figure 7-5. This peduncular shaped extra root is approximately 6 mm long.

FIGURE 7-4. Buccal aspect of two *unusual* maxillary third molars (top row) and five *unusual* mandibular molars (bottom row; left to right: third, second, two firsts, and third molar).

FIGURE 7-5. Mandibular left second molar with peduncular-shaped extra root; buccal view. (Courtesy of Drs. John A. Pike and Lewis J. Claman.)

B.   TYPE TRAITS OF MANDIBULAR MOLARS FROM THE *LINGUAL VIEW*

Refer to Figure 7-6 for similarities and differences of mandibular molars from the lingual view.

1.   CROWN TAPER OF MANDIBULAR MOLARS FROM THE *LINGUAL VIEW*

As with most teeth, mandibular first and second molar crowns taper from buccal to lingual and thus are narrower on the lingual side; this is more so on first molars where much of the taper is on the distal surface lingual to the distal cusp.

2.   RELATIVE SIZE OF MANDIBULAR CUSPS (AND THEIR ASSOCIATED GROOVES) FROM THE *LINGUAL VIEW*

Since the lingual cusps of *both* types of mandibular molars are both slightly longer and more pointed or conical than the buccal cusps, the buccal cusps are hidden behind them. Therefore, in most cases, only the mesiolingual and distolingual cusps of mandibular molars are visible from the lingual aspect (not true in Fig. 7-6, because of the camera angle). The mesiolingual cusp is often the slightly wider and longer of the two (noticeably wider on first molars). [On *mandibular first molars*, the mesiolingual cusp was wider on 58% of 256 teeth, while on 33% the distolingual cusp was wider. On mandibular *second* molars, the mesiolingual cusp was wider on 65% of 263 of these teeth, compared to only 30% with a wider distolingual cusp.] On sharpness, the lingual cusps were rated about even. [On first molars, 48% of the mesiolingual cusps were more pointed versus 47% distolingual cusps; on second molars, it was 44% versus 51%, respectively.]

The *lingual groove* separates the mesiolingual from the distolingual cusp. It may terminate occlusally or it may show up extending onto the lingual surface (usually occlusal third) with no pit.

3.   CERVICAL LINE OF MANDIBULAR MOLARS FROM THE *LINGUAL VIEW*

The cervical line on the lingual surface is relatively straight (mesiodistally) or irregular, and may dip cervically between the roots over the bifurcation as it also does on the buccal side of the crown.

4.   ROOTS OF MANDIBULAR MOLARS FROM THE *LINGUAL VIEW*

On *mandibular first molars*, the root trunk appears longer on the lingual than on the buccal side because the cervical line is more occlusal in position on the lingual than on the buccal surface. The roots are narrower on the lingual side than they are on the buccal side. From the lingual aspect, it is often possible to see the mesial surface of the mesial root owing to the way it is twisted on the trunk (seen on five *mandibular first molars* in Fig. 7-6). One can also see the distal side of the distal root because of its taper toward the lingual.

Mandibular Molars (Lingual)

Lefts   **Rights**

◄────────── **Distal** ──────────►

TRAITS TO DISTINGUISH MANDIBULAR FIRST MOLARS FROM SECOND MOLARS:
LINGUAL VIEW

MANDIBULAR FIRST MOLAR	MANDIBULAR SECOND MOLAR
Wider root spread, shorter trunk	Less root spread, longer trunk
Roots more curved	Straighter roots
More lingual side crown taper	Less lingual side crown taper

TRAITS TO DISTINGUISH MANDIBULAR RIGHT FROM LEFT MOLARS: ***LINGUAL VIEW***

MANDIBULAR FIRST MOLAR	MANDIBULAR SECOND MOLAR
Same outline traits as from buccal view are seen from the lingual view.	
Mesiolingual cusp is the longest.	
Distal marginal ridge is more cervical than the mesial marginal ridge.	

FIGURE 7-6. *Lingual views* **of mandibular molars** with traits to distinguish mandibular first from second molars and to help determine rights from lefts.

On first and second molars, the short root trunk has a depression between the cervical line and the bifurcation.

C. TYPE TRAITS OF MANDIBULAR MOLARS FROM THE *PROXIMAL VIEWS*

For proper orientation, as you study each trait, hold the crown so that the root axis line is in a vertical position as seen in Figure 7-7.

Recall that *both* types of mandibular molar crowns are relatively shorter cervico-occlusally compared to faciolingually, and that the crowns of *both* types of mandibular molars are tilted lingually from the root base. Remember that this slant is an arch trait characteristic of all mandibular posterior teeth and is nature's way of shaping them to fit beneath and lingual to the maxillary buccal cusps. The buccal outline is convex in the cervical third, then slightly curved and tapered occlusally in the middle and occlusal thirds.

1. HEIGHT (CREST) OF CONTOUR OF MANDIBULAR MOLARS FROM THE *PROXIMAL VIEWS*

As with all molars, the height of contour or bulge of the *buccal* surface is in the cervical third, close to the cervical line for second molars. The buccal crest of curvature is actually a ridge running mesiodis-

Right mandibular second molar   Right mandibular first molar

Mandibular Molars (Proximal)

Rights   Lefts

Firsts

Seconds

MESIAL SURFACES   DISTAL SURFACES
←— Buccal   Lingual —→   ←— Buccal   Lingual —→

TRAITS TO DISTINGUISH MANDIBULAR FIRST MOLARS FROM SECOND MOLARS: PROXIMAL VIEWS

MANDIBULAR FIRST MOLAR	MANDIBULAR SECOND MOLAR
Mesial root is wide F-L with blunt tip	Mesial root less wide FL with curved tip
Crown is wider faciolingually	Crown is less wide faciolingually

TRAITS TO DISTINGUISH MANDIBULAR RIGHT FROM LEFT MOLARS: PROXIMAL VIEWS

MANDIBULAR FIRST MOLAR	MANDIBULAR SECOND MOLAR

Mesial root broader buccolingually so D root not seen from mesial view.
Distal marginal ridge is more cervical than mesial marginal ridge.
Distal proximal contact is more cervical than mesial contact.

FIGURE 7-7. *Proximal views* of **mandibular molars** with traits to distinguish mandibular first from second molars and to help determine rights from lefts.

tally near the cervical line and is called the *buccal cervical ridge* (or buccal cingulum). It is more prominent on mandibular *second* molars than on first molars (actually seen better from the occlusal view in Fig. 7-9). The *lingual* outline of the crown of both molars appears nearly straight in the cervical third with its height of contour in the middle third. This trait is useful to tell buccal from lingual surfaces.

2. CUSP HEIGHT AND ASSOCIATED DISTAL TILT OF MANDIBULAR MOLARS FROM THE *PROXIMAL VIEWS*

In general, the lingual cusps of both mandibular first and second molars are more conical or pointed than the buccal. In review, the cusp length for mandibular molars is, from longest to shortest, mesiolingual, distolingual, mesiobuccal, distobuccal, and, when present, the smallest cusp found on 81% of first molars is the distal cusp. Due to the distal tilt to the crown and the sloping of the occlusal surface, much of the occlusal surface and all cusps can be seen from the distal aspect (as seen on the distal surfaces of all teeth in Fig. 7-7). Subsequently, on both first and second molars, from the distal aspect the tips of the mesiobuccal and mesiolingual cusps can be seen behind the distobuccal and distolingual cusps. On the first molar, the distobuccal cusp is seen above and somewhat buccal to the smaller, shorter distal cusp.

3. TAPER TO DISTAL OF MANDIBULAR MOLARS FROM THE *PROXIMAL VIEWS*

On *both* types of molars, the crown is more narrow on the distal side than on the mesial side. Therefore, from the distal aspect, some of the lingual and the buccal surfaces can be seen (noted especially on the distal views of mandibular *second* molars in Fig. 7-7). The distal contact is centered on the distal surface cervical to the distal cusp on *mandibular first molars*. There may be a wear facet here from proximal wear due to functional movements within the arch.

4. CERVICAL LINES OF THE MANDIBULAR MOLARS WHEN COMPARING *PROXIMAL VIEWS*

The *mesial* cervical line of *both* first and second molars slopes occlusally from buccal to lingual and curve toward the occlusal surface [0.5 mm on first molars, 0.2 mm on second molars]. The *distal* cervical line is nearly straight but slants occlusally from buccal to lingual.

5. MARGINAL RIDGES OF MANDIBULAR MOLARS WHEN COMPARING *PROXIMAL VIEWS*

Differences in mesial and distal marginal ridge heights are apparent on hand-held teeth when viewing from the lingual but rotating the tooth first just enough in one direction to see the *mesial* ridge height, and then enough in the opposite direction to compare the *distal* ridge height. For mandibular molars, as with all posterior teeth (EXCEPT the mandibular first premolar), the *distal* marginal ridges are more cervically located than the mesial marginal ridges. The *mesial* marginal ridge is concave buccolingually, usually longer on the mandibular *first* molar, and often sharply V-shaped on the *second* molar. It is occlusally positioned so that not much of the triangular ridges are visible from the mesial aspect. The *distal* marginal ridge of the *first* molar is short and V-shaped, located just lingual and distal to the distal cusp.

The *mesial* marginal ridges of mandibular molars are often crossed by a marginal ridge groove [68% of 209 first molars and 57% of 233 second molars]. The *distal* marginal ridges of mandibular molars are less likely to have a mesial ridge groove [48% of 215 first molars and 35% of 233 second molars].

6. ROOTS OF MANDIBULAR MOLARS FROM THE *PROXIMAL VIEWS*

From the mesial aspect, the *mesial* root of the **mandibular first molar** is broad buccolingually, hiding the distal root. It has a blunt and wide apex (Fig. 7-7, mesial views). It is less broad buccolingually on **mandibular second molars**, narrower in the cervical third, and more pointed at the apex. There is usually a deep depression on the mesial surface of the mesial root on *both* mandibular first and second molars extending from the cervical line to the apex, indicating the likelihood of *two* root canals in this broad root, one buccal and one lingual [as vividly seen later in cross-section views in Fig. 8-13). Sometimes this root is even divided into a buccal and lingual part[8] (as seen in the partially divided mesial root of one mandibular molar in Fig. 7-7). The depressions on the inner surfaces of the mesial and distal roots (that is, the surfaces between the mesial and distal roots) are often deeper than the depressions on the outer surfaces.

The *distal* root of *both* first and second mandibular molars is not quite as broad (buccolingually) nor as long as the mesial root, and it is more pointed at the apex. For this reason, the mesial root is usually visible behind the narrower distal root from the distal view (seen most clearly on all but one mandibular second molar from the distal view in Fig. 7-7). On some teeth the distal surface of the distal root is convex; on other teeth, there may be a shallow longitudinal depression. Although this root most often has *one* root canal, a distal root depression may indicate the presence of two root canals.

D. TYPE TRAITS OF MANDIBULAR MOLARS FROM THE *OCCLUSAL VIEW*

Refer to Figure 7-8 for similarities and differences of mandibular molars from the occlusal view.

1. LINGUAL INCLINATION OF MANDIBULAR MOLAR CROWNS FROM THE *OCCLUSAL VIEW*

To follow this description the tooth should be held in such a position that the observer is looking exactly along the root axis line. Because of the inclination lingually of the crown, more of the buccal surface should be visible than the lingual surface when the tooth is properly held in this position, similar to mandibular premolars.

2. OUTLINE SHAPE AND TAPER OF MANDIBULAR MOLARS FROM THE *OCCLUSAL VIEW*

As stated previously, *both* types of mandibular molars are wider mesiodistally than faciolingually [by 1.2 mm for 281 first molars; 0.9 mm wider for 296 second molars]. The **mandibular second molar** shape is roughly a four-sided rectangle, whereas the **first molar**, with the prominent buccal bulge of the distobuccal cusp and smaller distal cusp, is shaped more like a five-sided pentagon. The two major mesial cusps (mesiobuccal and mesiolingual) are larger than the two *major* distal cusps (see Fig. 7-10). (Recall, the first molar also has a minor distal cusp.) There are a couple of exceptions to this among the 10 *mandibular first molars* in Figure 7-8. Can you locate them?

The crown tapers two ways so that it is narrower buccolingually on the distal than mesial side, and is narrower mesiodistally on the lingual than on the buccal side (recall Appendix 7b and c). This distal taper is helpful in determining mesial from distal, and thus rights from lefts. This wider buccolingual dimension on the mesial half of the **mandibular second molar** is due primarily to a prominent mesial buccal bulge near the cervix called the **buccal cervical ridge** (Fig. 7-9). The widest buccolingual dimension of the crown is at this bulge, and spotting it should help you locate the mesial side on mandibular second molars (evident on all mandibular second molars in Fig. 7-8). However, the widest portion of the crown of the **first molar** (buccolingually) is at the distobuccal cusp, thereby giving it the pentagon shape (see height of contour or crest of curvature in Fig. 7-10).

The outline of the crown on the first molar is convex on the buccal, lingual, mesial, and distal (more so on the buccal). On the second molar, the mesial side outline is more nearly straight compared to the shorter distal side, which is convex.

3. RIDGES OF MANDIBULAR MOLARS FROM THE *OCCLUSAL VIEW*

On *both* first and second mandibular molars, the triangular ridges of the mesiobuccal and mesiolingual cusps meet to form a transverse ridge, and the triangular ridges of the distobuccal and distolingual cusps form a second transverse ridge (seen on the mandibular first molar in Fig. 7-10). Since lingual cusps are higher, the triangular ridges of the lingual cusps of first molars are longer than the triangular ridges of the buccal cusps.

4. FOSSAE OF MANDIBULAR MOLARS FROM THE *OCCLUSAL VIEW*

There are three fossae on *both* types of mandibular molars: the large central fossa (approximately in the center of the tooth), a smaller mesial triangular fossa (just inside the mesial marginal ridge), and the smallest distal triangular fossa (just inside the distal marginal ridge; it is very small on second molars). (These fossae are represented in Figs. 7-9 and 7-10.) There may be a pit at the junction of grooves in the deepest portion of any of these fossae.

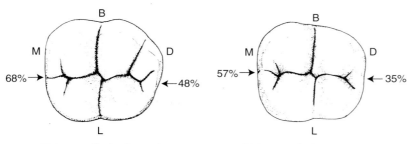

Right mandibular first molar

Right mandibular second molar

FIGURE 7-8. *Occlusal views* of **mandibular molars** with traits to distinguish mandibular first from second molars and to help determine rights from lefts. Percentages on drawings denote the frequency of occurrence of marginal ridge grooves on 233 unrestored teeth examined by Dr. Woelfel.

Mandibular Molars (Occlusal)

TRAITS TO DISTINGUISH MANDIBULAR FIRST MOLARS FROM SECOND MOLARS: OCCLUSAL VIEW

MANDIBULAR FIRST MOLAR	MANDIBULAR SECOND MOLAR
Usually five cusps (3 B and 2 L)	Usually four cusps (2 B and 2 L)
Less prominent buccal cervical ridge	Buccal ridge more prominent (mesially)
Pentagon shape likely	More rectangular shape
More crown taper from B to L	Less crown taper from B to L
Fewer secondary grooves	More secondary grooves
Central groove zigzags M-D'y	Central groove straighter
MB and DB grooves do not align with L groove	B and L grooves align to intersect with central groove like a "+"

TRAITS TO DISTINGUISH MANDIBULAR RIGHT FROM LEFT MOLARS: OCCLUSAL VIEW

MANDIBULAR FIRST MOLAR	MANDIBULAR SECOND MOLAR
Crown tapers to distal	Crown wider on mesial due to
Distal cusp smallest	buccal cervical ridge
Large mesiolingual and mesiobuccal cusps	

5. GROOVES OF MANDIBULAR MOLARS FROM THE *OCCLUSAL VIEW*

The typical groove pattern on **mandibular second molars** is simpler than that of the first molars. It is made up of three major grooves: a *central* groove running mesiodistally, plus a *buccal* and a *lingual* groove that intersect with the central groove in the central fossa (Fig. 7-9). The resultant groove pattern resembles a cross (or +) (Appendix 8, occlusal views of mandibular second molars). The *central groove* passes through the central fossa as it extends from the mesial triangular fossa to the distal triangular fossa. Its mesiodistal course is straighter than on *mandibular first molars*. The *buccal* groove separates the mesiobuccal and distobuccal cusps (often extending onto the buccal surface), and is usually continuous with the *lingual* groove which separates the mesiolingual and the distolingual cusps. Note this + pattern of grooves in the second molars in Figure 7-8.

Developmental marginal ridge grooves occur on the **mandibular second molar** more frequently on the mesial than the distal [57% and 35%, respectively, on 233 teeth as represented on the drawing at the top of Fig. 7-8]. There are sometimes supplemental grooves named according to their location and direction (mesiobuccal supplemental groove, distolingual supplemental groove, etc.). One author says that mandibular second molars have more secondary grooves and a more rectangular shape than first molars.[10] Supplemental ridges are located between supplemental and major grooves and serve as additional cutting blades. All grooves provide important escapeways for food as it is crushed. Without these ridges and grooves the teeth would be subject to unfavorable forces during mastication, as well as being inefficient crushers.

The grooves on the **mandibular first molar** separate the five cusps instead of four, so the pattern is slightly more complicated (Fig. 7-10). As on the second molars, there are several main grooves: the *central* groove passes through the central fossa from the mesial triangular to the distal triangular fossa. The central groove is more zigzag or crooked in its mesiodistal course. The *lingual* groove starts in the central fossa and extends lingually between the mesiolingual and the distolingual cusps onto the lingual surface.

Instead of one buccal groove, the mandibular first molar has two. The *mesiobuccal* groove, like the buccal groove of the second molar, starts from the central groove at or just mesial to the central fossa and extends between the mesiobuccal and the distobuccal cusps onto the buccal surface. This groove may be nearly continuous with the lingual groove, or it may not join with it. The *distobuccal* groove, unique to the first molar, starts from the central groove between the central fossa and the distal triangular fossa and extends between the distobuccal and the distal cusps onto the buccal surface.

The **mandibular first molar** has numerous minor supplemental ridges and grooves (named according to their direction and cusp). The *mesial* marginal ridge is often crossed by a groove [68% of 209 first molars] whereas the *distal* marginal ridge is less often crossed by a marginal ridge groove

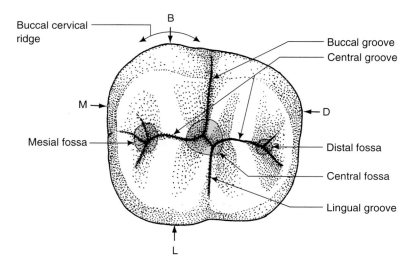

FIGURE 7-9. Mandibular right second molar with its **three fossae**. Notice the outline bulge on the mesial portion of the buccal surface formed by the **buccal cervical ridge**. Heights of contour (crests of curvature) are indicated by arrows. The mesial and distal crests of curvature would normally coincide with proximal contact areas in the mouth.

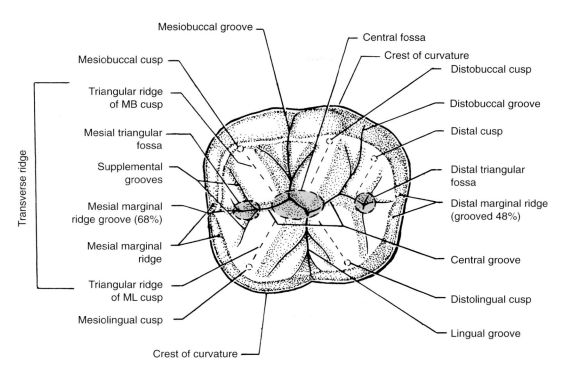

Mesiobuccal groove

Mesiobuccal cusp

Triangular ridge of MB cusp

Mesial triangular fossa

Supplemental grooves

Mesial marginal ridge groove (68%)

Mesial marginal ridge

Triangular ridge of ML cusp

Mesiolingual cusp

Transverse ridge

Crest of curvature

Central fossa

Crest of curvature

Distobuccal cusp

Distobuccal groove

Distal cusp

Distal triangular fossa

Distal marginal ridge (grooved 48%)

Central groove

Distolingual cusp

Lingual groove

FIGURE 7-10. Mandibular right first molar; occlusal view. Observe the **buccal crest of contour** is more in the center than on the second molar. There are **three fossae,** with the central fossa largest. Note that the central groove zigzags in its course from mesial to distal pit, and the mesiobuccal and lingual groove are *not* continuous from buccal to lingual. This pattern is quite common on first molars.

[48% of 215 first molars]. Seven of the ten *mandibular first molars* in Figure 7-8 have marginal grooves on the mesial, but only four have them on the distal ridge.

6. CONTACT AREAS OF MANDIBULAR MOLARS FROM THE *OCCLUSAL VIEW*

The *mesial* contact area of the mandibular *first* molar is about in the center buccolingually, whereas on the mandibular *second* molar it is slightly more buccal, near the junction of the middle and buccal thirds (Fig. 7-9). The *distal* contact of the mandibular *first* molar is just lingual to the distal cusp, whereas on the *second* molar, it is centered buccolingually.

7. VARIATIONS IN MANDIBULAR MOLARS FROM THE *OCCLUSAL VIEW*

As mentioned, on 874 casts of dental hygienists' dentitions at Ohio State University, 19% of the 1,327 *mandibular first molars* had only four cusps (no distal cusp). This four-cusp type of first molar does not taper as much from buccal to lingual as a four-cusp mandibular second molar (occlusal aspect); it often tapers from distal to mesial (recall Fig. 7-2), which is unusual and, of course, has only one groove, called the buccal groove.

Some *mandibular first molars* have a sixth cusp, which is named **tuberculum sextum** [too BUR kyoo lum SEKS tum] when located on the distal marginal ridge between the distal cusp and distolingual cusp; it is named **tuberculum intermedium** [too BUR kyoo lum in ter MEE di um] (Fig. 7-11) when located between the two lingual cusps.[11] A sixth cusp on the lingual aspect (and a third root) are common among the Chinese people.

The pattern of the grooves on the occlusal surface of the **mandibular molars** shows considerable variation. Studies have been made of the occlusal anatomy of these teeth, both in ancient and in modern man. Three principal types of occlusal groove patterns have been described: type Y, in which the zigzag central groove forms a Y figure with the lingual groove; type +, in which the central groove forms a + figure with the buccal and the lingual grooves (common in four-cusp type of first molars);

FIGURE 7-11. Mandibular first and second molars with three lingual cusps (**tuberculum inter-medium**). When an extra cusp is found on the distal marginal ridge, it is called **tuberculum sextum**.

and type X, in which the occlusal grooves are somewhat in the form of an X.[12] If you examine a collection of extracted mandibular molar teeth, you will see most of these variations.

It is reported that in the Bantu people in Africa, and sometimes in Eskimos, the mandibular molars often increase in size from first to third so that the third molar is the largest and the first molar is the smallest. This is reported to occur also in Pima Indians.[13] This is not the most frequent order of size found in American and European peoples.

Five-cusp mandibular second molars (shaped just like five-cusp first molars with a distal cusp) are not uncommon among the Chinese and Negroid populations.[11] In Figure 7-12, one is shown from a Caucasian dentition.

LEARNING EXERCISE

1. List all 19 ridges that circumscribe or make up the boundary of the occlusal surface of a mandibular *first* molar as represented in Figure 7-13A.

2. List all 17 ridges that circumscribe or make up the boundary of the occlusal surface of a mandibular *second* molar as represented in Figure 7-13B. In case you wondered, ridge 17 on the second molar is the buccal cervical ridge (sometimes evident, sometimes not).

FIGURE 7-12. *Unusual* mandibular second molar with *three* buccal cusps (buccal view above; occlusal view below with buccal side down).

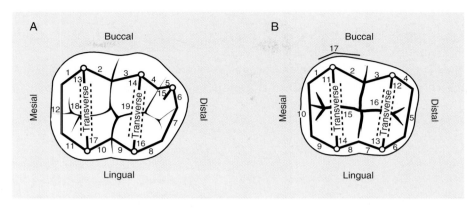

A. Name the ridges

B. Name the ridges

Ridges	Name		Ridges	Name
1.	_____		1.	_____
2.	_____		2.	_____
3.	_____		3.	_____
4.	_____		4.	_____
5.	_____		5.	_____
6.	_____		6.	_____
7.	_____		7.	_____
8.	_____		8.	_____
9.	_____		9.	_____
10.	_____		10.	_____
11.	_____		11.	_____
12.	_____		12.	_____
13.	_____		13.	_____
12.	_____		12.	_____
15.	_____		15.	_____
16.	_____		16.	_____
17.	_____		17.	_____
18.	_____			
19.	_____			

Answers: **A.** Mandibular First Molar ridges: 1. mesial cusp ridge of mesiobuccal cusp; 2. distal cusp ridge of mesiobuccal cusp; 3. mesial cusp ridge of distobuccal cusp; 4. distal cusp ridge of distobuccal cusp; 5. mesial cusp ridge of distal cusp; 6. distal cusp ridge of distal cusp; 7. distal marginal ridge; 8. distal cusp ridge of distolingual cusp; 9. mesial cusp ridge of distolingual cusp; 10. distal cusp ridge of mesiolingual cusp; 11. mesial cusp ridge of mesiolingual cusp; 12. mesial marginal ridge; 13. triangular ridge of mesiobuccal cusp; 14. triangular ridge of distobuccal cusp; 15. triangular ridge of distal cusp; 16. triangular ridge of distolingual cusp; 17. triangular ridge of mesiolingual cusp; 18. transverse ridge (mesial); 19 transverse ridge (distal).
B. Mandibular Second Molar ridges: 1. mesial cusp ridge of mesiobuccal cusp; 2. distal cusp ridge of mesiobuccal cusp; 3. mesial cusp ridge of distobuccal cusp; 4. distal cusp ridge of distobuccal cusp; 5. distal marginal ridge; 6. distal cusp ridge of distolingual cusp; 7. mesial cusp ridge of distolingual cusp; 8. distal cusp ridge of mesiolingual cusp; 9. mesial cusp ridge of mesiolingual cusp; 10. mesial marginal ridge; 11. triangular ridge of mesiobuccal cusp; 12. triangular ridge of distobuccal cusp; 13. triangular ridge of distolingual cusp; 14. triangular ridge of mesiolingual cusp; 15. transverse ridge (mesial) (mesiobuccal); 16. transverse ridge (distal); 17. mesial (mesiobuccal) cervical ridge.

FIGURE 7-13. A. Ridges on mandibular first molar with **five cusps** (circles indicate cusp tips). Name all 19 ridges. B. Ridges on mandibular second molar and on any first molars with **four cusps**. Name all 17 ridges.

LEARNING EXERCISE

Learning Exercise Related to Mandibular Molars:
Examine the mouth of a number of your associates to determine if they have first molars with five cusps and second molars with four cusps. Also, see if their first molars are bigger than their seconds, and seconds are bigger than their thirds.

LEARNING QUESTIONS

Answer the following questions about mandibular molars by circling the best answer(s). More than one answer may be correct.

1. Which of the following grooves radiate out from the central fossa in a mandibular second molar?
   a. central
   b. mesiobuccal
   c. distobuccal
   d. lingual
   e. buccal
2. Which cusp is the largest and longest on a mandibular second molar?
   a. mesiobuccal
   b. distobuccal
   c. mesiolingual
   d. distolingual
   e. distal
3. Which cusp may be absent on a mandibular first or third molar?
   a. mesiobuccal
   b. distobuccal
   c. mesiolingual
   d. distolingual
   e. distal
4. When this cusp is absent in question #3 above, which groove(s) would not be present?
   a. buccal
   b. lingual
   c. mesiobuccal
   d. distobuccal
   e. lingual
5. Which fossae are found on a mandibular first molar?
   a. mesial triangular
   b. distal triangular
   c. buccal
   d. lingual
   e. central

6. Which developmental groove connects with the lingual groove running in the same direction on a mandibular second molar?
   a. mesiobuccal
   b. distobuccal
   c. buccal
   d. mesiolingual
   e. distolingual

7. From which view is only one root visible on a mandibular first molar?
   a. mesial
   b. distal
   c. buccal
   d. lingual
   e. occlusal

8. Which root may occasionally be divided or bifurcated on a mandibular first molar?
   a. buccal
   b. lingual
   c. mesial
   d. distal
   e. mesiobuccal

9. Which cusp triangular ridge does *not* meet to form a transverse ridge on a five-cusp first molar?
   a. mesiobuccal
   b. distobuccal
   c. mesiolingual
   d. distolingual
   e. distal

10. Which ridges form the boundaries of the mesial triangular fossa of a mandibular molar?
    a. triangular ridge of mesiobuccal cusp
    b. triangular ridge of mesiolingual cusp
    c. mesial marginal ridge
    d. buccal cusp ridge of mesiobuccal cusp
    e. lingual cusp ridge of mesiolingual cusp

11. Which two pairs of cusp triangular ridges make up or join to form the two transverse ridges on a mandibular second molar?

12. List in sequential order the longest to shortest cusps on the mandibular first molar.

Answers: 1–a,d,e; 2–c; 3–e; 4–c,d; 5–a,b,e; 6–c; 7–a; 8–c; 9–c; 10–a,b,c; 11–mesiobuccal and mesiolingual PLUS distobuccal and distolingual, distolingual, distolingual, mesiobuccal, mesiobuccal, disto-buccal, then distal.

SECTION III. Type Traits That Differentiate Maxillary Second Molars from Maxillary First Molars

OBJECTIVES

This section prepares the reader to perform the following:

- Describe the type traits that can be used to distinguish the permanent maxillary *first* molar from the maxillary *second* molar.
- Describe and identify the buccal, lingual, mesial, distal, and occlusal surfaces for all maxillary molars.
- Assign a universal number to maxillary molars present in a mouth (or on a model) with complete dentition. If possible, repeat this on a model with one or more maxillary molars missing.
- Holding a maxillary molar, determine whether it is a *first* or a *second* and *right* or *left*. Then assign a universal number to it.

A.   TYPE TRAITS OF THE MAXILLARY FIRST AND SECOND MOLARS FROM THE *BUCCAL VIEW*

Examine a maxillary first and second molar as you read. Hold the roots up and the crowns down, with the two somewhat parallel roots toward you.

1.   RELATIVE CROWN SIZE AND SHAPE FROM THE *BUCCAL VIEW*

Refer to Figure 7-14 for similarities and differences of maxillary molars from the buccal view.

Maxillary first molars are the largest upper teeth (especially mesiodistally), followed closely by the second molars in the same mouth. (Third molars are generally the smallest molar.) [Studies on the variability in the relative size of molars revealed that maxillary *second* molars were larger than first maxillary molars in only 33% of a sample of an Ohio Caucasian population, and in 36% of a Pima Indian population.[23] In contrast, Dr. Woelfel found only two casts of young dental hygienists' mouths, from more than 600 sets of complete dentition casts, in which maxillary second molars were larger than the first molars.]

The crowns of *both* the first and second maxillary molars are broad near the junction of the occlusal and middle thirds and narrower near the cervical line. However, the **maxillary second molar** is less broad mesiodistally than the first molar, and is often tipped distally at the cervix on its root trunk so the occlusal surface slants cervically from mesial to distal. This distal tipping of the crown and the shortness of the distobuccal cusp make the buccal outline of the crown appear to be shorter on the distal than mesial, which is most helpful in determining rights from lefts.

On **maxillary first molars**, from the buccal aspect, the distal side of the crown is nearly flat in the cervical third. Occlusal to this flat region, the surface is convex.

2.   NUMBER AND SIZE OF CUSPS ON MAXILLARY MOLARS FROM THE *BUCCAL VIEW*

Both the first and second maxillary molars have four major cusps, but only two are prominently visible from the buccal view: the mesiobuccal cusp and the distobuccal cusp. The two lingual cusp tips (mesiolingual and distolingual) may show slightly from this view since they are positioned slightly to the distal of the buccal cusp tips.

Of the two buccal cusps, the mesiobuccal cusp is usually longer and wider than the distobuccal cusp, but not necessarily sharper. [Of 1,539 maxillary *first* molars, the mesiobuccal cusp was wider 64% of the time; on 1,545 *second* molars, this cusp was wider 92% of the time. On 468 *first* molars, the distobuccal cusp was sharper 72% of the time, whereas on 447 *second* molars, the sharpness of buccal cusps was equal.]

Right maxillary second molar

Right maxillary first molar

Maxillary Molars (Buccal)

Rights

Lefts

Firsts

Seconds

← Distal →

TRAITS TO DISTINGUISH MAXILLARY FIRST MOLARS FROM SECOND MOLARS: BUCCAL VIEW

MAXILLARY FIRST MOLAR	MAXILLARY SECOND MOLAR
Roots more spread out; shorter trunk	Root less spread out, longer trunk
Roots with less distal bend	Roots with more distal bend
Buccal groove longer, possible pit	Buccal groove shorter, no pit
Buccal cusps almost same size	MB cusp larger than DB

TRAITS TO DISTINGUISH MAXILLARY RIGHT FROM LEFT MOLARS: BUCCAL VIEW

MAXILLARY FIRST MOLAR	MAXILLARY SECOND MOLAR
Distobuccal cusp shorter than wider mesiobuccal cusp.	
Crown tilts distally on its root base with the occlusal surface shorter on distal.	

FIGURE 7-14. *Buccal views* of **maxillary molars** with traits to distinguish maxillary first from second molars and to help determine rights from lefts.

3. **BUCCAL GROOVE OF MAXILLARY MOLAR FROM THE *BUCCAL VIEW***

The buccal groove lies between the buccal cusps and may extend down the buccal surface to the middle third of the crown (less on second molars). Occasionally, there may be a pit at the end of this buccal groove.

4. **PROXIMAL CONTACTS OF MAXILLARY MOLARS FROM THE *BUCCAL VIEW* (SAME FOR ALL MOLARS)**

For **all** maxillary (and mandibular) first and second molars, the *mesial* contact is located at the junction of occlusal and middle thirds. The *distal* contact is located in the middle third of the tooth, near the middle. Sometimes you can observe a slightly worn spot (facet) in this location proximally where it contacted the adjacent molar.

5. **ROOTS OF MAXILLARY MOLARS FROM THE *BUCCAL VIEW***

At the cervical line the crown is attached to a broad, undivided base called the root trunk. Apical to the root trunk, the root separates into *three* parts (three roots): the mesiobuccal root, the distobuccal root, and the lingual root. The area of furcation is often near the junction of the cervical and middle thirds of the roots. This furcation is called a **trifurcation** since three roots come off the trunk. The furcation between the two buccal roots is a greater distance from the cervical line on **second** molars than on the **first** molars since the root trunks of the **second** molars are longer. [In Mongoloid peoples, the maxillary first molars often have a long root trunk; sometimes there is no furcation at all.[1] See the last maxillary first molar on the upper row, right side in Fig. 7-14.] The three roots are nearly the same length [within 1.5 mm] with the palatal (lingual) root the longest, followed by the mesiobuccal root, then the shortest distobuccal root.

There is much variation in the shapes of the roots. On **maxillary first molars**, the mesiobuccal and distobuccal roots are often well-separated (Appendix 8j) and may bend in such a way that they look like the handles on a pair of pliers, or the mesiobuccal and distobuccal roots often are curved distally. The mesiobuccal root bows out mesially in the cervical half before it curves toward the distal. This bend often places the apex of the mesiobuccal root distal to the line of the buccal groove on the crown. Both the mesiobuccal and distobuccal roots taper apically, with the apex of the mesiobuccal root usually more blunt. Characteristically, the spread of the middle third of the two buccal roots is nearly as wide as the crown.

In contrast, the **maxillary second molar** roots are often closer together, less curved, more nearly parallel, and with a longer root trunk. Often both roots bend toward the distal in their apical third. Find the two maxillary second molars in Figure 7-14 that are exceptions.

[In a Japanese study of root formation on 3,370 maxillary second molars, 50% had three roots, 49% were split equally between single and double roots, and 1% had four roots. In the three-rooted second molars, 75% had complete separation of roots, (no fusion). The tendency to fuse was higher in the roots of teeth extracted from females. Lingual roots were straight in half of the three-rooted teeth.[15]]

B. **TYPE TRAITS OF MAXILLARY MOLARS FROM THE *LINGUAL VIEW***

Refer to Figure 7-15 for similarities and differences.

1. **RELATIVE SIZE AND TAPER OF MAXILLARY MOLARS FROM THE *LINGUAL VIEW***

Little or no mesial or distal surfaces of **maxillary first molars** are visible from the lingual view since these teeth may be as wide or wider on the lingual half than on the buccal half (but not in the cervical third) due to a relatively wide distolingual cusp. This is an EXCEPTION, along with the three-cusp mandibular second premolar, to the normal taper towards the lingual for all other posterior teeth. This is not as likely on **second molars** which has a smaller or nonexistent distolingual cusp. The lingual surface of *both* types of maxillary molars is narrower in the cervical third than in the middle third, since the crown tapers to join the single palatal root (seen clearly in the maxillary molars in Fig. 7-15).

Maxillary Molars (Lingual)

TRAITS TO DISTINGUISH MAXILLARY FIRST MOLARS FROM SECOND MOLARS: LINGUAL VIEW

MAXILLARY FIRST MOLAR	MAXILLARY SECOND MOLAR
Buccal roots spread out behind lingual root	Buccal roots less spread out
Lingual cusps nearly the same length	Distolingual cusp much shorter

TRAITS TO DISTINGUISH MAXILLARY RIGHT FROM LEFT MOLARS: LINGUAL VIEW

MAXILLARY FIRST MOLAR	MAXILLARY SECOND MOLAR
Cusp of Carabelli present on ML [46%]	Cusp of Carabelli absent
Mesiolingual cusp larger than DL	ML even larger relative to smaller DL
The distal half of the crown is shorter than the mesial half.	

FIGURE 7-15. *Lingual views* **of maxillary molars** with traits to distinguish maxillary first from second molars and to help determine rights from lefts.

2. **NUMBER AND DESCRIPTION OF LINGUAL CUSPS ON A MAXILLARY MOLAR FROM THE *LINGUAL VIEW***

On the **maxillary first molar**, there are two well-defined cusps on the lingual surface, the larger mesiolingual cusp and the smaller, but still sizeable, distolingual cusp. The mesiolingual cusp is almost always the largest and highest cusp on any maxillary molar. Additionally, on the first molar there is often a small fifth cusp (or groove) on the lingual surface of the mesiolingual cusp [70 % of the time]. This cusp is called the cusp (or tubercle) of Carabelli, after the Austrian dentist, Georg von Carabelli

(1787–1842), who described it (recall Appendix 8i). It is a nonfunctioning cusp, even when large, because it is located about 2 mm short of the mesiolingual cusp tip.

There are two types of **maxillary second molars** based on the number of cusps (four and three). Slightly less than two-thirds of maxillary second molars have *four cusps*: two buccal and *two* lingual cusps, mesiolingual cusp (which is considerably larger) and a distolingual cusp. On *both* first and second molars with two lingual cusps, there is a groove extending between the mesiolingual and distolingual cusps that extends onto the lingual surface where it is called the *lingual groove*. This lingual groove may be continuous with the longitudinal depression on the lingual surface of the lingual root. It joins the distal oblique groove on the occlusal surface of the tooth.

Over one-third [38% of 1,396 unrestored second molars from 808 students' casts examined by Dr. Woelfel] of **maxillary second molars** have three cusps (tricuspid form) where the distolingual cusp is absent, leaving just one lingual cusp, which is large. This type has no lingual groove, and no distal (cigar-shaped) fossa. See if you can find five of these in Figure 7-15.

3. MAXILLARY MOLAR ROOTS FROM THE *LINGUAL VIEW*

On the **maxillary first molar**, the longest lingual root [averaging 13.7 mm on 308 maxillary first molars] is the third longest root on any maxillary tooth, after the maxillary canine and second premolar roots. The lingual root is not curved when seen from the lingual view, but it does taper apically to a blunt or rounded apex. There is usually a longitudinal depression on the *lingual* side of the lingual root of the first molar (seen in many lingual roots of maxillary first molars in Fig. 7-15). The characteristically wide mesiodistal spread of the curved buccal roots on the first molar is visible from this view.

The lingual root on the **maxillary second molar** is as long as, and resembles, the lingual root of the first molar. However, the buccal roots in the background bend somewhat more distally and are closer together and more parallel than on first molars.

C. CLASS TRAITS OF FIRST AND SECOND MAXILLARY MOLARS FROM THE *PROXIMAL VIEWS*

Refer to Figure 7-16 for similarities and differences of maxillary molars from the proximal views.

1. MAXILLARY MOLAR CUSPS FROM THE *PROXIMAL VIEWS*

The **maxillary first molar** crown appears short occlusocervically and broad faciolingually from the *mesial* view. Recall that the cusps of the first molar, in the usual order of their height, longest to shortest, are: mesiolingual, mesiobuccal, distobuccal, and distolingual, followed by the functionless fifth cusp (cusp of Carabelli). Since the mesial two cusps are longer than the distal, four cusps are visible from the *distal* view: the distobuccal cusp and smallest distolingual cusp in the foreground, and the cusp tips of the mesiobuccal and largest mesiolingual cusp behind them. When present on first molars, the Carabelli cusp can also usually be seen on the lingual surface from this view.

In contrast, only two (or three) cusps are seen from the *mesial* view: the mesiobuccal cusp, the long and large mesiolingual cusp, and, if present, the cusp of Carabelli (2–3 mm cervical to the mesiolingual cusp tip). The distobuccal and distolingual cusps are shorter and usually not seen when the tooth is examined from this side. Observe the number of cusps that are visible when comparing mesial with the distal views of maxillary first and second molars seen in Figure 7-16.

From the mesial and distal views, the crown of the **maxillary second molar** looks much like that of the first molar, except that there is no fifth cusp (Fig. 7-16). Also, the *distolingual* cusp is absent on more than one-third of these teeth.

2. HEIGHT OF CONTOUR FOR MAXILLARY MOLARS FROM THE *PROXIMAL VIEWS* (SAME FOR ALL POSTERIOR TEETH)

As on all other posterior teeth, the height of contour of the *buccal* side of *both* first and second maxillary molar crowns is in the cervical third, usually just occlusal to the cervical line. The height of contour of the *lingual* side of the crown is more occlusal, in or near the middle third of the crown. On teeth in which the fifth cusp is large, the lingual crest of curvature is located even more occlusally (Fig. 7-17).

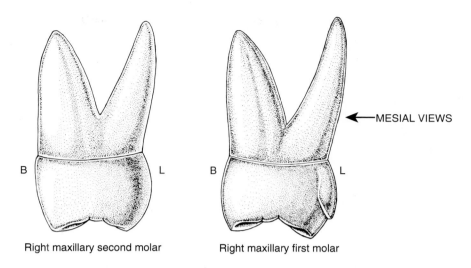

MESIAL VIEWS

B   L   B   L

Right maxillary second molar   Right maxillary first molar

Maxillary Molars (Proximal)

Lefts   Rights

Firsts

Seconds

DISTAL SURFACES   MESIAL SURFACES

⟵ Facial   Lingual ⟶

TRAITS TO DISTINGUISH MAXILLARY FIRST MOLARS FROM SECOND MOLARS: PROXIMAL VIEWS

MAXILLARY FIRST MOLAR	MAXILLARY SECOND MOLAR
More M marginal ridge tubercles [86%]	Fewer M marginal ridge tubercles [38%]
Parallelogram shape less twisted	Parallelogram shape more twisted
Some root flare beyond crown	Less root flare
Cusp of Carabelli on ML cusp [46%]	No cusp of Carabelli

TRAITS TO DISTINGUISH MAXILLARY RIGHT FROM LEFT MOLARS: PROXIMAL VIEWS

MAXILLARY FIRST MOLAR	MAXILLARY SECOND MOLAR
Cusp of Carabelli on ML cusp [46%]	Small or absent DL cusp

The distal marginal ridge is located more cervically than the mesial marginal ridge.
The distobuccal root is narrow so wider MB root is visible from distal view.

FIGURE 7-16. *Proximal views* of **maxillary molars** with traits to distinguish maxillary first from second molars, and to help determine rights from lefts.

FIGURE 7-17. Maxillary right first molar, mesial view, with an unusually **large cusp of Carabelli** and a lingual height of contour positioned quite occlusally. Also note that the wide mesiobuccal root hides the narrower distobuccal root.

3.   **TAPER TOWARD DISTAL OF MAXILLARY MOLARS FROM THE *DISTAL VIEW***

On *both* maxillary first and second molars, both the buccal surface and the lingual surface of the crown can be seen because the crown tapers toward the distal and is narrower buccolingually on the distal side than on the mesial side (Fig. 7-16).

4.   **MARGINAL RIDGES OF MAXILLARY MOLARS FROM THE *PROXIMAL VIEWS***

On *both* first and second maxillary molars, the concave *mesial* marginal ridge connects the mesiobuccal cusp and the mesiolingual cusp. It is longer buccolingually and located more occlusally than the distal marginal ridge. Consequently, little of the occlusal surface is visible from the mesial view.

Because the *distal* marginal ridge of these maxillary molars is both short and concave, and more cervically positioned than the mesial marginal ridge, more of the occlusal surface (including the triangular ridges) can be seen from the distal view. (Compare mesial and distal views in Fig. 7-16.) This marginal ridge height difference is very helpful in determining right from left sides.

In general, **marginal ridge grooves** are more common on the mesial marginal ridge than on the distal, and are more common on first molars than on seconds. [On **first** molars: 78% of 69 teeth had *mesial* marginal grooves, but only 50% of 60 had *distal* marginal grooves; on **second** molars, 67% of 75 teeth had *mesial* marginal grooves, but only 38% of 79 teeth had *distal* marginal ridge grooves.]

On the unworn marginal ridges of the maxillary molars, there will be one or more projections of enamel called **tubercles**. Like marginal ridge grooves, they are more common on mesial marginal ridges than on the distal, and more common on first molars than on seconds [on **first** molars: 86% of 64 teeth had mesial ridge tubercles but only 18% had distal ridge tubercles; on **second** molars: 38% of 79 teeth had mesial marginal ridge tubercles, but only 9% of 79 teeth had distal ridge tubercles]. These tubercles are seen most clearly on the mesial marginal ridges of the maxillary first and second molars in Figure 7-18.

5.   **CERVICAL LINES OF MAXILLARY MOLARS FROM THE *PROXIMAL VIEWS***

On *both* types of maxillary molars, the *mesial* cervical line has a slight occlusal curvature, [averaging only 0.7 mm on 308 first molars and 0.6 mm on second molars]. There is less curvature of the cervical line on the *distal* surface than on the mesial surface, but the difference is hardly discernible, since this cementoenamel junction is practically flat buccolingually.

6. ROOTS OF MAXILLARY MOLARS FROM THE *PROXIMAL VIEWS*

On **maxillary first molars** from the *mesial* view, two roots can be seen: the palatal root and the mesiobuccal root (broad buccolingually). The breadth of the mesiobuccal root is two-thirds of the faciolingual dimension, so it obscures the third distobuccal root. The apex of this mesiobuccal root is in line with the tip of the mesiobuccal cusp, whereas the convex buccal surface of this root often extends a little buccal to the crown. Observe this characteristic of maxillary first molars from the mesial view in Figure 7-16. The lingual outline of the mesiobuccal root is often more convex and, in the apical third, curves sharply facially toward the apex. The mesial surface of the mesiobuccal root has a longitudinal depression (and although they cannot be seen, there are *two* root canals in this root).

The lingual root is the longest of the three roots, is bent somewhat like a "banana," and on **maxillary first molars** extends conspicuously beyond the crown lingually. This feature alone should help you determine maxillary first from second molars. Compare the differences in Figure 7-16. The lingual root tapers apically and is usually curved buccolingually, being concave on its buccal surface. (It has only *one* root canal.)

From the *distal* view of the **first molar**, the distobuccal root is shorter and more narrow buccolingually than the mesiobuccal root. Therefore, the mesiobuccal root is visible behind the narrower distobuccal root. The distobuccal root does not extend as far buccally, and its apex is usually more pointed than the mesiobuccal root. The distal surface of the distobuccal root is convex, without a longitudinal depression (and it has only *one* root canal).

On the **maxillary second molars**, the roots are much *less* spread apart than the roots of the first molar (recall Appendix 8j). The banana-shaped lingual root is straighter than on first molars and is usually confined within the crown width from the proximal view, in contrast to first molars (Fig. 7-16). The mesiobuccal root of the maxillary second molar only rarely extends buccally beyond the buccal surface of the crown.

From the *distal* view, the mesiobuccal root, which is wider and longer than the distobuccal root, can be seen behind the distobuccal root. The apex of the lingual root of the **second molar** is often in line with the tip of the distolingual cusp.

FIGURE 7-18. Dental stone casts of the maxillary dentition demonstrating **decreasing size from first to third molars**. Both *second* molars are *three-cusp types* with only one lingual cusp (tricuspid form). Also note the **tubercles** on the mesial marginal ridges of the first molars.

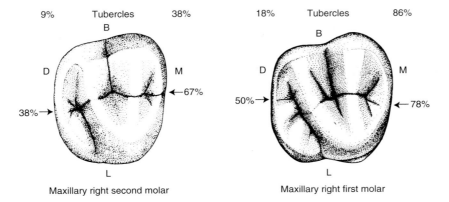

9% Tubercles 38%   18% Tubercles 86%

B   B

D   M   D   M

←67%   50%→   ←78%

38%→

L   L

Maxillary right second molar   Maxillary right first molar

FIGURE 7-19. *Occlusal views* **of maxillary molars** with traits to distinguish maxillary first from second molars and traits to distinguish rights from lefts. Percentages in drawings indicate the frequency of marginal ridge tubercles and marginal ridge grooves observed by Dr. Woelfel.

Maxillary First Molars (Occlusal)

←— Mesial

Lefts

Rights

Mesial —→

Maxillary Second Molars

←— Mesial

Lefts

Rights

Mesial —→

TRAITS TO DISTINGUISH MAXILLARY FIRST MOLARS FROM SECOND MOLARS: OCCLUSAL VIEW

MAXILLARY FIRST MOLAR	MAXILLARY SECOND MOLAR
Distolingual cusp slightly smaller than mesiolingual cusp	Distolingual cusp much smaller than mesiolingual or absent
Crowns often wider on lingual half	Crowns narrower on lingual half
Crown outline nearly square	Crown outline more twised
Crown larger (in same mouth)	Crowns smaller (in same mouth)
More prominent oblique ridge	Smaller oblique ridge
Fewer supplemental grooves	More supplemental grooves (wrinkled)
Less prominent MB cervical ridge	More prominent MB cervical ridge

TRAITS TO DISTINGUISH MAXILLARY RIGHT FROM LEFT MOLARS: OCCLUSAL VIEW

MAXILLARY FIRST MOLAR	MAXILLARY SECOND MOLAR
Cusp of Carabelli is on ML cusp [46%]	Distolingual cusp is smaller than ML

Mesiobuccal and distolingual angles of crown are more acute.
Distolingual cusp is smaller than mesiolingual cusp (or absent).
A mesiobuccal cervical ridge is visible.
The distal half of the crown is smaller faciolingually.
Oblique ridge goes from largest mesiolingual diagonally to distobuccal cusp.

D. CLASS TRAITS OF MAXILLARY MOLARS FROM THE *OCCLUSAL VIEW*

Refer to Figure 7-19 for similarities and differences. To follow the description of traits from the occlusal view, the tooth should be held in such a position that the observer is looking exactly perpendicular to the plane of the occlusal surface. Because of the spread of the first molar roots, some of each of the three roots (particularly the lingual root) may be visible when the tooth is in this position (characteristic of **first** molars only seen in Figure 7-20). In studying these teeth, it must be remembered that the morphology is variable.

1. OUTLINE OF FIRST MOLAR FROM *OCCLUSAL VIEW*

On the **maxillary first molar**, the outline of the occlusal surface is not quite square, but it gives the general impression of squareness when compared to other teeth. Actually, it is more like a parallelogram, with two acute (sharper) and two obtuse (blunter) angles (Appendix 8k). The acute angles are the mesiobuccal and distolingual. The parallelogram is larger buccolingually than mesiodistally (arch trait for the maxillary molars). The oblique ridge traverses diagonally across the tooth between the obtuse outline angles, that is, from mesiolingual to distobuccal (Appendix 8d). Also, on many maxillary *first* molars, the lingual side of the crown is slightly wider mesiodistally than the buccal side. Try to locate one or two maxillary first molars in Figure 7-19 that are not wider on the lingual than on the buccal sides. They are a minority.

The **maxillary second molar** crown is also wider buccolingually than mesiodistally, but tapers more from buccal to lingual due to the smaller or absent distolingual cusp. There is much variation in the morphology of *maxillary second molars*, particularly in the size of the distolingual cusp. When the distolingual cusp is absent (about one-third of the time), the tooth has only three cusps (six maxillary second molars in Fig. 7-19 have no distolingual cusps). The three-cusp type is somewhat triangular or heart-shaped, the blunt apex of the triangle being the lingual cusp.

The more common *four-cusp* type of **maxillary second molars** is less square in appearance than the first molar. Even when the distolingual cusp is present, it is not very large. Therefore, second maxillary molars taper to the lingual and so are noticeably narrower on the lingual side than are first molars (Appendix 8h). The fact that the crown of the second molar tapers from buccal to lingual and from mesial to distal is helpful in differentiating rights from lefts. The parallelogram shape of second molars is twisted more than on first, with the more acute angle at the mesiobuccal corner due in part to a prominent *mesial (or mesiobuccal) cervical ridge* on second molars, visible from this view (all 20 second molars in Fig. 7-19). These traits are helpful in differentiating rights from lefts and are vividly apparent on all maxillary second molars in Figure 7-19.

2. NUMBER AND SIZE OF CUSPS ON MAXILLARY MOLARS FROM THE *OCCLUSAL VIEW*

Most *first* maxillary molars usually have four larger cusps plus the fifth cusp (cusp of Carabelli), and most *second* molars have four larger cusps (without a cusp of Carabelli) *or* have three cusps (when the distolingual cusp is absent).

The cusp size on the *four-cusp* type of *both* maxillary first and second molars are, from largest to

FIGURE 7-20. Two maxillary right first molars comparing the difference in the mesiolingual cusp: one has a very large **cusp of Carabelli**, but the other has a slight depression in the same location. Also notice the prominent **lingual root** showing from this view due to the large spread of roots on the maxillary first molars.

FIGURE 7-21. Maxillary first and second molars, each with a Carabelli cusp. It is *unusual* to have this Carabelli cusp on the second molar. (Courtesy of Dr. Jeff Warner.)

smallest: the conspicuous mesiolingual [largest 95% of 1469 first molars on stone casts], mesiobuccal, distobuccal, and distolingual [smallest 72% of the time]. The **first molar** has the smallest fifth (minor) cusp of Carabelli (or a depression) [present about 70% of the time], whereas the second molar does not have this cusp (see exceptions in Fig. 7-21.) On **second molars**, there is usually a greater difference in the size of the buccal cusps, with the mesiobuccal noticeably larger (Fig. 7-22).

The cusp of Carabelli varies greatly in shape and size. It may be a conspicuous, well-formed cusp, or, at the other extreme, it may be barely discernible, absent, or there may even be a depression in this location (both extremes are seen in Fig. 7-20). Some of the variations in shape and size are seen in the upper two rows of Figure 7-15. [As seen in Table 7-4, 46.5% of 1558 maxillary first molars had some form of Carabelli cusp (large or small), 24% had a depression in this location, and 29.5% were without any type of Carabelli formation.] The cusp of Carabelli is *rarely* found on **maxillary second molars** or third maxillary molars.

[A number of studies have been done concerning the occurrence and size of the cusp of Carabelli.[16-20] One investigator reports that it is extremely rare in the East Greenland Eskimo. In European people, it is usually present. The Carabelli trait was absent on 35.4% of the teeth in 489 Hindu children.[21] The groove form was more common (35%) than tubercles (26%) on the first molars.[21]]

3. RIDGES OF MAXILLARY MOLARS FROM THE *OCCLUSAL VIEW*

On the four-cusp type **maxillary first molar**, each of the four major cusps has at least one definite triangular ridge. The triangular ridges of the mesiolingual cusp and the distobuccal cusp meet and form

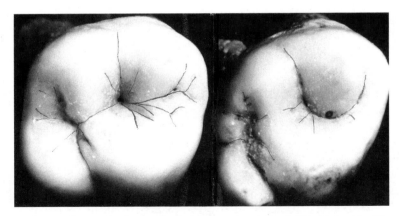

FIGURE 7-22. Left: Maxillary right *first* molar (without cusp of Carabelli). Right: Maxillary right *second* molar. Note how the *first* molar is much wider on the lingual half with a relatively large distolingual cusp, whereas the *second* molar tapers more toward the lingual surface, is twisted slightly, and has more **acute mesiobuccal and distolingual angles** than the first molar.

Table 7-4		
FREQUENCY OF OCCURRENCE AND TYPE OF CARABELLI CUSP FORMATION ON 1558 MAXILLARY FIRST MOLARS*		
Large Carabelli cusp	19%	
Small Carabelli cusp	27.5%	
		70.5% some type of Carabelli formation
Slight depression (groove)	24%	
Nothing	29.5%	
Same type on right and left	76%	
Different on each side	24%	
(835 comparisons on casts)		

* Observations from dental stone casts of Ohio dental hygienists made by Dr. Woelfel and his students, 1971–1983.

a diagonal ridge called the *oblique ridge* (an arch trait of most maxillary molars) (Appendix 8d). The largest mesiolingual cusp usually has a *second* triangular ridge mesial to the one that forms the oblique ridge (Fig. 7-23). This second triangular ridge meets the triangular ridge of the mesiobuccal cusp to form a *transverse ridge*. The groove between the two triangular ridges on the mesiolingual cusp is called the Stuart groove (named after the late Dr. Charles E. Stuart).

The oblique ridge is smaller on second molars than on first molars.[22]

4. FOSSAE OF MAXILLARY MOLARS FROM THE *OCCLUSAL VIEW*

On *four-cusp* type maxillary molars, there are *four* fossae on the occlusal surface (Fig. 7-23). The largest *central* fossa is near the center of the occlusal surface. It is bounded distally by the elevation of the oblique ridge, mesially by the mesial transverse ridge, and buccally by the buccal cusp ridges. The second largest *distal* fossa is an elongated fossa (cigar-shaped) extending between the mesiolingual and the distolingual cusps. A smaller, *mesial* triangular fossa is just within the mesial marginal ridge. The fourth minute, *distal triangular fossa* is just mesial to the distal marginal ridge. (Recall Fig. 3-18.)

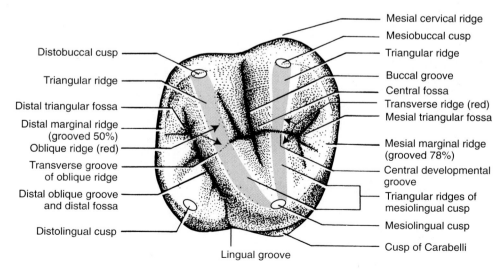

FIGURE 7-23. Occlusal surface of a maxillary right *first* molar (four-cusp type) with all of the major landmarks named. The landmarks are the same for maxillary four-cusp type maxillary *second* molars, except seconds do not normally have a cusp of Carabelli.

On *three-cusp type* maxillary (second) molars, when the distolingual cusp is missing, the distal fossa is also missing and there are only three fossae remaining (one large central and two very small triangular ones).

5. GROOVES ON MAXILLARY MOLARS

Refer to Figure 7-23 while studying these grooves. On the *four-cusp type* of **maxillary first or second** molar, the prominent oblique ridge plays an important role in defining developmental grooves. This type of maxillary molar has five major grooves: the central, buccal, distal oblique, lingual, and sometimes the transverse groove of the oblique ridge. Unlike the mandibular molar where the central groove extends from the mesial fossa to the distal fossa, the *central* groove of the maxillary molar extends from the mesial fossa over the mesial transverse ridge and ends in the central fossa. Distal to the central groove is the prominent oblique ridge which usually has no groove crossing it, but when it does, the groove appears to be a continuation of the central groove and is called the *transverse groove of the oblique ridge*. (One author calls these two grooves the mesial and distal groove, respectively,[10] while another combines these grooves and calls them the central groove.[26])

Distal to the oblique ridge, grooves parallel the direction of the oblique ridge and extend onto the lingual surface of the crown. The *distal oblique groove* extends lingually from the distal triangular fossa between the distolingual cusp and the mesiolingual cusp (along the distal fossa), and continues onto the lingual surface as the *lingual* groove. (One author calls these two grooves combined the distolingual groove.[10]) The *buccal* groove in the central fossa extends buccally from the central fossa and may continue onto the buccal surface of the crown (Fig. 7-23). The *fifth cusp groove* separates the fifth cusp (Carabelli) from the mesiolingual cusp. The pit and groove pattern on **maxillary second molars** may have more supplemental grooves and pits than on the first molar.[22]

On the *three-cusp type* of **second molar**, the distolingual cusp and cigar-shaped distal fossa are absent, so the grooves normally found within that fossa are also missing: namely, the distal oblique and lingual grooves.

All of these grooves are often fissured, so they can become the sites of dental decay. However, since the transverse groove of the oblique ridge is usually *not* fissured, decay on the occlusal surfaces of maxillary molars normally occurs mesially and distally to the oblique ridge. The result is two *separate* occlusal fillings (restorations) similar to decay pattern on the mandibular first premolar where the prominent transverse ridge seems to separate mesial and distal pit decay. An example of this decay pattern is seen later in the maxillary molar in Figure 12-13.

6. PROXIMAL CONTACTS OF MAXILLARY MOLARS FROM THE *OCCLUSAL VIEW*

Mesial and distal contacts of maxillary molars are near the center buccolingually. The mesial contact is more buccal than the distal contact on maxillary molars, especially on first molars.

LEARNING EXERCISE

1. Examine the teeth of your associates and notice the variation in the cusp of Carabelli. This little cusp has intrigued many people. It may be somewhat prominent and pointed, small and blunt, absent, or you may even see a slight depression in that part of the mesiolingual cusp where the cusp of Carabelli would be found.

2. Name each of the 17 ridges in Figure 7-24.

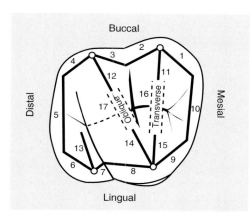

Name the ridges

Ridges	Name	Ridges	Name
1. _____		10. _____	
2. _____		11. _____	
3. _____		12. _____	
4. _____		13. _____	
5. _____		12. _____	
6. _____		15. _____	
7. _____		16. _____	
8. _____		17. _____	
9. _____			

Answers: Maxillary Molar ridges: 1. mesial cusp ridge of mesiobuccal cusp; 2. distal cusp ridge of mesiobuccal cusp; 3. mesial cusp ridge of distobuccal cusp; 4. distal cusp ridge of distobuccal cusp; 5. distal marginal ridge; 6. distal cusp ridge of distolingual cusp; 7. mesial cusp ridge of distolingual cusp; 8. distal cusp ridge of mesiolingual cusp; 9. mesial cusp ridge of mesiolingual cusp; 10. mesial marginal ridge; 11. triangular ridge of mesiobuccal cusp; 12. triangular ridge of distobuccal cusp; 13. triangular ridge of distolingual cusp; 14. (distal) triangular ridge of mesiolingual cusp; 15. (mesial) triangular ridge of mesiolingual cusp; 16. transverse ridge; 17. oblique ridge.

FIGURE 7-24. Maxillary molar, first or second (circles denote cusp tips).

LEARNING QUESTIONS

LEARNING QUESTIONS on Maxillary Molars. Circle the correct answer(s) that apply. More than one answer may be correct.

1. Which three grooves radiate out from the central fossa in a maxillary first molar?
   a. central
   b. mesial
   c. transverse groove of oblique ridge (when present)
   d. buccal
   e. lingual

2. Which cusp has two triangular ridges on the maxillary first molar?
   a. mesiobuccal
   b. mesiolingual
   c. distobuccal
   d. distolingual
   e. cusp of Carabelli

3. Which cusp is the largest and longest on a maxillary second molar?
   a. mesiobuccal
   b. mesiolingual
   c. distobuccal
   d. distolingual
   e. cusp of Carabelli

4. Which cusp is most likely to be absent on a maxillary second (or third) molar?
   a. mesiobuccal
   b. mesiolingual
   c. distobuccal
   d. distolingual
   e. distal

5. When the cusp is absent in question 4 above, which groove(s) would not be present?
    a. central
    b. buccal
    c. distal oblique
    d. lingual
    e. distal

6. Of the four fossae on a maxillary first molar, which is the largest?
    a. mesial triangular
    b. distal triangular
    c. central
    d. distal

7. From which view are only two roots visible on a maxillary first molar?
    a. mesial
    b. distal
    c. buccal
    d. lingual

8. Which grooves are likely to radiate out of the mesial triangular fossa on the maxillary first molar?
    a. mesiobuccal fossa groove
    b. mesiolingual fossa groove
    c. mesial marginal ridge groove (when present)
    d. central
    e. buccal

9. Which two cusps have the triangular ridges that make up or join to form the oblique ridge on a maxillary molar?
    a. mesiobuccal
    b. distobuccal
    c. mesiolingual
    d. distolingual
    e. cusp of Carabelli

10. Which two cusps have the triangular ridges that make up or join to form a transverse ridge on most maxillary molars?
    a. mesiobuccal
    b. distobuccal
    c. mesiolingual
    d. distolingual
    e. cusp of Carabelli

11. List in sequential order the largest to smallest cusp area on the maxillary first molar (occlusal view).

Answers 1. a,c,d; 2. b; 3. b; 4. d; 5. c,d; 6. c; 7. a; 8. a,b,c,d; 9. b,c; 10. a,c; 11. mesiolingual, mesiobuccal, distobuccal, distolingual, cusp of Carabelli (if even present).

SECTION IV. Maxillary and Mandibular Third Molar Type Traits

OBJECTIVES

After studying this section, you should be able to perform the following:
- List the type traits that are unique to all third molars that can be used to distinguish them from first or second molars.
- From a selection of all types of molars, select the mandibular and maxillary third molars and assign each a universal number.
- In mouths (or casts) of mandibular and maxillary arches with only one or two molars per quadrant, identify which molars are present and which are absent based on crown anatomy and position in the arch. (Remember that second or third molars can drift forward and take up the arch position normally occupied by lost first or second molars, respectively, so arch position should not be the only way to confirm which molars are present.)

A. TYPE TRAITS OF ALL THIRD MOLARS (DIFFERENT FROM FIRST AND SECOND MOLARS)

The mesial surfaces of third molars contact the distal surfaces of second molars, but the distal surface of third molars are *not* in proximal contact with any tooth. The *maxillary* third molars occlude with only the mandibular third molars; all other teeth have the potential for occluding with two teeth EXCEPT mandibular central incisors.

Third molars, also known by many as wisdom teeth, have gotten a bad reputation. Due to the posterior location of third molars in the mouth making them more difficult to keep clean, and their wrinkled, fissured occlusal surface, these teeth may be more prone to developing decay than other teeth. Further, mandibular third molars often erupt so far distally that they emerge near the vertical mandibular ramus with compromised gingival health, so dentists often suggest that these teeth be removed to prevent future problems. Inflammation of the tissue around these teeth (called pericoronitis) can be a cause of acute pain and spread of infection, resulting in the need for gingival surgery or extraction. However, it is *not* true that third molars have soft enamel, are useless, or should be routinely extracted. If the dental arches are of sufficient length to permit full eruption of third molars and a person's oral hygiene is good, third molars can function for a lifetime without problems. Also, healthy third molars can serve as the posterior attachment (abutment) when replacing lost or missing first or second molars.

Some oral surgeons recommend that when third molars have to be extracted, they be removed at an early age (under 25 years old) to facilitate an easier, less traumatic removal, and a quicker, more comfortable recovery period than when they are extracted later in life.[25] Since many third molars are extracted before the roots are completely formed, you can easily look into the open ends of the root canals at the apices of the roots.

Many third molars never form or develop. [Among 710 Ohio State University dental hygiene students, there were 185 *maxillary* third molars and 198 *mandibular* third molars congenitally absent. Many students were missing more than one third molar, so the percentage of the population missing one or more third molars might be close to 20%.]

Although third molars may resemble first *or* second molars, they all have certain type traits in common that set them apart from the first and second molars in their arches. These third molar traits include the following:

1. Normally, third molars are smaller than first or second molars in the same mouth (Fig. 7-25). A common exception is the *five-cusp* third molar, which may have a crown somewhat larger and more bulbous than the second molar.
2. Third molar crowns are bulbous.
3. Occlusal surfaces of third molars are relatively small compared to first and seconds (that is, the buccal cusp tips are closer to the lingual cusp tips than on first and second molars).
4. Occlusal surfaces of third molars are quite *wrinkled* due to numerous supplemental grooves and ridges (Fig. 7-26).
5. A third molar crown may have a number of traits in common with the first *or* second molar within its arch.

FIGURE 7-25. Dental stone casts of maxillary and mandibular teeth (facial view) showing the decrease in size of molars from first to third molar that is *typical* in most people. (Model courtesy of Ms. Colleen Seto.)

6. Third molar roots are short (with small root to crown ratio) compared to first and second molars in the same mouth (Fig. 7-27).
7. Roots are frequently fused together, subsequently with long root trunks (Fig. 7-27).
8. Roots are pointed and frequently curve distally in the apical third.

B. SIZE AND SHAPE OF THIRD MOLARS

Maxillary third molars vary considerably in size, but they are usually the *shortest* of the permanent teeth and are therefore smaller than the first or second molar. The roots of maxillary third molars are ordinarily shorter [by 2.0 mm, average of 920 teeth] and the root trunks are proportionally longer than the root trunks of the first and second molars.

Similarly, **mandibular third molars** are usually the shortest of the mandibular teeth [averaging 18.2 mm], although these teeth also vary considerably in size and can be either large or small.

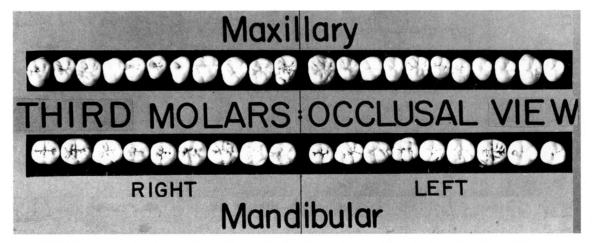

FIGURE 7-26. *Occlusal views* of **maxillary and mandibular third molars**. The lingual surfaces of the maxillary teeth face down, and those of the mandibular teeth face up. All mesial surfaces face the centerline. Observe the **wrinkled** occlusal designs in both and try to recognize the similarities to first and second molars in each arch. For example, most of the maxillary third molars are largest faciolingually in contrast to the mandibular third molars whose greater dimension is mesiodistally.

FIGURE 7-27. *Buccal views* of maxillary and mandibular third molars. Notice the **fused roots** and **long root trunks**. The mesial surfaces all face toward the centerline. Notice the tremendous variation among the maxillary third molars. Observe the differences between maxillary and mandibular anatomy. Also, note the similarity of each to the first and second molars found within their respective arches. (Method of comparison and teeth furnished by Kelli Whapham, first-year O.S.U. dental hygiene student, 1978.)

C. SIMILARITIES AND DIFFERENCES OF *THIRD MOLARS CROWNS* COMPARED WITH FIRST AND SECOND MOLARS IN THE SAME ARCH

Maxillary third molars have the *greatest* morphologic variance of all teeth. The great amount of variation in *maxillary third molars* also makes a general description difficult. The crown may have only one cusp or as many as eight,[24] but it also may resemble a small maxillary first molar (complete with cusp of Carabelli) or second molar (without the cusp of Carabelli, and perhaps without the distolingual cusp). As with the mandibular third molar, the *maxillary third molar* can be distinguished from the first or second molar in its arch because it has more numerous supplemental grooves, a small occlusal surface, and ridges, giving it a *wrinkled* appearance, and its roots are shorter, thin, or often fused.

Sometimes the form of the **maxillary third molar** crown is so irregular that it is difficult to identify the mesiobuccal, the distobuccal, and the lingual cusps. However, the usual relative cusp size from largest to smallest is the same as in the first and second molars: first the mesiolingual cusp is largest and longest, followed by the mesiobuccal cusp which is wider and usually longer than the distobuccal cusp, and the smallest distolingual cusp (if present). The oblique ridge is poorly developed and often absent (maxillary molars in Fig. 7-26).

From the occlusal view, the maxillary third molar crown usually tapers from buccal to lingual, being narrower on the lingual side, and tapers from mesial to distal, being considerably larger faciolingually in their mesial half due to a prominent mesiobuccal cervical ridge and large mesiolingual cusp. This latter trait is a great help in identifying rights from lefts from the occlusal view (Fig. 7-26). Also, the buccal surface can be distinguished from the lingual because it is relatively more flat.

The **mandibular third molar** also exhibits great variance in size and shape as seen in Figure 7-28. However, quite often, its crown resembles the crown of the mandibular second molar (with four cusps) or the crown of the mandibular first molar (with five cusps), or it may bear little resemblance to either. As with mandibular first and second molars, the crown may appear tipped distally on the root base, so from the buccal aspect, the distal half of the crown is usually noticeably shorter than the mesial half.

The lingual cusp of the **mandibular third molar** is often larger and longer than the buccal cusps, with the mesiolingual cusp being the largest of all. The mesiobuccal cusp is often the widest and usually highest of the two or three buccal cusps. This difference in cusp height aids in determining mesial from distal sides and therefore, rights from lefts.

FIGURE 7-28. *Buccal view* of six *unusual* **mandibular third molars** and occlusal view (left side) of one with a small tooth (called a paramolar) fused to its buccal surface. Two in the lower row are double or fused teeth.

The occlusal outline of a **mandibular third molar** crown is rectangular or oval and wider mesiodistally than buccolingually. The crown of the *four-cusp* type tapers from mesial to distal, but only slightly from buccal to lingual (occlusal aspect). [It was wider mesiodistally than faciolingually by 1.2 mm on 262 teeth.] The buccal crown outline is often relatively flat compared to the more curved lingual outline (occlusal view).

D. SIMILARITIES AND DIFFERENCES OF *THIRD MOLARS ROOTS* COMPARED WITH FIRST AND SECOND MOLARS IN THE SAME ARCH

As on maxillary first and second molars, **maxillary third molars** usually have three roots: mesiobuccal, distobuccal, and lingual, which may be separated, as in the first and second molars, but more commonly are *fused* most of their length. This results in a *long root trunk* with the furcation located only a short distance from the apices of the roots. Often the roots are entirely fused from the cervix to the apices as seen in 10 maxillary teeth in Figure 7-27. The roots are noticeably *shorter* than on the first and second molars [303 teeth averaged 2 mm shorter on their buccal roots and 2.5 mm shorter on their lingual roots]. The roots, fused or not, are often very crooked, and the majority of them curve distally in their apical third.

As with first and second mandibular molars, **mandibular third molars** have two roots, mesial and distal, but often these are fused together. If the roots are separate, the root trunk is long and the roots are usually more pointed at the apex than on the other molars (Fig. 7-27). Often they curve more distally than the roots of first and second molars. They may have one or more extra roots. The mandibular third molar roots are normally significantly shorter than those on the second molar [averaging over 2 mm shorter on 839 mandibular molars]. The roots on mandibular third molars are only about half again as long as the crown, and the root-to-crown ratio is noticeably different from that of mandibular first and second molars [1.6:1 compared to 1.8:1 on 839 teeth].

LEARNING EXERCISE

Learning Exercises for All Molars:
1. First, review all arch traits that differentiate the maxillary from the mandibular molars in Table 7-3. Then, review the summary tables in this chapter of type traits that differentiate the maxillary first from second molars, maxillary right from left molars, mandibular first from second molars, and mandibular right from left molars.

2. Assign a Universal number to a hand-held molar.

Suppose a patient just had all of their permanent teeth extracted. Imagine being asked to find tooth #14 from among a pile of 32 extracted teeth on the oral surgeon's tray because you wanted to evaluate a lesion seen on the x-ray on a root of that molar. How might you go about it? Try the following steps:

- From a selection of all permanent teeth (extracted teeth or tooth models) select only the molars (based on class traits).
- Determine whether each molar is maxillary or mandibular. *You should never rely on only one characteristic difference* between teeth to name them; rather, make a list of many traits which suggest the tooth is a maxillary molar as opposed to only one trait that makes you think it belongs in the mandible. This way you can play detective and become an expert at recognition at the same time.
- If you determine that the tooth is maxillary, position the roots up; if it is mandibular, position the roots down.
- Next, using type traits, determine the type of molar you are holding (first or second or third).
- Use characteristic traits for each surface to identify the buccal surface. This will permit you to view the tooth as though you were looking into a patient's mouth.
- Finally, determine which surface is the mesial. While viewing the molar from the facial, and picturing it within the appropriate arch (upper or lower), the mesial surface can be positioned toward the midline in only one quadrant, the right or left.
- Once you have determined the quadrant, assign the appropriate universal number for the molar in that quadrant. For example, the first molar in the upper left quadrant would be tooth #14.

REFERENCES

1. Tratman EK. A comparison of the teeth of people. Indo-European racial stock with Mongoloid racial stock. Dent Record 1950;70:31–53, 63–88.
2. Masters DH, Hoskins SW. Projection of cervical enamel into molar furcations. J Periodontol 1964;35:49–53.
3. Dahlberg AA. The evolutionary significance of the protostylid. Am J Phys Anthropol 1950;8:NS:15.
4. Dahlberg AA. Geographic distribution and origin of dentitions. In Dent J 1965;15:348–355.
5. Hellman M. Racial characters of human dentition. Proc Am Philosoph Soc 1928;67:No.2.
6. Everett FG, Jump EG, Holder TD, Williams GC. The intermediate bifurcation ridge: a study of the morphology of the bifurcation of the lower first molar. J Dent Res 1958;37:162.
7. Scott JH, Symons NBB. Introduction to Dental Anatomy. London: E & S Livingstone, Ltd., 1958.
8. Tratman EK. Three-rooted lower molars in man and their racial distribution. Br Dent J 1938;64: 264–274.
9. Turner CG. Three-rooted mandibular first permanent molars and question of American Indian origin. Am J Phys Anthropol 1971;34:239–242.
10. Brand RW, Isselhard DE. Anatomy of Orofacial Structures. 6th ed. St. Louis: C.V. Mosby, 1998: 438.
11. Jordan R, Abrams L. Kraus's Dental Anatomy and Occlusion. St. Louis: Mosby Year Book, 1992.
12. Jorgensen KD. The Dryopithecus pattern in recent Danes and Dutchmen. J Dent Res 1955; 34:195.
13. Garn SM, Lewis AB, Kerewsky RS. Molar size sequence and fossil taxonomy. Science 1963; 142:1060.
14. Dahlberg AA. The dentition of the American Indian. In: Laughlin WS, ed. The Physical Anthropology of the American Indian. New York: The Viking Fund, 1949.
15. Matsumoto Y. Morphological studies on the roots of the Japanese maxillary second molars. Shikwa Gukuho 1986;86:249–276.
16. Carbonelli VM. The tubercle of Carabelli in the Kish dentition, Mesopotamia, 3000 B.C. J Dent Res 1960;39:124.

17. Garn SM, Lewis AB, Kerewsky RS, Dahlberg AA. Genetic independence of Carabelli's trait from tooth size or crown morphology. Arch Oral Biol 1966;11:745–747.

18. Kraus BS. Carabelli's anomaly of the maxillary molar teeth. Observations on Mexican and Papago Indians and an interpretation of the inheritance. Am J Hum Genet 1951;3:348.

19. Kraus BS. Occurrence of the Carabelli trait in the Southwest ethnic groups. Am J Phys Anthropol 1959;17:117.

20. Meredith HV, Hixon EH. Frequency, size, and bilateralism of Carabelli's tubercle. J Dent Res 1954;33:435.

21. Joshi MR, Godiawala RN, Dutia A. Carabelli trait in Hindu children from Gujurat. J Dent Res 1972;51:706–711.

22. Brand RW, Isselhard DE. Anatomy of the Orofacial Structures. St. Louis: C.V. Mosby, 1982:159, 163.

23. Garn SM, Lewis AB, Kerewsky RS. Molar size sequence and fossil taxonomy. Science 1963; 142:1060.

24. Jordan R, Abrams L. Kraus's Dental Anatomy and Occlusion. St. Louis: Mosby Year Book, 1992.

25. Chiles DG, Cosentino BJ. Third molar question: report of 522 cases. J Am Dent Assoc 1987; 115:575–576.

26. Bath-Balogh M, Fehrenbach MJ. Illustrated Dental Embryology, Histology, and Anatomy. Philadelphia: W.B. Saunders, 1997.

General References

Oregon State System of Higher Education. Dental Anatomy. A Self-instructional Program. East Norwalk: Appleton-Century-Crofts, 1982:403–414.

Proskaves C, Witt F. Pictorial History of Dentistry. (Cave P, trans.) Koln: Verlag M. Dumont Schauberg, 1962.

Renner RP. An Introduction to Dental Anatomy and Esthetics. Chicago: Quintessence Publishing, 1985.

Ring ME. Dentistry: An Illustrated History. St. Louis: C.V. Mosby, 1985.

Clinical Application of Root Morphology

I. Periodontal considerations related to external morphology and surrounding structures
   A. Definitions of basic periodontal terms
   B. The healthy periodontium
   C. Anatomy of diseased periodontium
   D. Periodontal measurements: indicators of disease and conditions
   E. Relationship of periodontal disease and restorations (fillings)
   F. Relationship of tooth support and root morphology
   G. Influence of root anatomy and anomalies on periodontal disease
   H. Periodontal therapy

II. Internal pulp cavity morphology related to endodontic and restorative therapy
   A. The shape of pulp cavities and configuration of pulp canals
   B. Shape of pulp cavities in sound young teeth
   C. Why pulp cavities get smaller in older teeth
   D. Clinical application of pulp morphology related to restorative dentistry
   E. Clinical application of pulp morphology related to endodontics

III. Location of root and cervical crown concavities, furcations, depressions, and canals
   A. Maxillary central incisors
   B. Maxillary lateral incisors
   C. Mandibular central and lateral incisors
   D. Maxillary canines
   E. Mandibular canines
   F. Maxillary first premolars
   G. Maxillary second premolars
   H. Mandibular first premolars
   I. Mandibular second premolars
   J. Mandibular first and second molars
   K. Maxillary first and second molars

SECTION I. Periodontal Considerations Related to External Morphology and Surrounding Structures[a]

OBJECTIVES

This section is designed to prepare the learner to perform the following:
- List the functions of gingiva, the periodontal ligament, alveolar bone, and cementum.
- Describe and recognize the signs of gingivitis, periodontitis, and gingival recession.

---

[a] Section I of this chapter was written by Lewis Claman, D.D.S., M.S., Associate Professor, Section of Periodontology, The Ohio State University.

- Describe the periodontal measurements that can be used to differentiate periodontal diseases from the healthy periodontium, and be able to record these findings on a dental chart.
- Describe the relationship of periodontal disease with restorations placed close to the gingival attachment.
- Describe the relationship of tooth support with root morphology.
- List contemporary methods of periodontal therapy.

While the anatomy of the crown is significant to tooth function from an occlusal standpoint, the root morphology and healthy surrounding structures determine the actual support for the teeth. This section focuses on how external root morphology affects the progression of disease of the periodontium, and why the periodontium, which seems so perfect in health, may be challenged when periodontal disease affects tooth support and stability. An emphasis is placed on periodontal disease initiation, the measurements and descriptions that can be used to differentiate periodontal health from disease, and the therapies that can be used to stop or prevent the disease. As this is a basic text on dental anatomy, the important relationship of periodontal disease relative to sound restorative dentistry involving the placement of fillings and crowns is also introduced. Before reading this chapter, you should review the descriptions of the normal periodontium presented in Chapters 1 and 2.

A. DEFINITIONS OF BASIC PERIODONTAL TERMS

The following definitions are important to the understanding of periodontal disease and related therapy.

- **Periodontium:** The tissues that invest (surround, envelop, or embed) the teeth: that is, the gingiva, cementum, periodontal ligament, the alveolar and supporting bone, and the alveolar mucosa. (Refer to Fig. 8-1 to locate these surrounding structures.)
- **Gingivitis:** Inflammation (disease) of the gingiva.
- **Periodontitis:** Inflammation (disease) of the supporting tissues of the teeth; a spread of inflammation of the gingiva into the adjacent periodontium (bone and periodontal ligament) usually resulting in a progressively destructive change involving loss of bone and periodontal ligament.
- **Periodontal diseases:** Those pathologic processes affecting the periodontium, most often gingivitis and periodontitis.
- **Dental plaque:** A layer containing microorganisms that adheres to teeth and contributes to the development of gingival and periodontal diseases, as well as to tooth decay (dental caries).
- **Dental calculus (tartar):** A hard concretion that forms on teeth or dental prostheses through calcification of bacterial plaque.
- **Periodontics:** That specialty of dentistry that encompasses the prevention, diagnosis and treatment of diseases of the supporting tissues of the teeth or their substitutes; the maintenance of the health, function and esthetics of these structures and tissues; and the replacement of lost teeth and supporting structures by grafting or implantation of natural and synthetic devices and materials.
- **Periodontist:** A dental practitioner who by virtue of special knowledge and training limits his/her practice or activities to periodontics.

B. THE HEALTHY PERIODONTIUM

1. FUNCTIONS OF HEALTHY GINGIVA

In health, the gingiva provides support, protection, and esthetics to the dentition.

a. Support:

The gingiva somewhat *supports* the tooth by means of attachment coronal to the crest of the alveolar bone that form a dentogingival junction near the cementoenamel junction from tooth to gingiva. It includes the **junctional epithelium** [average width = 0.97 mm] and the **connective tissue attachment** [average = 1.07 mm] (Fig. 8-1). The more coronal band (junctional

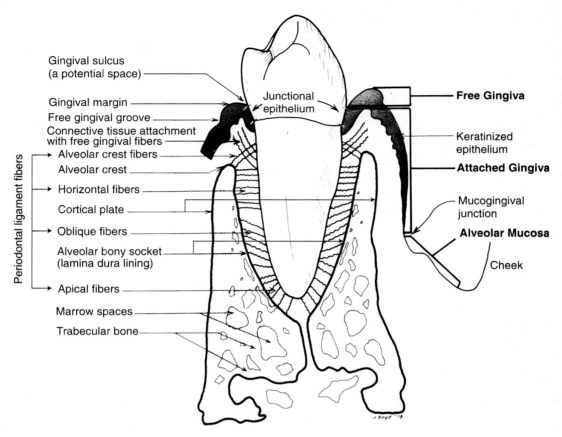

FIGURE 8-1. Cross-section of tooth within periodontium. Mesial side of a mandibular left first premolar suspended in its alveolus by groups of fibers of the periodontal ligament. Periodontal ligament fibers include the apical, oblique, horizontal, and alveolar crest fibers. Other fibers include free gingival fibers, and a sixth group (not visible in this view) called transseptal fibers that run directly from the cementum of one tooth to the cementum of the adjacent tooth at a level between the free gingival and alveolar crest fibers. The fibers of the periodontal ligament are *much* shorter than depicted here, averaging only 0.2 mm long.

epithelium) attaches gingiva to the tooth by cell junctions [called hemidesmosomes, or half desmosomes], while the more apical band (connective tissue) attaches gingiva to cementum by several gingival fiber groups made up of connective tissue called collagen.

b. **Esthetics:**

In health, gingiva covers the roots of teeth, and the gingival papillae normally fill the gingival embrasure areas between adjacent teeth (Fig. 8-2). The shape of healthy gingiva contributes to what we consider to be an esthetic smile. It is pink (or has masking pigmentation), firm in consistency, has a stippled (orange-peel) or matte surface texture, and does not bleed, even when probed.

c. **Protection:**

The gingiva generally protects underlying tissue because it is comprised of dense fibrous connective tissue covered by a relatively tough tissue layer called **keratinized epithelium**. It is resistant to bacterial, chemical, thermal, and mechanical irritants. Keratinized gingiva helps prevent the spread of inflammation to deeper underlying periodontal tissues. However, the sulcular lin-

FIGURE 8-2. Healthy gingiva, close up. Note the ideal scalloped contours and stippled (orange peel) surface texture that is usually most noticeable on the maxillary labial attached gingiva.

ing (epithelium) and junctional epithelium of the marginal gingiva and interdental papillae provide less protection. Since these areas are *not* keratinized, they are more permeable to bacterial products, providing only a weak barrier to bacterial irritants, and may even allow bacterial penetration in aggressive forms of periodontal diseases.

Healthy gingiva is somewhat protected by ideally positioned and contoured natural teeth and well-contoured restorations. The protection provided by ideal contours, including appropriate heights of contour, helps to minimize injury from food during mastication (chewing) since food is diverted away from the thin gingival margin and the non-keratinized sulcus. However, poor tooth or restoration contours, especially over-contoured restorations, contribute to the retention of bacteria-laden dental plaque that may predispose to gingival and periodontal diseases, and will be described in more depth later. Ideal *proximal* tooth contours and contacts help prevent food from impacting between teeth and damaging the interdental papilla or contributing to periodontal disease interproximally. Be aware, however, that even ideal tooth contours do *not prevent* the formation of bacterial plaque.

2. FUNCTIONS OF THE HEALTHY PERIODONTAL LIGAMENT, ALVEOLAR BONE, AND CEMENTUM

The entire periodontal ligament consists of thousands of collagen fiber bundles, which attach the cementum of the tooth root to the alveolar bony sockets. In that sense the periodontal ligament is analogous to a ligament which attaches one bone to another. These fibers, from apex to free gingiva, include apical, oblique, horizontal, and alveolar crest fibers. Transseptal and free gingival fibers attach the free gingiva to the cementum (refer back to Fig. 8-1). The periodontal ligament provides the majority of *support* for the teeth and resistance to forces such as those encountered during chewing (mastication). It is a viable structure that, in health, is capable of adaptation and remodeling.

As with the gingiva, the periodontal ligament, bone, and cementum are at risk for breakdown during inflammation with resultant loss of bone height and periodontal ligament. This disease process can, in turn, result in exposure of the cementum on the root surface, which is less mineralized than enamel, making it more susceptible to the effects of pathogenic bacteria and their products, which contribute to root caries (decay) formation.

C. ANATOMY OF DISEASED PERIODONTIUM

1. GINGIVITIS

Traditionally, periodontal disease (the inflammation in the periodontium) begins as **gingivitis**, an inflammatory condition confined to, and altering the gingival tissues. Alterations in the gingiva may reflect gingivitis alone, active slight periodontitis, more advanced disease, or evidence of previous disease that has been arrested. Gingival inflammation results from the metabolic products of bacterial colonies within dental plaque that are in close proximity to gingival tissues over time. The earliest indication of gingivitis on a *microscopic* level involves an increase in inflammatory cells and breakdown of the connective tissue (collagen) in the gingiva. This leads to an increase in tissue fluids (edema), proliferation of small blood vessels, and some loss of the integrity of the epithelium (ulceration). As this breakdown progresses, changes in the tissues can be clinically observed.

Clinically, gingival characteristics that should be evaluated as indicators of gingival health (versus disease) include: its shape and size, color, consistency, surface texture, and the presence or absence

FIGURE 8-3. Gingivitis. A. A periodontal probe is inserted into the gingival sulcus and gently swept or "walked" around the tooth. **B.** The examiner looks for **gingival bleeding** that occurs within 30 seconds. (Note the generalized physiologic melanin pigmentation (dark regions) on the attached gingiva common in persons with some ethnic heritages.) **C. Inflamed gingiva:** Note the contour changes (bulbous papillae, rolled margins), increased size, and glazed surface texture. Clinically, the papillae and margins are red and bleed easily when probed. The gingiva separates (retracts) from the teeth easily when air is directed at it.

of bleeding and/or suppuration (purulence or pus). Visually, the inflammation and edema of *mild* gingivitis is seen as slight redness, rolled margins, smooth and shiny surface texture (loss of stippling) and loss of resiliency (tissues can be depressed or free gingiva can be deflected from the tooth when a stream of air is directed toward it). In *moderate or severe* gingivitis, these changes become more pronounced and the proliferation of small vessels and ulcerations results in bleeding upon probing. Moderate to severe gingivitis is evident in Figure 8-3. Additionally, in severe inflammation, especially with periodontitis, *suppuration*, or expressing of pus (also known as purulent exudate), may occur. See Table 8-1 for normal gingival characteristics compared to descriptions of tissue exhibiting gingivitis.

2. PERIODONTITIS

In the classic progression of disease, gingivitis, if untreated, may progress to **periodontitis**, when inflammatory breakdown extends from the gingiva to the periodontal ligament and bone and when the junctional epithelium, which attaches to tooth at the cementoenamel junction, migrates apically onto the root. This occurs because the connective tissue attachment has broken down, allowing the epithelium to migrate apically. Periodontitis associated with alveolar bone loss is best appreciated in dental radiographs (Fig 8.4). The bone height (crestal bone) is no longer at pre-disease levels. Although the immune system protects the periodontium, bone resorption occurs when **osteoclasts** (bone-resorbing cells) are stimulated by the host and by bacterial products.

Factors Contributing to Periodontitis:

In addition to the primary role of bacteria in the pathogenesis, there are many factors that contribute to periodontal disease development and progression. To date, the only two risk factors that are proven to increase the c ʲds of periodontal disease progression are smoking and diabetes.

Table 8-1

CHARACTERISTICS OF NORMAL GINGIVA COMPARED TO DISEASED GINGIVA

GINGIVAL CHARACTERISTICS	NORMAL (EXAMPLES)	NOT NORMAL/DISEASE (EXAMPLES)
SIZE AND SHAPE:		
Papillae:	Fill embrasures, thin	Blunted; bulbous; cratered
Margins:	Knife-edged in profile	Rolled (thickened) in profile
Scallops:	Present & normal, parabolic	Flattened; exaggerated; reversed; clefted
COLOR	Coral pink, or pink with masking melanin pigmentation	Red, bluish-red cyanotic
CONSISTENCY	Resilient, firm, non-retractable with air	Soft & spongy, air-retractable
SURFACE TEXTURE	Stippled (orange peel); matte (dull)	Smooth & shiny (glazed); pebbled (coarse texture)
BLEEDING	None	Upon probing or spontaneous
MUCOGINGIVAL DEFECT	None (adequate zone of keratinized gingiva)	Pockets traverse mucogingival junction; lack of keratinized gingiva; Frenum inserts on marginal gingiva
SUPPURATION (PURULENT EXUDATE OR PUS)	None	Exudate is expressed when the gingival pocket wall is compressed; exudate streams out of the pocket after probing

Other factors that may *contribute to* this disease include specific bacterial pathogens, alterations in the tooth form and surface which influence the accumulation and retention of dental plaque, systemic illnesses or conditions (including genetics) which modify or impair the immune response, and injury to the periodontium resulting from heavy forces during tooth function (occlusion).

FIGURE 8-4. Radiographic bone loss. This radiograph shows advanced periodontal disease as indicated by loss of bone (especially around teeth numbers 29 and 31; note tooth number 30 is missing) which would normally be surrounding all teeth to a level much closer (within 2 mm) to the cementoenamel junction.

Breakdown of the periodontium resulting in attachment loss and bone loss usually begins in an inaccessible area (such as adjacent to a root concavity or an exposed furcation) that is neither self-cleansing nor easy for a patient to reach with oral hygiene aids. Therefore, it is paramount that both the dentist and the dental hygienist be thoroughly familiar with root anatomy as they perform a periodontal examination in order to detect periodontal disease at these inaccessible locations that are at greatest risk to breakdown. Further, an essential objective in treating periodontal disease involves using special instruments to remove deposits (plaque and calculus) and cementum on root surfaces that have become affected by periodontal disease. Knowledge of root morphology also helps when identifying sites that are difficult or impossible to reach, or ones that have not responded to treatment during root cleaning (debridement which includes root planing), and when providing instructions to patients for the appropriate use of oral hygiene aids.

Periodontitis itself may be a risk factor or contributing factor for several systemic diseases including cardiovascular disease, stroke, and diabetes, as well as contributing to low birth weight and pre-term babies when the pregnant mother has periodontal disease.

3. GINGIVAL RECESSION

Gingival recession is a loss of gingival tissue (usually with underlying loss of bone) resulting in the exposure of more root surface (Fig 8.5). In gingival recession, the gingival margin is apical to the cementoenamel junction, and the papillae may be blunted or rounded, and no longer fill the interproximal embrasure. Gingival recession is often seen in older individuals, hence the reference to an older person as being "long in the tooth." It may be part of an active process of periodontal disease, or may reflect previous disease that is now under control. However, destruction of the periodontium (including gingival recession) should *not* be regarded as a natural consequence of aging.[1]

Conditions that contribute to gingival recession around individual teeth, especially in the presence of plaque, are poorly aligned teeth within an arch resulting in abnormal tooth and root prominence (Fig. 8-5B and 8.6), a lack of attached gingiva,[2] or aggressive tooth brushing. Abnormal tooth positions do not necessarily indicate disease; but they do contribute to other tissue alterations such as flattened or exaggerated contours, and variations in tissue thickness.

D. PERIODONTAL MEASUREMENTS: INDICATORS OF DISEASE AND CONDITIONS

Several clinical measurements are critical when evaluating overall periodontal status. These measurements can be used to describe a tooth's stability and loss of support, and a patient's degree of inflammation and pattern of disease. They help to establish a diagnosis, guide the development of a treatment plan,

FIGURE 8-5. Gingival Recession and Mucogingival Defects. A. Area of gingival recession (clefting). The gingiva no longer covers the cementoenamel junction and the root surface is exposed. **B.** Severe gingival recession. The prominent canine root and lack of attached gingiva are factors that may have contributed to the recession. Note the blunted papillae (arrows). Both figures show marginal depths where there is a diminished zone of keratinized gingiva, and probe depths reach or transverse the mucogingival junction indicating a mucogingival defect. (Courtesy of Alan R. Levy, D.D.S.)

FIGURE 8-6. Effects of tooth position (alignment) within the arch on gingival shape: Examples of contour variations caused by tooth malpositions. Tooth #11 is too labial, showing exaggerated escalloping and thin gingiva. Tooth #10, which is in lingual version, has flattened gingival contours and thicker tissue. Rotated tooth #7 shows V-shaped gingival margin contour on the labial gingiva.

and document changes following active therapy. Throughout this discussion, references will be made to documenting this information using the clinic chart obtained from the Ohio State University College of Dentistry (Fig. 8-7).

1. TOOTH MOBILITY

Tooth mobility is the movement of a tooth in response to applied forces. Teeth may become mobile due to repeated excessive occlusal forces, inflammation, and weakened periodontal support (often associated with a widened periodontal ligament as noted on radiographs). The healthy periodontal ligament (PDL) is about 0.2 mm wide, decreasing to only 0.1 mm with advanced age. Tipping movements are minimal at the rotational center of the tooth and greater at either the cervical or apical end of the root. Thus, there is a functional difference in the width of the periodontal ligament in these three regions. At any age it is wider around both the cervix and the apex than around the middle of the root, depending upon the amount of rotational movements to which the tooth is subjected. Further, the periodontal ligament of a natural tooth in occlusal function is slightly wider than in a nonfunctional tooth because it does not have an antagonist to stimulate the periodontal ligament and bone cells to remodel.[3]

Injury to the periodontium from occlusal forces is known as **occlusal trauma**. It may contribute to destructive changes in the bone, widening of the periodontal ligament, and root shortening (resorption), all of which may contribute to increased tooth mobility. Many of the changes are reversible, meaning that the periodontium can accommodate.[4] Occlusal trauma is a disorder that does *not* initiate, but can influence the course of inflammatory periodontal disease under specific circumstances.[5]

Technique to Document Mobility:

First, the patient's head should be stabilized to minimize movement. Next, view the occlusal surfaces and observe movement of the marginal ridges of the tooth being tested relative to adjacent teeth as you use two rigid instruments (such as the mirror and probe handles) to apply reciprocating forces first one way, then another. The forces should be fairly light and alternate fairly rapidly. Observe the tooth for movement in a buccolingual or mesiodistal direction, as well as for vertical "depressibility." Numbers assigned to denote the extent of mobility are presented in Table 8-2.

Fremitus is the vibration or movement of a tooth during occlusal contact or excursive movements. It is determined by placing the nail of the index finger at right angles to the facial tooth surface using a light force. The patient is asked to tap his/her teeth or clench and move the mandible from right to left (excursive movements). If definite vibration is felt or tooth displacement is detected, fremitus is confirmed and could be noted as an "F" on a patient's chart for that tooth. See Figure 8-7 for charting examples of mobility and fremitus.

2. PROBE DEPTHS

Determining (probing) the depth of the potential space between the tooth and gingiva (called the **gingival sulcus or crevice**) is a critical periodontal finding that is routinely performed in dental

FIGURE 8-7. Charting periodontal findings (on a partial reproduction of the form used at The Ohio State University College of Dentistry). This form provides a logical method for documenting periodontal findings (as well as other findings). **A.** The left column provides the key for recording the following: **Fremitus** is recorded as F as on tooth #5; **Mobility** is denoted by 1 for tooth #2; **2** for tooth #5; **Probe depths** (six per tooth) are recorded during the initial examination (Initial Probe Depths) in the three boxes for three facial depths and three boxes for three lingual depths. After initial periodontal therapy has been completed, they should be recorded again (as Post Initial Preparation or PIP Probe Depths). This permits easy comparison to identify sites that respond to treatment and those that do not respond. **Bleeding on probing (BOP)** is denoted by a red dot over the probe depth readings as on the *facial* surfaces of teeth #2 (mesial, midfacial and distal), #3 (distal), and #5 (mesial and distal); and *lingually* all mesial and distal surfaces. **Gingival margin position** is recorded as numbers in red on the root of teeth as follows: +1 (1 mm *apical* to the cementoenamel junction or CEJ) on the facial of teeth #2 and #3; +2 on the facial of tooth #5; -1 (1 mm *occlusal* to the cementoenamel junction) on the lingual of teeth #3 and #4; and 0 (located at the level of the cementoenamel) on all other surfaces. **Furcation Classes** are seen as red triangular shapes (incomplete, outlined, or solid). Class I involvement is evident on the midfacial of tooth #3. Class II involvement is noted midfacial on #2, as well as on the mesial (from the lingual) on #2, and the distal (from the lingual) on #3. Class III involvement is noted on a mandibular molar discussed below). A **Mucogingival defect** is recorded as a red wavy line seen on the facial of tooth #5. **B.** A mandibular molar (#30) showing a **Class III furcation** evident from the facial and lingual views. Note that the triangle point is directed *up* toward the furcation in the mandibular arch, but was directed *down* toward the furcation in the maxillary arch as shown in A. **C. Calculation of Plaque Index % and Bleeding on Probing (BOP) %.** The **Plaque Index %** can be calculated by dividing the number of surfaces with plaque by the total number of surfaces (four per tooth). When considering only the four teeth in this figure, 9 surfaces had plaque divided by 16 possible surfaces = 56%. The **BOP %** is the number of tooth surfaces that bleed on probing divided by the total number of surfaces (six per tooth). When considering only the four teeth in this figure, 14 surfaces bled divided by 24 total surfaces = 58%.

Table 8-2

NUMBERS ASSIGNED TO MOBILITY CATEGORIES

MOBILITY CATEGORY	CLINICAL OBSERVATION	MAGNITUDE
0	No observed movement	
1	Slight movement	Less than 1 mm
2	Moderate movement	Greater than 1 mm
3	Extreme movement	Depressible

offices and may indicate the presence of periodontal disease. A blunt tipped instrument with millimeter markings called a **periodontal probe** is inserted into the gingival sulcus (Fig. 8-8). In the presence of periodontal disease, this sulcus may be called a **pocket**. **Probing depth** (referred to as *pocket* depth if periodontal disease is present) is the distance from the gingival margin to the apical portion of the gingival sulcus. Probing depths *greater than 3 mm* are a possible cause for concern. However, if gingival tissues are overgrown (as may result as a side effect from some medications), a pocket depth reading of 4 mm or greater (called a **pseudopocket**) may be present even in the absence of periodontitis. On the other hand, if there is gingival recession (described below), there may be shallow probing depths in the presence of true periodontal disease. Therefore, the critical determinant of whether periodontitis has occurred is the presence of attachment loss (to be described later).

Probing Technique:

The probe should be "walked around" the tooth with a light force to ensure a tactile sense and to minimize probing beyond the base of the pocket. That is, the probe should be directed apically within the sulcus along the root surface (to prevent it from engaging or being impeded by the pocket wall). The intent is to probe apically within the sulcus just to the attachment, although in reality the probe usually broaches (impinges on) some of the attachment. When the depth of the sulcus/pocket has been reached, resilient resistance is encountered. Probing depths are generally recorded as the deepest measurement for each of the six areas around each tooth. Three areas are recorded while moving around within the sulcus from the buccal (mesiobuccal, midbuccal, and distobuccal), and three areas are recorded from the lingual (mesiolingual, midlingual, and distolingual). Interproximally, the probe should aim for and engage the most interproximal point by angling it approximately 10° to 15° buccal (or lingual) to the tooth axis line when teeth have contacts.

3. **GINGIVAL MARGIN LEVEL (GINGIVAL RECESSION OR NON-RECESSION)**

Before any periodontal disease has occurred, the gingival margin level of a young healthy person is slightly coronal to the cementoenamel junction, which is the reference point. If the gingival margin

FIGURE 8-8. Periodontal probe in place in the gingival sulcus. **A.** Interproximal probing. **B.** Facial probing. In health, the area probed is the gingival sulcus. If periodontal disease is present, it is called a pocket.

is apical to the cementoenamel junction, there has been gingival recession and the root is exposed (Fig. 8-5B).

By convention, the following denotes the gingival margin level:

- negative (−) numbers denote that gingiva is coronal to the cementoenamel junction.
- zero (0) denotes that the gingiva is at the cementoenamel junction.
- positive (+) numbers denote recession (the gingival level is apical to the cementoenamel junction).

Technique to Determine the Gingival Margin Level:

If recession has occurred, the distance between the cementoenamel junction and the gingival line can be visually measured with the periodontal probe. If the gingival margin covers the cementoenamel junction, the distance from the gingival margin to the cementoenamel junction may be estimated by inserting the probe in the sulcus and feeling for the cementoenamel junction. If this junction is difficult to detect or is subgingival, the probe should be at a 45° angle. The overlap between enamel and cementum will stop the probe at their junction. Gingival margin levels are charted in Figure 8-7.

4. CLINICAL ATTACHMENT LEVEL (INDICATORS OF ATTACHMENT LOSS)

Clinical attachment level refers to the distance from the cementoenamel junction to the apical extent of the periodontal pocket. It is a measurement that indicates how much support has been lost and is therefore a critical determinant of whether periodontal disease has occurred.

Technique to Determine Clinical Attachment Loss:

Add the probing depth and the gingival margin level measurements together to obtain the clinical attachment level. A patient with a 3 mm pocket and a gingival level of +2 (2 mm of recession) has 5 mm of attachment loss. A patient with a 3 mm pocket and a gingival level of −2 mm (the gingiva covers the CEJ by 2 mm) has only 1 mm of attachment loss. Clinical attachment loss may be severe with minimal pocket depths if there is considerable gingival recession. There may be no attachment loss with deep pockets if pseudopockets are present.

5. BLEEDING ON PROBING

Bleeding on probing occurs when bacterial plaque effects the gingival sulcular epithelium, resulting in inflammation in the underlying connective tissue. Bleeding visible from the gingival margin when probing is an important indicator of inflammation (Fig. 8-3B).

Technique to Document Bleeding on Probing:

When bleeding is noted after probing several teeth, teeth that exhibit bleeding can be recorded at each probing site on the chart as a red dot above the probe depth. The percentage of sites that bleed can be calculated by dividing the number of bleeding sites by the number of total sites (where total sites equal the number of teeth present times six probe sites per tooth). Bleeding sites are charted in Figure 8-7, and a percentage has been calculated for four teeth.

6. FURCATION INVOLVEMENT:

A furcation is the branching point on a multi-rooted tooth. Normally, furcations cannot be clinically probed because they are filled in with bone and periodontal attachment. With advancing periodontal disease, however, attachment loss and bone loss may reach a furcation area resulting in a **furcation involvement**. Pockets that extend into the furcation create areas with difficult access for the dentist and dental hygienist to clean during regular office visits, and are a real challenge for patients to reach and clean during their normal home care. Therefore, these areas of furcation involvement readily accumulate soft plaque deposits and mineralized calculus. These deposits frequently become impossible to remove and may provide a pathway for periodontal disease to continue to progress (Fig. 8-9).

FIGURE 8-9. **Calculus in the furcation area and root depressions**: **A.** Extracted molar with mineralized deposits (calculus) extending into the furcation. Once disease progresses into the furcation area, access for removal by the dentist or hygienist becomes exceedingly difficult. **B.** Calculus deposit (arrow) in the longitudinal depression on the mesial side of the root of a maxillary first premolar.

    With advancing periodontal disease, attachment loss and bone loss may reach the furcation area. At that point there may be an incipient (initial or beginning) furcation involvement. As disease progresses into the inter-radicular (furcation) area, attachment loss and bone loss will change directions and begin to progress horizontally between the roots. At that point, a furcation probe (a blunt curved instrument) can be used to detect the concavity between roots (Fig 8.10). The first sign of detectable furcation involvement is termed Grade I, and can progress to a Grade II involvement when the probe can hook the furcation roof (the part of the root forming the most coronal portion of the furcal area). In the most extreme circumstances, the furcation probe may actually extend from the furcation of one tooth aspect to the furcation on another tooth aspect. This is referred to as a through-and-through (Grade III) furcation involvement. (A summary of the grades of furcation involvement is presented in Table 8-4.)

    The location of the furcation is an important consideration (Table 8-3). Recall that mandibular molar furcations are located near the midbuccal and midlingual (between mesial and distal roots); maxillary molar furcations are located midbuccal (between mesiobuccal and distobuccal roots), mesially (between palatal and mesiobuccal roots), and distally (between palatal and distobuccal roots). Clinically, more coronal furcations will become involved with periodontal disease more readily than more apically positioned furcations since less bone destruction is required to expose the

FIGURE 8-10. **Probing to check for furcation involvement**: Severe buccal furcation involvement on a mandibular second molar. The furcation probe is able to engage far into the interradicular area because of periodontal destruction. (Note the arrow pointing to an abscessed area indicating infection.)

Table 8-3

NORMAL LOCATION OF FURCATIONS

TOOTH TYPE	POTENTIAL FURCATIONS
MAXILLARY MOLARS	Mid-buccal
	Mesial (accessed from the lingual)
	Distal (accessed from the lingual)
MANDIBULAR MOLARS	Mid-buccal
	Mid-lingual
MAXILLARY PREMOLARS	Middle of mesial
(with buccal and lingual roots)	Middle of distal

more cervical furcation. However, more coronally positioned furcations are more easily treated by traditional periodontal therapy due in part to improved access. Recall that the furcation is closer to the cementoenamel junction on first molars (their root trunks are shorter) than on second molars, and closer to the cementoenamel junction on second molars than on thirds (Fig. 8-11). The more apical the furcation, the more complex the treatment will become. The maxillary first premolar provides a good example of a furcation that is located nearer to the apex (Fig. 8-9B). *Proximal* furcations, once they are involved with disease, are particularly difficult to gain access to because of vertical longitudinal depressions coronal to the furcation and close approximation to adjacent teeth (Fig. 8-12).

Technique to Document Furcation Involvement

When probing into a potential furcation area, the furcation probe should be positioned at the gingival line at the location around the tooth where the furcation is suspected. The probe should first be directed apically. When the bottom of the pocket is reached, the probe should be directed toward the tooth to engage the roof of the furcation. The notation used to record each grade of furcation is summarized in Table 8-4, and examples of charting furcation involvement are presented in Figure 8-7.

7. MUCOGINGIVAL DEFECTS:

A width of **keratinized gingiva** (recall Fig. 8-1) normally surrounds each tooth, extending from the gingival line to the mucogingival line. Mucosa apical to the mucogingival junction is more moveable,

FIGURE 8-11. Variations in furcation location for maxillary molars. a. Divergent roots with the furcation in the coronal one third of the root with a short root trunk. **b.** Convergent roots with the furcation in the middle one half of the root with a longer root trunk. **c.** Very convergent roots. **d.** Fused roots with the furcation in the coronal one-third of the root.

FIGURE 8-12. Radiograph showing close root approximation between the distal root of the maxillary first molar and the mesial root of the second molar (arrows). Furcations and concavities like these are virtually inaccessible when destruction occurs at those locations.

Table 8-4

NOTATIONS FOR THREE CATEGORIES OF FURCATION INVOLVEMENT

FURCATION GRADE	NOTATION	BONE/ATTACHMENT LOSS	CLINICAL FINDING	CLINICAL EXPLANATION
Grade I: incipient	Caret: ∨ or ∧	No real bone loss No attachment loss in furcation	Probe engages concavity	Probe locks horizontally; doesn't catch furcation roof.
Grade II: moderate	Open triangle: △ or ▽	Definite bone loss or attachment loss	Probe catches furcation roof	Probe hooks onto roof of furcation and must be rotated to disengage but probe cannot be passed to another tooth aspect
Grade III: (through-and through)	Solid triangle: ▲ or ▼	Complete bone loss with clinical attachment loss under the furcation roof	Probe can pass from one tooth aspect to another	

more vascular (redder), less firm, and non-keratinized. In health, a width of **attached gingiva** is that portion of the keratinized gingiva that is firmly bound to the underlying tooth and/or bone.

A **mucogingival defect** (Fig. 8.5A and B) is present in the following three circumstances:

a. Keratinized gingiva is present but there is a lack of *attached* gingiva. This condition is confirmed when the periodontal probe depth of the gingival sulcus reaches or exceeds (traverses) the external mucogingival junction indicating an absence of attached gingiva. In this case keratinized gingiva may form part of the pocket wall, but it is not attached to the underlying structures.

b. There is a lack of keratinized gingiva.

c. A frenum inserts onto the marginal tissues so that when tension is applied there is movement or blanching at the margins.

Mucogingival defects are most likely to be present on the aspects of teeth where the normal keratinized attached gingiva is adjacent to the movable alveolar mucosa; in other words, on the facial aspects of maxillary teeth, and the facial and lingual aspects of mandibular teeth (examples are presented in Fig. 8-5 A and B). It is very unusual for mucogingival defects to be present on the palatal aspects of maxillary teeth where the entire palate is keratinized to the midline. The only exception is when teeth are positioned so far posteriorly that they are near the *soft* palate. Mucogingival defects may place a tooth at risk for progressive gingival recession.

Technique for Determining Mucogingival Defects

Both visual observations and measurements are required for detecting mucogingival defects. The width of keratinized gingiva should first be measured. If the periodontal probe depth reaches or exceeds the mucogingival junction, a mucogingival defect is noted on the chart as a horizontal wavy line placed over the root apical to recession readings. See the charting example in Figure 8-7.

8. THE PLAQUE INDEX:

Bacterial dental plaque is a thin layer containing organized microorganisms which loosely adheres to teeth, but can be removed with proper tooth brushing. It is an almost *invisible* layer which accumulates on teeth in the absence of excellent oral hygiene. Therefore, applying a mechanism to identify the location of this nearly invisible plaque can be helpful when teaching plaque removal techniques, and when monitoring a person's success using specific oral hygiene techniques designed to reduce and eliminate their plaque.

The metabolism of these attached, organized colonies of microorganisms contributes to the inflammation of gingival tissue associated with gingivitis, the destruction of bone and periodontal ligament associated with periodontitis, as well as the destruction of mineralized tooth structure during the formation of dental decay (dental caries). Many factors contribute to plaque retention, including tooth malpositions and malformations, the irregular surface of advancing dental caries (decay), defective restorations, and accumulation of calculus (tartar).

Technique to Determine Plaque Index (Score)

Plaque can be stained with *disclosing solution*, a dye that is absorbed by bacterial plaque. When this solution is swished in the mouth, four tooth surfaces of each tooth are usually evaluated for the presence of the stained plaque: mesial, facial, distal and lingual. The **plaque index** is calculated as the percentage of sites with plaque divided by the total sites (number of teeth times 4). Note: Disclosing solutions should not be used until periodontal measurements and the oral physical exam have been made and reviewed since the color change to oral tissues from the solution may influence the ability to observe the initial findings. A charting example is presented for four teeth in Figure 8-7.

E. RELATIONSHIP OF PERIODONTAL DISEASE AND RESTORATIONS (FILLINGS)

A healthy **biologic width** of attached gingiva (known as the dentogingival junction) includes the junctional epithelium (about 1 mm wide) as well as a band of connective tissue fibers (about 1 mm wide) attaching the gingiva to the cementum. Care must be taken when restoring teeth to protect this biological width of attachment. If a restoration encroaches into the attachment, it could be a factor in initiating periodontal disease (periodontitis/bone loss/attachment loss), gingival recession, or chronically inflamed gingival tissue. Therefore, if a restoration is to be placed to restore an area of decay that has destroyed tooth structure very close to bone, it is advisable to perform a surgical procedure (called **crown lengthening**) to ensure the restoration does not encroach on the biologic width. Crown lengthening is a procedure that increases the extent of supragingival tooth structure by causing surgical recession through removal of gingival tissue, or apical positioning gingival tissue and usually removing supporting bone.

Further, a defective restoration, especially one that is overcontoured or is not flush with the tooth structure, may retain bacterial plaque more readily, so it could be an initiating factor for periodontal disease. Therefore, it is always important to keep in mind that when teeth must be restored, ideal tooth contours, as have been discussed in the earlier chapters of this text, should be reproduced.

F. RELATIONSHIPS OF TOOTH SUPPORT AND ROOT MORPHOLOGY

The area of root attachment is of primary importance to the stability and health of a tooth. Root attachment area depends on root length, the number of roots, and the cross-sectional diameter of the root from the cementoenamel junction to the apex (Fig. 8-13). It also depends on the presence or absence of concavities and other root curvatures. These features greatly influence the resistance of a tooth to occlusal and other forces, particularly when they are applied in a lateral (buccolingual) direction.

In health, prior to periodontal disease, connective tissue fibers insert into cementum on the entire root surface. This attachment represents insertion of the *gingival fibers* (supracrestal) near the cementoenamel junction, and *periodontal ligament fiber* insertions for the majority of the root. Long roots and wide cross-sectional tooth diameters increase support. Concavities and other root curvatures increase periodontal support in two ways. First, they augment the total surface area. Secondly, the concave configuration provides multidirectional fiber orientation, which makes the tooth more stable and resistant to occlusal forces. For example, a root with a mesial concavity is more resistant to buccolingual forces than a tooth that is conical or convex (Fig. 8-13). Vertical and longitudinal depressions and concave areas occur commonly on the mesial and distal root surfaces of many anterior and most posterior teeth (see Section III of this chapter for a detailed summary of these root depressions). More coronally located root

FIGURE 8-13. **Series of stained cross-sections of a root** of a lower first molar from crown to near apices. For each section, the mesial aspect is left, the lingual aspect is above, the distal aspect is right, and the buccal aspect is below. There is a 10-mm scale between the top and the middle section on the left. **A.** Cross-section through the crown showing enamel, dentin, and pulp. (Caries is evident distally—on the right.) **B.** Cross-section near the cementoenamel junction. Note the shape of the pulp chamber. **C.** Cross-section of the root trunk slightly coronal to the bifurcation (furcation). Buccal and lingual depressions are coronal to the entrances to the bifurcation. **D.** Cross-section of mesial and distal roots slightly apical to the bifurcation. Note the root canals. Thickened cementum (darkly stained) is apparent on the furcal aspect (between the roots). **E.** Cross-section of roots 4 mm apical to the bifurcation. There are pronounced concavities on the mesial aspect of the mesial root and the furcal aspects of both roots. **F.** Cross-section of the roots near the apex. The mesial (left) root is longer. The complex shape of molar roots helps provide a greater surface area of attachment and greater tooth stability, but becomes a problem to treat during progressive periodontal disease.

depressions are also found on the mesial surface of maxillary first premolars (both on the root and crown), and on molar root surfaces just coronal to furcations.

Likewise, multirooted teeth have increased support and force resistance. For those teeth, the location of the furcation is important; the more coronal it is, the more stability is afforded. Additionally, convergence or divergence of roots influences support. Divergent roots increase stability and allow for more interradicular bone support (Fig. 8-11).

Another important factor for determining tooth stability is the degree of root taper. Teeth with conical roots, such as mandibular first premolars, tend to have the majority of their root area (greater than 60%) in the coronal half of the root, and much less area (only about 40%) in the apical half of the root (Fig. 8-14).[6] The degree of root taper influences the support once periodontal disease has occurred. *A conical root may have lost more than 60% of the periodontal ligament, even though it has lost only 50% of the bone height.* This is because a small proportion of the root area is present near the apex. For severely conical roots, the apical half of the root may account for even less attachment area than seen in Figure 8-14.

MEAN RELATIONSHIP BETWEEN AREA OF ATTACHMENT AND ROOT HEIGHT

FIGURE 8-14. Relationship between the area of attachment and root length for a lower first premolar. Approximately 60% of the root area is present in the coronal one-half of the root, with only 40% of the area present in the apical one-half of the root. These determinations were made by measuring the areas of many serial cross-sections of tooth roots as shown in Figure 8-13. (Courtesy of Alan R. Levy, D.D.S.)

Based on root area alone, one would generally expect to find the maxillary canine to be the most stable single-rooted tooth, and the mandibular central incisors to be the least stable. For posterior teeth, one would expect the maxillary first molar, with its three divergent roots, to be more stable than the third molars, which frequently have fused roots. While these rules generally apply, additional factors, such as the presence or absence of inflammatory periodontal disease and excessive occlusal forces, may greatly influence tooth stability. Also, the density and structure of the supporting bone have an influence on tooth stability.

G. INFLUENCE OF ROOT ANATOMY AND ANOMALIES ON PERIODONTAL DISEASE

Although furcations, concavities, vertical grooves, and other root curvatures tend to increase the area of attachment, making the tooth resistant to occlusal forces, these root anatomy features may also become foci where forces are concentrated. These foci occur because the root curvatures, and the corresponding bone and periodontal ligaments that conform to it, permit the tooth to compress against periodontal ligament and bone in a variety of directions. Furthermore, these foci are more plaque retentive and more difficult to clean once periodontal disease progression reaches them.

There are several types of defects in the root structure that weaken periodontal attachment and are potential areas for periodontal disease to develop. Enamel extensions frequently occur on mandibular molars, and enamel pearls often are present on maxillary molars (Fig. 8-15). Both prevent a normal connective tissue attachment and may channel disease into the furcation area. Palatal gingival grooves occur on maxillary incisors and readily collect and retain plaque, which can frequently lead to periodontal destruction (Fig. 8-16). Root fractures also predispose periodontal destruction (loss of attachment of the periodontal ligament) along the fracture line.

H. PERIODONTAL THERAPY

Currently there is a wide range of techniques available to treat periodontal problems. Non-surgical periodontal therapy is traditionally centered around effective root planing (debridement), oral hygiene instructions, and the use of systemically administered antibiotics. More recently, sustained release antimicrobial and antibiotic agents are being locally administered to affected sites. Additionally, agents that prevent breakdown in connective tissue (anticollagenases) are being prescribed for systemic use.

Conservative surgical therapy is designed to gain access to the root surface for debridement.[7] Resective periodontal surgery is performed to correct some of the results of periodontal diseases by removal of soft and hard tissue components of the pocket wall. Resective techniques include gingivectomy (both through the conventional scalpel and the more recent use of the laser),[8] root resection to remove periodontally involved roots on multi-rooted teeth,[9] and periodontal flaps with osseous surgery.[10] Resective periodontal surgery usually results in gingival recession with enhanced access to previously diseased sites. Regenerative periodontal surgery is intended to attain new cementum, new bone, and a new functionally

FIGURE 8-15. Anomalies on roots that may contribute to increased plaque retention and subsequent bone loss and furcation involvement. A. Enamel pearl in the mesial furcation of a maxillary molar. B. Enamel extension (arrow) downward into the buccal furcation of a lower second molar. (Courtesy of Charles Solt, D.D.S., and Todd Needham, D.D.S.)

FIGURE 8-16. Palatal gingival groove. A. Indentation on the lingual surface of both maxillary lateral incisors. B. Periodontal probe in place showing a deep periodontal pocket formed where the groove extends apically on the root. C. Groove extending apically on the midpalatal aspect of a maxillary canine. The tooth was extracted because of severe periodontal disease on the palatal aspect. (Courtesy of Leonard K. Ebel, D.D.S.)

oriented periodontal ligament. Recent advances in the area of periodontal regeneration involve three basic strategies. In guided tissue regeneration, a resorbable or non-resorbable membrane (barrier) is placed over bone and the periodontal defect and beneath the gingiva to exclude epithelium and allow for regenerative cells to migrate from the periodontal ligament and bone. Bone grafting materials, both synthetic and from the patient or from donors, create a scaffolding for new bone and may provide growth factors that induce bone regeneration. Chemical treatment of the root detoxifies the root surface and may allow the application of growth factors that induce the formation of new cementum. Periodontal plastic surgery includes soft tissue reconstructive techniques such as connective tissue grafts designed to treat mucogingival defects and cover roots which have been exposed through gingival recession[11] and clinical crown lengthening techniques to create esthetic tooth lengths, ideal gingival contours and allow for restoration.

LEARNING QUESTIONS

Learning Questions About Periodontal Considerations

Unless stated otherwise, each item may have more than one correct answer.

1. Which of the following descriptors apply (applies) to normal, healthy gingiva?
   a. coral pink or pink with masking melanin
   b. resilient
   c. stippled
   d. spongy
   e. knife edged in profile

2. Which of the following locations is likely to have a root furcation?
   a. buccal of the root of the maxillary molar
   b. buccal of the root of the mandibular molar
   c. mesial of the root of a maxillary molar
   d. distal of the root of a mandibular molar
   e. lingual of the root of a mandibular molar

3. Which one maxillary tooth has its furcation closest to the cervical line of the tooth?
   a. first premolar
   b. second premolar
   c. first molar
   d. second molar
   e. third molar

4. What is the clinical attachment loss of a tooth with +2 mm of gingival recession and a 4 mm pocket?
   a. +2 mm
   b. +6 mm
   c. −6 mm
   d. −2 mm

5. Which of the following periodontal fibers attach to cementum and alveolar bone?
   a. horizontal
   b. oblique
   c. transseptal
   d. apical
   e. alveolar crest

ANSWERS: 1–a, b; c, e; 2–a, b, c, e; 3–c; 4–b; 5–a, b, d, e.

SECTION II. Internal Pulp Cavity Morphology Related to Endodontic and Restorative Therapy[b]

OBJECTIVES

This chapter is designed to prepare the learner to perform the following:
- Describe the four types of root canal configurations I-IV.
- Describe the shape and location of the pulp chamber for each class of tooth.
- Identify the number of canals most likely to be found within the roots of each type of secondary (adult) tooth.
- Describe the scope of responsibility for an endodontist.
- Describe endodontic therapy.

A.   THE SHAPE OF PULP CAVITIES AND CONFIGURATION OF PULP CANALS

The **pulp cavity** is the cavity in the central portion of the tooth containing the nerves and blood supply to the tooth. It is divided into the pulp chamber (more coronal) and the root canals (in the roots).

1.   PULP CHAMBER

The **pulp chamber** is the most occlusal or incisal portion of the pulp cavity. It may be located partly in the crown of anterior teeth, but is mostly in the cervical part of the root of posterior teeth. Its walls are the innermost surface of the dentin. There is one pulp chamber in each tooth. Each pulp chamber has a *roof* at its incisal or occlusal border often with projections called **pulphorns**, and the pulp chambers of multirooted teeth have a *floor* at the cervical portion with an opening (orifice) for each root canal (Fig. 8-17).

2.   ROOT CANALS (PULP CANALS)

Root canals (pulp canals) are the portions of the pulp cavity located within the root(s) of a tooth. Root canals connect to the pulp chamber through **canal orifices** on the floor of the pulp chamber, and open to the outside of the tooth through openings called **apical foramen** (plural foramina) most commonly located at or near the root apex (Fig. 8.17). The shape and number of root canals in any one root have been anatomically divided into four major configurations (Fig. 8-18). The Type I configuration has one canal, whereas Types II, III, and IV have either *two* canals, or one canal which is spilt into *two* for part of the root. The four canal types are defined as follows:

Enamel —
Dentin —
Pulp chamber —
Root (pulp) canals —
Apical foramen —

— Roof of pulp chamber
— Pulp horn
— Floor of pulp chamber
— Orifice from chamber to canal
— Accessory canal

FIGURE 8-17. Parts of a pulp cavity. The pulp cavity of this mandibular second molar is made up of a coronal pulp chamber and two root (pulp) canals.

---

[b] This section was provided by Al Reader, D.D.S., M.S., Professor, Department of Restorative Dentistry, Prosthodontics & Endodontics, The Ohio State University.

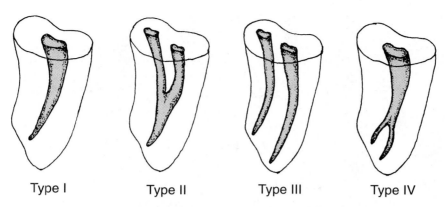

Type I   Type II   Type III   Type IV

FIGURE 8-18. Types of Canal Configurations occurring in one root.

Type I—*one canal* extends from the pulp chamber to the apex.

Type II—*two separate canals* leave the pulp chamber but they join short of the apex to form one canal apically, and one apical foramen.

Type III—*two separate canals* leave the pulp chamber and remain separate, exiting the root apically as two separate apical foramina.

Type IV—one canal leaves the pulp chamber but divides in the apical third of the root into *two separate canals* with two separate apical foramina.

Accessory (or lateral) canals also occur, located most commonly in the apical third of the root (Fig. 8-19) and, in maxillary and mandibular molars, in the furcation area [64% of the time[12]].

FIGURE 8-19. Accessory canals. A. A scanning electron photomicrograph of an instrumented (cleaned) root canal of a maxillary central incisor. After cleaning the root canal, the tooth was split and mounted for viewing with the scanning electron microscope. This view shows the apex of the tooth at the top of the picture and includes the apical third of the root. Near the bottom of the picture (right wall of canal), an accessory canal can be seen. This canal contains blood vessels. (Bar = 1 μm.) *(continued)*

FIGURE 8-19. *(continued)* **B.** A scanning electron photomicrograph at a higher power of the accessory canal observed in **A.** The blood vessel can be seen emerging from the dentin. This vessel appears to be a vein due to its thin walls and large size. The adherent "stringy" extensions around the blood vessels are supporting collagen fiber bundles. The dentinal tubules can be observed on the right side of photomicrograph. (Bar = 125 mm.) (Courtesy of Dr. Dennis Foreman, Department of Oral Biology, College of Dentistry, Ohio State University.)

B.   SHAPE OF PULP CAVITIES IN SOUND YOUNG TEETH

LEARNING EXERCISE

Section extracted teeth to expose the pulp cavity: The size, shape, and variations or pulp cavities are best studied by the interesting operation of grinding off one side of an extracted tooth. Wearing a mask and gloves, you can use a dental lathe equipped with a fine-grained abrasive wheel about 3 inches in diameter and 3/8-inch thick to remove any part of the tooth. Simply decide which surface is to be removed, hold the tooth securely in your fingers, and apply this surface firmly to the flat surface of the abrasive wheel. Operating the lathe at a fairly high speed is less apt to flip the specimen from your fingers than operating it at a low speed. If you can devise an arrangement by which a small stream of water is run onto the surface of the wheel as the tooth is ground, you will eliminate flying tooth dust and the bad odor of hot tooth tissue. If such an arrangement is not feasible, keep the tooth moist by frequently dipping the surface being ground in water or by dripping water onto the wheel with a medicine dropper. Look often at the tooth surface you are cutting and adjust your applied pressure to attain the plane in which you wish the tooth to be cut. A high-speed dental handpiece and bur will greatly facilitate your exploration of the insides of teeth.

Extracted teeth should always be kept moist or wet with buffered neutral formalin as described in the introduction of this text. As you remove different sides of each kind of tooth, notice how the inside shape has irregularities similar to the external morphology. On incisors and canines, either the mesial or distal side should be removed from some teeth, and the facial or lingual side removed from others. This way, the shape of the pulp cavity can be seen from both the mesiodistal and labiolingual planes.

On premolars and molars, the removal of either the mesial or distal side will expose the outline of the roof of the pulp chamber, which has pulp horns extending beneath the cusps (see Figs. 8-23, 8-24, and 8-25). When the buccal or lingual sides are removed to the level of the buccal and lingual cusp tips, the shape of the pulp cavities in a mesiodistal plane seen in Figure 8-28 (A and B) is similar to that seen on a dental radiograph. Also, on molars, the removal of the occlusal surface will reveal the openings (orifices) to the root canals on the floor of the pulp chamber (Fig. 8-27).

1. **PULP SHAPE IN ANTERIOR TEETH (INCISORS AND CANINES)**

a. **Pulp Chamber of Anterior Teeth**

When cut mesiodistally and viewed from the facial (or lingual) (similar to the view on dental radiographs), the pulp chambers of incisors are broad and may have a suggestion of mesial and distal horns. (See the maxillary central incisors in Fig. 8-20.) A young tooth may show the configuration of mamelons at the incisal border of the pulp wall (roof of chamber). When cut labiolingually and viewed from the proximal, the pulp chambers of anterior teeth taper to a point toward the incisal edge (Fig. 8-21). In maxillary and mandibular canines, the incisal wall or roof of the pulp chamber is often rounded (Fig. 8-22).

FIGURE 8-20. **Maxillary central incisors sectioned mesiodistally.** A. Maxillary central incisor (young tooth), facial side removed. The high pulp horns and the broad root canal indicate that this is a young tooth. This outline of the pulp cavity may be seen on a dental radiograph. B. Maxillary central incisor (old tooth), facial side removed. The pulp chamber of this older tooth is partially filled with secondary dentin and the root canal is narrower than in the tooth shown in B. Also, the incisal edge is worn to a straight line. (The damage to the cervical part of the root on the distal (left) side of the tooth has been there for some time because the underlying dentin has been altered by a defense mechanism of the pulp tissues.)

FIGURE 8-21. Incisors sectioned faciolingually. A. Maxillary central incisor, mesial side removed. There is attrition on the incisal edge, and secondary dentin has begun to fill in the incisal part of the pulp chamber. The root canal is moderately wide. As commonly occurs, much of the pulp chamber is located in the cervical third of the root. It is *not* possible to see this view of the pulp cavity on a dental radiograph. **B.** Mandibular lateral incisor, mesial side removed (young tooth). Curvature of the root prevented cutting the pulp cavity in one plane so that the apical portion was lost. Notice how the pulp cavity extends in a narrow point toward the incisal edge. Even extensive attrition on the incisal edge would not expose the pulp since secondary dentin would form in the incisal part of the pulp chamber and the pulp would be additionally protected.

FIGURE 8-22. Canines sectioned faciolingually. A. Maxillary canine, mesial side removed (young tooth). There is no attrition evident on the incisal edge and the pulp cavity is still large. **B.** Mandibular canine, mesial side removed (young tooth). The pulp cavity is large. Only at the incisal tip is there a little evidence of secondary dentin formation. The cementum is extremely thin at the cementoenamel junction, only 50 μm thick (about half as thick as this page). Care must be taken not to remove this thin lining when using scalers or pumice on teeth in this vicinity. The roof of the chamber is slightly more rounded than on incisors.

b. Root Canal(s) of Anterior Teeth

Recall that all anterior teeth are most likely to have one root. *The number of root canals in each type of anterior tooth is also most frequently one.* *Maxillary* central incisors, lateral incisors, and canines *almost always* have one canal (Type I) as seen in Figure 8-18, whereas *mandibular* anterior teeth, although *most likely* to have one canal (60% of the time), may have two canals with the frequency varying depending on the study cited.[13–15] For example, **mandibular central incisors** may have two canals with two separate apical foramina (Type III) 3% of the time, and two canals converging to one foramen (Type II) from 17 to 43% of the time. **Mandibular lateral incisors** may have two canals from 20 to 45% of the time (usually Type II with one foramen, or Type III with two separate foramina about 3% of the time). **Mandibular canines** may have two canals from 4 to 22% of the time.

2. PULP SHAPE IN PREMOLARS

a. Pulp Chambers in Premolars

When premolars are cut mesiodistally and viewed from the facial (or lingual) similar to the view on dental radiographs, the occlusal border or roof of the pulp chamber is curved beneath the cusp similarly to the curvature of the occlusal surface. When cut buccolingually and viewed from the proximal, the pulp chamber often has the general outline of the tooth surface, sometimes including a constriction near or apical to the cervix. The pulp horns on the roof are visible beneath each cusp, and their relative lengths are similar to the relative heights of the cusps. Thus, the buccal horn is longer than the lingual horn (Fig. 8-23).

b. Root Canal(s) of Premolars

Maxillary first premolars *most often have two roots and two canals.* Approximately 57% of these first premolars have two roots but only 37% have one root.[16] The average incidence of two canals, one in the buccal root and one in the lingual root, is 90%. [When two roots are present, the canals in both roots exhibit a Type I configuration, and, when one root is present, the canal configuration is either a Type II or Type III.[17]] The incidence of three canals is approximately 3%.[17] The dentist must know the location of each canal opening on the pulp chamber floor in order to remove diseased pulpal tissue from the *entire* pulp cavity. The buccal canal orifice in the maxillary first premolar (viewed with the roof of the pulp chamber removed) is located just lingual to the buccal cusp tip. The lingual canal orifice is located just lingual to the central groove (Fig. 8-26).

Maxillary second premolars most often have *one root,* but may have one or two canals. The average incidence of two canals is about 50% [Type II or Type III, as seen in Fig. 8-18].[17] Three

FIGURE 8-23. Maxillary First Premolar Sectioned Faciolingually. Mesial side removed (young tooth). The curvature of the tips of the roots prevented cutting the root canals in one plane. The pulp horns are sharp, there is little, if any, secondary dentin, and the floor of the pulp chamber is rounded. The buccal pulp horn is considerably longer than the lingual horn. Notice the floor of the pulp chamber, which has two openings, one for each canal. Also note the constriction of the pulp chamber near the cervix.

canals occur about 1% of the time.[17] When there is one canal, its orifice on the pulp chamber floor is located in the exact center of the tooth (Fig. 8-26). If the orifice is located toward the buccal or the lingual, it probably means there are two canals in the root.

Mandibular first and second premolars most frequently have *one root* and *one root canal* (Type I) about 70% of the time in first premolars and 96% in second premolars. Mandibular first premolars may have two canals (Type IV) 24% of the time, but mandibular second premolars have two canals only 2.5% of the time[18] (Fig. 8-24). The canal orifice is located on the floor of the pulp chamber just buccal to the center of the occlusal surface (see Fig. 8-26).

3. PULP SHAPE IN MOLARS

The pulp chamber of **maxillary first and second molars** is broader buccolingually than mesiodistally (like the crown) and is often constricted near the floor of the chamber. On **mandibular first and second molars**, the chamber is broader mesiodistally than buccolingually. As in all cusped teeth, pulp horns on molars are located in the roof of the pulp chamber well beneath each cusp. The pulp chamber is normally deep to, or some distance from, the occlusal surface (Fig. 8-25). Surprisingly, the pulp chamber on maxillary molars often is not penetrated by the dentist until the drill reaches the level of the gum line. One exception might be the pulp horn of the prominent mesiolingual cusp of the maxillary molars. The floor of the pulp chamber is considerably apical to the cervical line; it is located in the root trunk. The pulp floor has multiple openings, one for each root canal. The floor is level or flat in young teeth. It may become convex in older teeth with the deposition of additional dentin over time.

Maxillary first molars most frequently have *three roots, but four canals*; one each in the distobuccal and palatal root; two in the mesiobuccal root. In the **palatal root**, the canal is larger and more easily accessible from the floor of the pulp chamber than for the other two roots, but this root and its canal often curve toward the buccal in the *apical* third, requiring skillful procedures to clean and treat it. The **mesiobuccal root** of the maxillary first molar has two canals 90% of the time [one located more buccally within this root called *mesiobuccal canal*, and one located more lingually within this root called the *mesiolingual canal*.[19] Type III canal systems have been reported to occur 33–60% of the time.[19]]

On maxillary first molars, there are four orifices on the floor of the pulp chamber: one for each canal (Figs. 8-26 and 8-27). Opening into the palatal root, the palatal orifice on the floor of the pulp chamber is located beneath the mesiolingual cusp. Opening into the mesiobuccal root, the mesiobuccal ori-

FIGURE 8-24. Mandibular First Premolars Sectioned Faciolingually. A. Mandibular first premolar, distal side removed. Root curvature prevented cutting the root canal in one plane. The pulp horn in the buccal cusp is large; in the lingual cusp it is small. It is unusual to observe much of a pulp horn beneath the nonfunctional lingual cusp on mandibular first premolars. **B.** Mandibular first premolar, mesial side removed, with root and root canal divided near the apex (Type IV).

FIGURE 8-25. Maxillary First Molars Sectioned Buccolingually. A. Young tooth with mesial side removed; lingual side (with cusp of Carabelli) is on the right. The tooth is sectioned through the center of the lingual root canal, but not through the center of the mesiobuccal canal. The pulp chamber is seen to open into the lingual root canal. The floor of the pulp chamber is relatively flat as it often is on young teeth. **B.** Young tooth with mesial side removed; lingual side is on the left. There is an area of dental caries in the groove where the small cusp of Carabelli is attached to the mesiolingual cusp. The tooth is sectioned through the mesiobuccal and lingual root canals. The pulp chamber is mostly in the root trunk. Only mesiobuccal and mesiolingual pulp horns extend a little into the part of tooth we define as the anatomic crown (covered with enamel).

Endodontic access openings

Maxillary teeth | Mandibular teeth

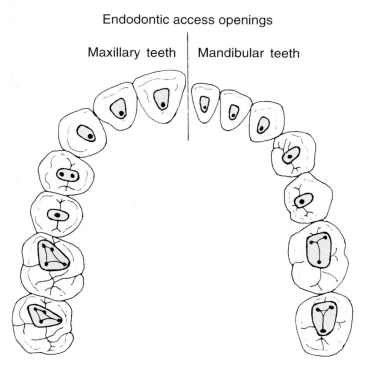

FIGURE 8-26. Access Preparations Into Pulp Chambers. Ideally shaped openings providing access into the pulp chamber for endodontic treatment. Pulp canal orifices on the floor of each pulp chamber correspond with the number and location of pulp canals in each tooth. The left half of the arch shows maxillary teeth; the right half shows mandibular teeth.

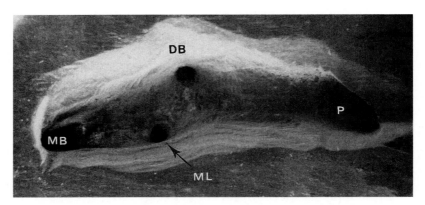

FIGURE 8-27. Scanning electron photomicrograph of the pulp chamber floor of a maxillary molar with four canal orifices. The palatal (P), mesiobuccal (MB), distobuccal (DB), and mesiolingual (ML-arrow) orifices are identified for orientation. (Original magnification x20.) (Courtesy of Dr. James Gilles and Dr. Al Reader.)

fice is located slightly mesial to and beneath the mesiobuccal cusp tip. The mesiolingual orifice is located slightly to the palatal aspect of the mesiobuccal orifice. Usually, this orifice is difficult to locate because of an overhanging dentinal shelf. Opening into the distobuccal root, the distobuccal canal orifice is located on a line between the palatal orifice and the buccal developmental groove at a point just short of the angle formed by the buccal and distal walls of the pulp chamber.

Maxillary second molars, like maxillary first molars, most frequently have *three roots and four canals*. The distobuccal and palatal roots each have one canal. The mesiobuccal root has two canals 70% of the time.[19] The location of the orifices in the maxillary second molar is similar to the maxillary first molar, except that they are closer together (Fig. 8-26).

Both mandibular first and second molars most frequently have *two roots* (mesial and distal) and *three canals* (two in the wider mesial root and one in the distal root). The roof of the pulp chamber is often about at the same level as the cervical border of the enamel, with only the pulp horns extending into the anatomic crown (Fig. 8-28). Most of the pulp chamber is located within the root trunk. The

FIGURE 8-28. Mandibular first molars sectioned mesiodistally. A. Buccal side removed (old tooth). The apical foramen of the distal root is on the distal side of the root, not at the root tip. The unusual thickening of cementum on the roots is hypercementosis. B. Old tooth (exhibiting occlusal wear) with lingual side removed. Again, notice that the roof of the pulp chamber is about at the level of the cervical line. The pulp horns extend occlusal to the cervical line. The rest of the pulp chamber is in the root trunk. The floor of the pulp chamber is convex (a condition founded in older teeth) because of the deposition of secondary dentin. (There appears to be caries in the enamel above the mesiolingual pulp horn, but it has penetrated only slightly into the dentin.)

mesial root usually has two canals: *mesiobuccal* and *mesiolingual*. [The mesial root of mandibular *first* molars have two canals virtually all of the time: a Type III canal system is present 60% of the time and a Type II canal system is present 40% of the time.[17,20] The mesial roots of mandibular *second* molars have two canals 64% of the time: a Type II canal system 38% of the time and a Type III canal system 26% of the time, but one canal 27% of the time.[18]] The **distal root** of mandibular first and second molars usually have one canal [but on mandibular first molars there are two canals approximately 35% of the time, usually Type II configuration,[21] whereas the distal roots of mandibular second molars have one canal 92% of the time[18]].

In both mandibular first and second molars, the mesiobuccal canal orifice on the chamber floor is located slightly mesial and close to the *mesiobuccal* cusp tip (Fig. 8-26). The *mesiolingual* canal orifice is just lingual to the mesial developmental groove of the mesial marginal ridge. It is not under the mesiolingual cusp tip, but is in a more central location. If the distal root has one canal, the *distal canal orifice* is large and located just distal to the center of the crown. When two canals are present, the distolingual orifice is small and is located centrally just lingual to the central fossa. Careful inspection of the chamber floor toward the buccal will successfully locate the distobuccal orifice.

Maxillary third molars usually have three root canals and **mandibular third molars** usually have two. However, they do vary considerably in form with some teeth having only two root canals. Third molars are 9–11 years younger biologically than first molars, completing their development later in life than first and second molars. Therefore, on radiographs (x-ray films), their pulp chambers and root canals are generally larger than in the other molars in the same mouth, especially for patients between the ages of 15 and 35 years. Teeth, other than third molars, exhibiting unusually large pulp chambers on dental radiographs are immediately suspected to have necrotic pulps, which are a possible source of infection. Without vital pulp tissue, dentin formation ceases, and the pulp chamber size remains constant (once the pulp died) rather than continuing to decrease in size as is normal for vital teeth.

4. PULP SHAPE IN DECIDUOUS TEETH

The shape of the pulp chamber in **deciduous teeth** will be discussed in detail in the next chapter. Briefly, these teeth generally have thinner amounts of dentin and enamel so their pulp cavities are proportionally much larger than on secondary teeth and their pulp horns are closer to the occlusal surface.

C. WHY PULP CAVITIES GET SMALLER IN OLDER TEETH

In a young tooth, the pulp chamber is large and resembles the shape of the crown surface. It has projections called horns extending beneath the cusps or mamelons in the roof of the chamber and is usually constricted somewhat at the cervix. In old teeth, the pulp chamber becomes smaller and is more apically located because of deposits of secondary dentin produced by specialized cells called odontoblasts lining the pulp chamber. Dentin formation normally continues as long as the pulp is intact or vital. Dentin forms on the wall of the pulp cavity, thickening the dentin and making the pulp chamber and canals smaller. Dentin formation over a lifetime may be stimulated to occur *more rapidly* or in greater quantity when the tooth is subjected to attrition, trauma, or caries (i.e., tooth decay), or when calcium hydroxide dental cement is applied on the pulp (direct pulp cap).

The deposition of dentin over time results in reduction in size of the pulp chamber. In some cases, it may become entirely filled. Reduction in size makes endodontic access openings difficult since there is no chamber to "fall into" as in young teeth. The floor of the pulp chamber is nearly flat in young teeth, later becoming convex. In a radiographic study of 259 children in England, from their eleventh to fourteenth birthdays, the mesiodistal and roof-to-floor pulp dimensions were recorded with a Lysta-Dent Digitizer. Mesiodistal reduction in size in mandibular first molars over 3 years was minimal [1–3.5%] compared to a considerable height reduction [15%] of the pulp chambers. This was mostly the result of secondary dentin deposition on the floor, not the roof, of the chamber.[22]

The diameter of the root canal also decreases in size with age, getting small in older teeth because of the gradual addition of dentin of the internal wall over the years. The canal may be round, flat, or ribbon-shaped.

D. CLINICAL APPLICATION OF PULP MORPHOLOGY RELATED TO RESTORATIVE DENTISTRY

The dentist's knowledge of normal pulp shape and size and depth beneath the enamel is important to a successful practice because, when removing dental decay, the dentist must prepare the teeth in such a way that the pulpal soft tissues in the teeth are not disturbed or injured. For the same reason, the dentist always tries to avoid overheating or desiccating the tooth during preparation, and attempts to leave some sound (undecayed) dentin on the floor of the cavity preparation to provide support for the restoration (such as a filling using composite resin or amalgam). The dentist normally tries to avoid exposing any part of the pulp cavity when restoring the tooth with a cutting bur or hand instrument because of the danger of pulpal inflammation. This is accomplished through a knowledge of the shape of the pulp chamber and canals, and a careful evaluation of the patient's radiographs to determine the location of the pulp relative to the external surface of the tooth. The implications of dental anatomy on restorative dentistry are discussed in more detail in Chapter 12.

E. CLINICAL APPLICATION OF PULP MORPHOLOGY RELATED TO ENDODONTICS

1. ENDODONTICS DEFINED

Endodontics is a specialty branch of dentistry concerned with the morphology, physiology, and pathology of human dental pulp and periapical tissues. Its study and practice encompasses related basic and clinical sciences, including biology of the normal pulp, the etiology, diagnosis, prevention, and treatment of diseases and injuries of the pulp, and resultant pathologic periradicular conditions (that is, pathosis around the root).[23]

An **endodontist** is a dentist who specializes in endodontics (root canal therapy). An endodontist is specially trained to treat difficult and complex endodontic situations that may be referred from a general dentist. Treatment may involve difficult root canal anatomy, medically compromised patients, and/or surgical treatments of periapical pathosis and infection.

2. DIAGNOSIS OF PULPAL AND PERIAPICAL DISEASE

Irreversible pulpitis (inflammation of the pulp that cannot be healed) is a condition of the pulp tissue where root canal treatment is indicated. The tooth is unusually sensitive to cold or hot, and sometimes either stimuli may cause an exaggerated response (prolonged pain). The patient may also experience *spontaneous* pain in the tooth (that is, pain felt without provocation, such as heavy chewing, or exposure to hot or cold). The usual cause of irreversible pulpitis is deep caries (decay), although deep or poorly adapted restorations may also contribute. The proximity of caries to the pulp can often be evaluated best using dental radiographs (Fig. 8-29). As the caries approaches the pulp,

FIGURE 8-29. Dental Decay (Caries) Exposing the Pulp. Radiograph of a lower left first molar with a distal carious lesion (seen as an area of lost enamel and darkened dentin) that has exposed the pulp. There is also mesial caries on this tooth and on the second molar.

a normal defense reaction will occur involving inflammation and formation of reparative dentin. However, when the caries exposes the pulp, bacteria will overwhelm the defenses, and the tooth usually becomes painful. This prompts the patient to seek emergency dental treatment. Access to, and removal of, affected pulp tissue will provide relief from the pain. The pulp tissue *cannot* be successfully treated with medications alone once the pulp is *irreversibly* damaged.

Periapical disease occurs when the pulp has died (becomes necrotic). When the pulp has been overwhelmed by the disease process in the crown, the pulp tissue in the root canals gradually dies. The bacteria and products of pulpal breakdown contained within the root canals cause the periapical tissue around the tooth to react to this insult. A chronic inflammatory response ensues in the bone with the formation of a granuloma (that is, a mass of chronic inflammatory tissue enclosed within a fibrous capsule). Since a granuloma is less dense than bone, a radiograph will usually reveal a radiolucency (dark area at end of the root; Fig. 8-30). In some cases, the granuloma undergoes degeneration and a cyst is formed. A cyst is an epithelium lined sac filled with liquid or semiliquid material. The difference between a granuloma and cyst cannot be determined on a radiograph.

When the bacteria from the root canal overwhelm the defenses of the periapical tissues, or the patient's immune system is compromised, bacteria invade the surrounding bone and soft tissue, resulting in severe pain and/or facial swelling. Cleaning the root canals and draining the area of infection will usually provide relief within 2 to 3 days.

3. ENDODONTIC THERAPY

The *goal* of endodontic therapy is to relieve pain, control infection, and preserve the tooth so it may function normally during mastication. Endodontic treatment is normally preferred to extraction because if the tooth was extracted, the patient would be without the tooth throughout the healing process, and during the time required to construct and place the replacement tooth. Further, endodontic therapy is less expensive than having a tooth extracted and subsequently replaced with a dental prosthesis (bridge) or an implant.

Endodontic Treatment: The first step of the endodontic procedure is for the dentist to gain access to the pulp chamber and the root canals of teeth through an **access opening** in the crown of the

FIGURE 8-30. Periapical Radiolucency. Radiograph of a maxillary right canine with the dark area on the distal aspect of the root apex indicating the pulp has become necrotic and a granuloma or cyst has developed in the bone, probably as a result of the exposure of the pulp by a large distal carious lesion (seen as an area of lost enamel and darkened dentin).

tooth. On anterior teeth, the opening is made on the lingual surface and on posterior teeth through the occlusal surface. These access openings vary considerably from cavity preparations used in operative dentistry. The shape (outline form), size, and position of the access opening are determined by studying ideal openings of maxillary and mandibular teeth shown in Figure 8-26, and then modifying them to conform to what is present on the initial radiograph of the tooth. Finding the pulp may be difficult in older teeth or teeth that have large or deep restorations, since the formation of secondary or reparative dentin may obliterate the pulp chamber making endodontic access difficult. Further, if the tooth is covered with a metal crown, the pulp chamber will not be visible on the radiograph.

Once the access opening is complete, the dentist locates the root canal orifices on the floor of the pulp chamber. A knowledge of the number of root canals present in teeth is *critically important* to successful endodontic treatment. Not locating and cleaning all the canals may result in continued discomfort for the patient or unsuccessful endodontic treatment with ensuing periapical disease. When the canal orifices have been located, endodontic files are used to remove the diseased pulpal tissue, and to refine and clean the canals. The files are carefully inserted into the root canals after the file length is approximated by measuring the length of the corresponding root and crown on the preoperative radiograph. A radiograph is then made with the files in the root (Fig. 8-31). The positions and length of the files are adjusted to extend to approximately 1 mm short of the radiographic apex of the root (which corresponds to the natural constriction of the canal at the cementodentinal junction). The canals are then cleaned and shaped at this length with incrementally larger diameter files until the root canal system is clean.

Following this cleaning procedure, the root canals are filled with gutta percha (a rubber-type material) and a zinc oxide eugenol sealer (Fig. 8-32). When there is sufficient tooth structure remaining, the opening through the crown used to access the pulp may be restored with a tooth-colored composite or silver amalgam restorative material. Since teeth requiring endodontic treatment usually have large restorations or are weakened by extensive decay, tooth structure may be restored with a crown. In some instances, a post placed into the prepared root canal space is used in order to provide sufficient retention for the artificial crown.

Once a tooth has had endodontic therapy and the pulp has been removed, it should not be con-

FIGURE 8-31. Endodontic files in radiograph. Radiograph of a lower left first molar where endodontic files have been placed within the root canals to the cementodentinal junction apically.

FIGURE 8-32. Radiograph of completed endodontic Treatment. A lower left first molar where the root canals have been filled with gutta percha and sealer. The part of the crown that was lost has also been restored with a temporary filling. Both the gutta percha and the temporary filling appear whiter than enamel or dentin on the radiograph.

sidered a "dead tooth." Although it cannot respond to stimuli like hot or cold, and cannot form reparative dentin, the periodontal support is the same as if it never had endodontic treatment. Therefore, if the periodontium remains healthy, the treated tooth generally will last for the lifetime of the patient.

SECTION III. Location of Root and Cervical Crown Concavities, Furcations, Depressions, and Canals

OBJECTIVES

The purpose of this section is to summarize the shape of the external root surface, and the internal pulp shape at the level of the cementoenamel junction, and halfway down the root toward the apex. The following tooth drawings are labeled:

M = Mesial; D = Distal; F = Facial; and L = Lingual

A. MAXILLARY CENTRAL INCISORS

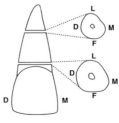

Tooth #8

- Cross-section of the root at the cervix is somewhat triangular with the mesial side longer than the distal side, consistent with the slight distal placement of the cingulum.

- There are no prominent root grooves (depressions) on this incisor, though the *mesial* surface may be flattened or have a *slight* longitudinal depression. The *distal* root surface is convex.
- It has one root canal close to 100% of the time.

B. MAXILLARY LATERAL INCISORS

Tooth #7

- The cross-section of the root at the cervix is "egg-shaped" or ovoid, with the widest mesiodistal portion on the labial.
- A shallow longitudinal root depression is often found on the middle of the *mesial* root surface extending about half of the root length, but *not* on the distal surface.
- There is one root canal close to 100% of the time.

C. MANDIBULAR CENTRAL AND LATERAL INCISORS

Tooth #25   Tooth #26

- In cross-section, the cervical portion of the root is ovoid, considerably broader labiolingually than mesiodistally [by about 2 mm].
- Longitudinal root depressions are present on *both* proximal sides with the distal depression more distinct than the mesial.
- Most commonly there is one root canal [about 70% of the time for centrals and 55% for laterals].

D. MAXILLARY CANINES

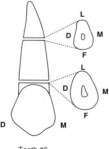

Tooth #6

- The cervical cross-section is broad labiolingually and appears ovoid.
- Developmental grooves (depressions) are present on *both* the mesial and distal sides providing better anchorage. The groove may be more distinct on the distal.
- As in other maxillary anterior teeth, there is one root canal almost 100% of the time.

E.   MANDIBULAR CANINES

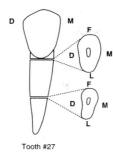

Tooth #27

- Roots are wide labiolingually in the cervical half.
- Longitudinal root depressions are present on *both* sides, often deeper on the distal.
- Variations in double-root depressions include clearly separated roots labiolingually to deep proximal grooves.
- There is most often one root canal [70% of the time].

F.   MAXILLARY FIRST PREMOLARS

Tooth #5

- There are most often two canals [90% of the time].
- Most have two roots and two canals, or when one root is present, two pulp canals are usually found.
- *M*esial and *distal* root depressions occur on both one- and two-rooted first premolars.
- The prominent *mesial* developmental depression of the crown continues across the cervical line to join the deep mesial root depression (between the buccal and lingual roots or between the buccal and lingual halves of a single root).
- When considering all premolars, it has the only root where the *mesial root depression is deeper* than a distal root depression.
- When two roots are present, the bifurcation occurs in the apical third to half of the root.

G.   MAXILLARY SECOND PREMOLARS

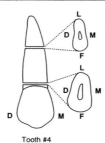

Tooth #4

- Although there is normally only one root, there may be two roots 11% of the time.
- There may be a shallow developmental groove on the *mesial* side of the root, but it does not extend onto the crown, as on the first premolar. A root depression can usually be found on the *distal* side, often deeper than on the mesial.
- There is most often one root canal [50% of the time].

H. MANDIBULAR FIRST PREMOLARS

Tooth #28

- In cross-section, the cervical portion of the root is ovoid, and is widest buccolingually.
- Longitudinal depressions are often present on *both* sides, deeper on the distal. Sometimes these depressions may be quite deep and end in a bucco-lingual apical bifurcation.
- There is usually one root canal [70% of the time].

I. MANDIBULAR SECOND PREMOLARS

Tooth #29

- Cross-section of the cervical portion of the root is ovoid buccolingually.
- Longitudinal depressions are *not* common on the mesial root surface, but are frequent on the *distal* surface in the middle third.
- The cervical cross-section of the root of the three-cusp premolars is particularly wide on the lingual, more so than on two-cusp types.
- The root is rarely bifurcated, and normally has one root canal [96% of the time].

J. MANDIBULAR FIRST AND SECOND MOLARS

Tooth #30   Tooth #31

- Mandibular molars normally have two roots: mesial (broader and longer) and distal. Both roots are broad buccolingually.
- Mandibular first *and* second molars normally have three root canals, two in the mesial root and one in the distal root.
- The *mesial root* of both molars commonly has prominent root depressions on the mesial and distal surfaces, and there are usually two root canals [nearly 100% of the time]. This root may even be divided into a buccal and lingual part. The *distal root* surface contours are more variable, but may be convex.
- The *distal roots* in the mandibular first and second molars usually have one canal [65% of the time in the first molar and 92% of the time in the second molar.]
- Access to the root bifurcations is located near midbuccal and midlingual.

- Enamel of buccal and lingual cervical lines may extend into the bifurcation (Fig. 8-15).
- The root trunk is shorter on first molars than on second molars; the furcation is nearest to the cervical line on the buccal of first molars. The cervical line is more occlusal on the lingual of first molars. Buccal and lingual depressions are seen on the relatively short root trunk, extending from the cervical lines to buccal and lingual furcations.
- First molar roots are broader and more widely separated than second molar roots, which may exhibit a distal inclination.

K. MAXILLARY FIRST AND SECOND MOLARS

Tooth #3   Tooth #2

- There are normally three roots: mesiobuccal, distobuccal (shortest), and lingual (longest).
- Maxillary first *and* second molars usually have four root canals: two in the wide mesiobuccal root, and one each in the distobuccal and lingual roots.
- The *mesiobuccal root* has mesial and distal side root depressions (and usually has *two root canals*).
- The distal contour of the *distobuccal root* varies but is normally convex (and normally has *one canal*).
- There is usually a slight longitudinal depression on the lingual side on the *lingual root* (which has *one canal*).
- Access to furcations between the roots is located in the cervical third of the root: on the buccal surface near the center mesiodistally and on the mesial and distal surfaces, located slightly lingual to the center buccolingually.
- Often a depression extends from the trifurcation to the cervical line and sometimes into the enamel of the crown on first molars.
- Separation between roots is more pronounced on first molars than on second molars; on second molars, the buccal roots are more nearly parallel and inclined distally in their apical third.
- The root trunk is broader (longer) than on mandibular molars, so the furcation between mesiobuccal and distobuccal root may be at the junction of the cervical and middle thirds of the mesiobuccal root, especially on second molars.

LEARNING QUESTIONS

Each of the following questions may have more than one correct answer.
1. Which of the following are possible indications of periodontal disease?
    a. bleeding gums
    b. loss of bone
    c. type IV mobility
    d. mucogingival stress
    e. gingival sulcus readings of 3 mm
2. The furcations are likely to be farther away from the cervical portion of the tooth in which ONE of the following teeth?
    a. mandibular first molar
    b. mandibular second molar

    c.   mandibular third molar

    d.   maxillary first molar

    e.   maxillary second molar

3. A depression associated with a furcation between roots on a maxillary first molar might be detectable on which of the following surfaces?

    a.   buccal surface

    b.   lingual surface

    c.   mesial surface

    d.   distal surface

4. Which teeth are NOT likely to have root depressions on both the mesial and distal root surface?

    a.   maxillary central and lateral incisor

    b.   maxillary canine

    c.   maxillary second premolar

    d.   mandibular second premolar

5. Maxillary anterior teeth are most likely to have how many root canals?

    a.   one

    b.   two

    c.   three

    d.   one or two

6. Maxillary first molars are most likely to have __ roots and __ root canals?

    a.   two . . . two

    b.   two . . . three

    c.   two . . . four

    d.   three . . . three

    e.   three . . . four

7. The one premolar most likely to have two roots (and two root canals) is the:

    a.   maxillary first premolar

    b.   maxillary second premolar

    c.   mandibular first premolar

    d.   mandibular second premolar

8. The two roots of a maxillary first premolar are called:

    a.   mesial and lingual

    b.   mesial and distal

    c.   buccal and mesial

    d.   buccal and lingual

    e.   mesiobuccal and distobuccal

ANSWERS: 1–a, b, c, d; 2–c; 3–a, c, d; 4–a, d; 5–a; 6–e; 7–a; 8–d.

REFERENCES

1. Burt BA. Periodontitis and aging: reviewing recent evidence. JADA 1994;125(Mar):273–279.
2. Kennedy J, Bird W, Palcanis K, Dorfman H. A longitudinal evaluation of varying widths of attached gingiva. J Clin Periodontol 1985;12:667.

3. Renner RP. An introduction to dental anatomy and esthetics. Chicago: Quintessence Publishing, 1985:162.

4. Zander H, Polson A. Present status of occlusion and occlusal therapy in periodontics. J Periodontol 1977;48:540.

5. Ericsson I, Lindhe J. Effect of long-standing jiggling on experimental marginal periodontitis in the beagle dog. J Clin Periodontol 1982;9:497.

6. Levy A, Wright W. The relationship between attachment height and attachment area of teeth using a digitizer and digital computer. J Periodontol 1978;49:483.

7. Ramfjord SP, Nissie R. The modified Widman flap. J Periodontol 1974;45:601.

8. Zakariasen KL. New and emerging techniques: promise, achievement and deception. JADA 1995;126(Feb):163.

9. Basaraba N. Root amputation and tooth hemisection. Dent Clin North Am 1969;13:121.

10. Oschenbein C. Current status of osseous surgery. J Periodontol 1977;48:577.

11. Langer B, Langer L. Subepithelial connective tissue flap for root coverage. J Periodontol 1985;56:15.

12. Perlich MA, Reader A, Foreman DW. A scanning electron microscopic investigation of accessory foramens on the pulpal floor of human molars. J Endodontics 1981;7:402–406.

13. Benjamin KA, Dowson J. Incidence of two root canals in human mandibular incisor teeth. Oral Surg 1974;38:123–126.

14. Rankine-Wilson RW, Henry P. The bifurcated root canal in lower anterior teeth. JADA 1965;70:1162–1165.

15. Bellizzi R, Hartwell G. Clinical investigation of in vivo endodontically treated mandibular anterior teeth. J Endodontics 1983;9:246–248.

16. Vertucci FJ, Gegauff A. Root canal morphology of the maxillary first premolar. JADA 1979;99:194–198.

17. Bellizzi R, Hartwell G. Radiographic evaluation of root canal anatomy of in vivo endodontically treated maxillary premolars. J Endodontics 1985;11:37–39.

18. Vertucci FJ. Root canal anatomy of the human permanent teeth. Oral Surg 1984;58:589–599.

19. Gilles J, Reader A. An SEM investigation of mesiolingual canal in human maxillary first and second molars. Oral Surg Oral Med Oral Path 1990; 70:638-643.

20. Neaverth EJ, Kotler LM, Kaltenbach RF. Clinical investigation (in vivo) of endodontically treated maxillary first molars. J Endodontics 1987;13:506–512.

21. Skidmore AE, Bjorndal AM. Root canal morphology of the human mandibular first molar. Oral Surg 1971;32:778–784.

22. Shaw L, Jones AD. Morphological considerations of the dental pulp chamber from radiographs of molar and pre-molar teeth. J Dent 1984;12:139–145.

23. The American Association of Endodontists. Web site 2000.

General References

GENERAL REFERENCES ON PERIODONTAL CONSIDERATIONS RELATED TO EXTERNAL MORPHOLOGY AND SURROUNDING STRUCTURES

Resources and Authorities for Periodontics

The American Academy of Periodontology, Suite 800, 737 North Michigan Avenue, Chicago, Illinois 60611-2690. Website: <http://www.perio.org>
The American Dental Association. 211 East Chicago Avenue, Chicago, Illinois. 60611. Website: <www.ada.org>

Resource for Periodontal Terms

Glossary of Periodontal Terms, 3rd edition. 1992. The American Academy of Periodontology, Chicago.

Basic Textbook

Carranza F, and Newman M. Clinical Periodontology, 8th Edition. Philadelphia: W.B. Saunders Company, 1996.

Resource for the pathogenesis, diagnosis, and risk factors for periodontal diseases and periodontal therapy

Proceedings of the 1996 World Workshop in Periodontics, 1996. The Annals of Periodontology. The American Academy of Periodontology, Chicago.
Periodontal Literature Reviews: a summary of current knowledge. 1996. The American Academy of Periodontology, Chicago

Resource for Periodontal Disease Classification

Amitage G. Development of a classification system for periodontal disease and conditions. Annals of Periodontology 1999; 4(1):1-6.

OTHER GENERAL REFERENCES

Estrela C, Pereira HL, Pecora JD. Radicular grooves in maxillary lateral incisor: case report. Braz Dent J 1995;6(2):143–146.

Pecora JD, Saquy PC, Sousa Neto MD, Woelfel JB. Root form and canal anatomy of maxillary first premolars. Braz Dent J 1991;2(2):87-94.

Pecora JD, Sousa Neto MD, Saquy PC, Woelfel JB. In vitro study of root canal anatomy of maxillary second premolars. Braz Dent J 1992;3(2):81–85.

Pecora JD, Woelfel JB, Sousa Neto MD. Morphologic study of the maxillary molars. Part I: External anatomy. Braz Dent J 1991;2(1):45–50.

Pecora JD, Woelfel JB, Sousa Neto MD, Issa EP. Morphologic study of the maxillary molars. Part II: Internal anatomy. Braz Dent J 1992;3(1):53–57.

Walton RE, Torabinejad M. Principles and Practice of Endodontics, Second Edition. Philadelphia: W.B. Saunders Company, 1996.

Web site: American Association of Endodontists (with information for the professional and for media/public) <http://www.aae.org/media/index.html>

Primary (and Mixed) Dentition

I. Background information
   A. Definitions
   B. Dental formulae
   C. Functions of the primary dentition
II. Developmental data for primary and secondary teeth
   A. Important times for tooth emergence
   B. Crown and root development
III. Dentition traits of all primary teeth
IV. Class and type traits of primary teeth
   A. Primary incisor traits
   B. Primary canine traits
   C. Primary molar traits
V. Pulp cavities of primary teeth

OBJECTIVES

This chapter is designed to prepare the learner to perform the following:
- Describe the important functions of the primary dentition and the problems that can occur from premature loss of primary teeth.
- List the time ranges for primary and secondary tooth eruption.
- List the time ranges for crown and root formation for primary and secondary teeth.
- Give the order of emergence of primary and secondary teeth.
- Describe the dentition (set) traits that differentiate primary from secondary teeth.
- Describe class and type traits that distinguish the primary incisors, canines, and molars from all views.
- Describe the size and shape of primary tooth pulp chambers.
- Using the universal identification system, identify permanent and primary teeth present in the mouth with mixed dentition.
- Establish the expected "dental age" of a person by studying their mixed dentition.

SECTION I. Background Information

A. DEFINITIONS

Primary teeth are often called **deciduous** (dee SIJ oo es) **teeth**. Deciduous comes from the Latin word meaning to fall off. Deciduous teeth fall off or are shed (like leaves from a deciduous tree) and are replaced by the adult teeth that succeed them. Common nicknames for them are "milk teeth," or "temporary teeth," which, unfortunately, denote a lack of importance. The dentition that follows the primary teeth may be called the **permanent dentition**, but since so many of the so-called permanent teeth are lost due to disease, trauma, or other causes, the authors have chosen to call it the **secondary dentition** (or **adult dentition**). [There are millions of people in the United States who have lost all of their "permanent teeth" (are edentulous).]

B. DENTAL FORMULAE

As stated in Chapter 1, the number and type of primary teeth in each half of the mouth is represented by this formula:

$$\text{Incisors}\frac{2}{2} \qquad \text{Canines}\frac{1}{1} \qquad \text{Molars}\frac{2}{2} = \frac{5 \text{ maxillary teeth per side}}{5 \text{ mandibular teeth per side}}$$

Compare this formula to that for the secondary dentition and you will be able to draw some interesting conclusions:

$$\text{Incisors}\frac{2}{2} \quad \text{Canines}\frac{1}{1} \quad \text{Premolars}\frac{2}{2} \quad \text{Molars}\frac{3}{3} = \frac{8 \text{ maxillary teeth per side}}{8 \text{ mandibular teeth per side}}$$

Notice that there are no primary premolars. When primary teeth are replaced by teeth of the secondary dentition, the *primary molars* are replaced by *premolars*. The 20 secondary teeth that succeed their primary tooth predecessors are called **succedaneous** (suck si DAY nee ous) **teeth**. The 12 secondary molars, however, have no predecessors in the primary dentition and erupt distal to the primary molars. Therefore, in the strict sense, secondary molars are *not* succedaneous teeth.

Primary teeth exhibit an arch form similar to permanent teeth (Fig. 9-1). Recall from Chapter 3 that

Primary dentition

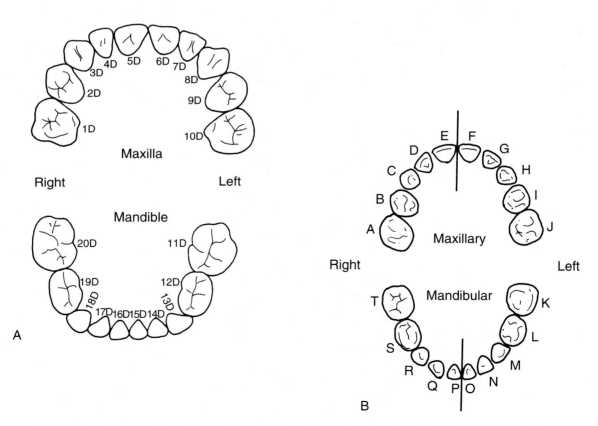

FIGURE 9-1. Diagram of maxillary and mandibular **primary dental arches**. Two methods of identifying these primary teeth are shown. On the right diagram, the Universal System of assigning letters to each tooth is shown, while on the left diagram, a numbering system 1 through 20 followed by "D" for deciduous is shown.

the 20 primary teeth can be identified using the universal identification system by assigning letters A (for the primary right maxillary second molar) through T (for the primary right mandibular second molar). Another method that can be used to identify these teeth uses a "D" to denote deciduous followed by numbers 1 (D1 for the primary right maxillary second molar) through 20 (D20 for the primary right mandibular second molar). Both of these systems are seen in Figure 9-1. (Two other methods for numbering deciduous teeth were presented in Table 3.1.)

C. FUNCTIONS OF THE PRIMARY DENTITION

Some parents do not consider the care of the primary teeth of their children to be a priority since they consider them as "temporary" or "baby" teeth, but remember that primary teeth are the *only* teeth that children have until approximately their 6th birthday, and some remain functioning until age 12. Primary teeth are actually in the mouth functioning for almost 6 years for mandibular central incisors to almost 10 years for maxillary canines [the average being 8 years for maxillary teeth and 7.6 years for mandibular teeth[1]]. When people live to be 70 years of age, they will have spent 6% of their life masticating solely with primary teeth. This small proportion of time should not infer a lack of importance of primary teeth, however, because they play a very important role in "reserving" space for the permanent teeth, which assures proper alignment, spacing, and occlusion of the permanent teeth. Consider the following functions of primary teeth in order to confirm the importance of keeping them healthy:

- Primary teeth are needed for efficient mastication of food.
- They provide support for the cheeks and lips maintaining a normal facial appearance and smile.
- They are necessary for the formulation of clear speech.
- They are critical for maintaining the space and arch continuity required to provide room for the emergence of secondary teeth.

When primary teeth are lost prematurely, or are not shed as succedaneous teeth emerge, the results on tooth alignment can be devastating (Figs. 9-2 and 9-3). Correction of tooth alignment and deformities in these children would require extensive orthodontic therapy (involving placement of orthodontic appliances, or braces, which can be used to improve tooth alignment). Further, maintenance of a proper diet and good oral hygiene are necessary to avoid dental decay of primary teeth which can cause infection with concomitant pain possibly making the child reject difficult to chew foods. Finally, an abscess

FIGURE 9-2. A crowded mandibular secondary dentition caused by the premature loss of deciduous molars. Notice that the left lateral incisor almost contacts the right central incisor and that the left first premolar is only 2.5 mm from contacting the first molar.

FIGURE 9-3. Extreme crowding of a maxillary permanent dentition in a 12-year-old child. The left deciduous canine (arrow) was not shed because its successor emerged labially to it. Both 12-year molars (three-cusp type) are in the process of emerging.

from the infection of the pulp of a primary tooth can cause dark spots (Turner's spots) on the developing secondary tooth beneath it (seen later in Fig. 11-36).

SECTION II. Developmental Data for Primary and Secondary Teeth

Dental students and dental hygiene students should become familiar with the emergence dates of primary and secondary teeth in order to adequately and correctly inform worried parents and patients about the normal times when teeth emerge or erupt above the gingiva (gums). Expected eruption patterns for primary and secondary teeth from one study are presented in Table 9-1A; eruption patterns from another study of only primary teeth are presented in Table 9-1B. An emergence time for *primary* teeth can be within 4 to 5 months (early or late) of the dates in Table 9-1A and still be considered normal. *Secondary* tooth emergence can be within 12 to 18 months (early or late) of those dates and still be of no real concern. Early emergence of these teeth usually presents no problems other than a concern about instituting oral hygiene measures.

Dental radiographs (x-ray films) are the best means for determining what is covered up (unerupted) or missing in a dentition when the expected teeth have not emerged, particularly when they are considerably overdue (See Fig. 9-7).

A. IMPORTANT TIMES FOR TOOTH EMERGENCE

Instead of memorizing the specific times of eruption of each tooth (which would be a daunting task), first consider this overview of the development of permanent and primary teeth based on their normal eruption patterns. If you learn the following time ranges, you will be well on your way to understanding the schedule of tooth eruption for both dentitions.

- **Birth to 6 (or 8) months old:** There are no teeth visible within the mouth.
- **6 (or 8) months to 2 (or 2½) old:** All twenty primary teeth emerge into the child's mouth over this period.
- **2 (or 2½) to 6 (or 5¾) years old:** All primary teeth are present; no permanent teeth are yet visible in the mouth.

Table 9-1A

DECIDUOUS AND SECONDARY TOOTH FORMATION AND EMERGENCE TIMES

		TOOTH	HARD TISSUE FORMATION BEGINS	CROWN COMPLETED	EMERGENCE	ROOT COMPLETED
Deciduous dentition	Maxillary teeth	Central incisor	4 mos. in utero	4 mos.	7½ mos.	1½ yrs.
		Lateral incisor	4½ mos. in utero	5 mos.	9 mos.	2 yrs.
		Canine	5 mos. in utero	9 mos.	18 mos.	3¼ yrs.
		First molar	5 mos. in utero	6 mos.	14 mos.	2½ yrs.
		Second molar	6 mos. in utero	11 mos.	24 mos.	3 yrs.
	Mandibular teeth	Central incisor	4½ mos. in utero	3½ mos.	6 mos.	1½ yrs.
		Lateral incisor	4½ mos. in utero	4 mos.	7 mos.	1½ yrs.
		Canine	5 mos. in utero	9 mos.	16 mos.	3 yrs.
		First molar	5 mos. in utero	5½ mos.	12 mos.	2¼ yrs.
		Second molar	6 mos. in utero	10 mos.	20 mos.	3 yr.
Permanent dentition	Maxillary teeth	Central incisor	3–4 mos.	4–5 yrs.	7–8 yrs.	10 yrs.
		Lateral incisor	10–12 mos.	4–5 yrs.	8–9 yrs.	11 yrs.
		Canine	4–5 mos.	6–7 yrs.	11–12 yrs.	13–15 yrs.
		First premolar	1½–1¾ yrs.	5–6 yrs.	10–11 yrs.	12–13 yrs.
		Second premolar	2–2¼ yrs.	6–7 yrs.	10–12 yrs.	12–14 yrs.
		First molar	birth	2½–3 yrs.	6–7 yrs.	9–10 yrs.
		Second molar	2½–3 yrs.	7–8 yrs.	12–15 yrs.	14–16 yrs.
		Third molar	7–9 yrs.	12–16 yrs.	17–21 yrs.	18–25 yrs.
	Mandibular teeth	Central incisor	3–4 mos.	4–5 yrs.	6–7 yrs.	9 yrs.
		Lateral incisor	3–4 mos.	4–5 yrs.	7–8 yrs.	10 yrs.
		Canine	4–5 mos.	6–7 yrs.	9–10 yrs.	12–14 yrs.
		First premolar	1¾–2 yrs.	5–6 yrs.	10–12 yrs.	12–13 yrs.
		Second premolar	2¼–2½ yrs.	6–7 yrs.	11–12 yrs.	13–14 yrs.
		First molar	birth	2½–3 yrs.	6–7 yrs.	9–10 yrs.
		Second molar	2½–3 yrs.	7–8 yrs.	11–13 yrs.	14–15 yrs.
		Third molar	8–10 yrs.	12–16 yrs.	17–21 yrs.	18–25 yrs.

* Logan and Kronfeld (slightly modified by McCall and Schour)

Table 9-1B

TOOTH DEVELOPMENT AND ERUPTION: PRIMARY TEETH

		HARD TISSUE FORMATION BEGINS (WEEKS IN UTERO)	ENAMEL COMPLETED (MONTHS AFTER BIRTH)	ERUPTION (MONTHS)	ROOT COMPLETED (YEAR)
Maxillary	Central incisor	14	1½	10 (8–12)	1½
	Lateral incisor	16	2½	11 (9–13)	2
	Canine	17	9	19 (16–22)	3¼
	First molar	15½	6	16 (13–19 boys) (14–18 girls)	2½
	Second molar	19	11	29 (25–33)	3
Mandibular	Central incisor	14	2½	8 (6–10)	1½
	Lateral incisor	16	3	13 (10–16)	1½
	Canine	17	9	20 (17–23)	3¼
	First molar	15½	5½	16 (14–18)	2¼
	Second molar	18	10	27 (23–31 boys) (24–30 girls)	3

From Lunt R. C., and Law, D. B., A review of the chronology of deciduous teeth. J. Am. Dent. Assoc. 89;872. October 1974.

- **6 (or 5¾) years old:** Secondary teeth start to appear, beginning with the first molars (also called **six-year molars**) just distal to the second primary molars. This is followed closely by the loss of the primary mandibular central incisors, which are quickly replaced by the secondary mandibular central incisors.
- **6 to 9 years old:** All secondary incisors replace primary incisors that are exfoliated (shed).
- **9 to 12 years old:** All eight premolars and four canines replace primary molars and canines.
- **12 years old:** Second molars (also called **12-year molars**) emerge distal to the permanent first molars.
- **17 to 21 years old:** Third molars (if present) emerge.

B. CROWN AND ROOT DEVELOPMENT

With these basic time periods in mind, one must not forget that much more is taking place during the development of these teeth than just their eruption and/or exfoliation. Prior to eruption, tooth crowns are forming from lobes and are calcifying within the jawbones. After **crown calcification** is completed, the tooth root starts to form which results in the movement of the tooth through bone toward the surface (**eruption process**) and eventually through the oral mucosa into the oral cavity (**emergence**). After emergence, the root continues to form until **root formation** is completed.

The process of *primary* tooth formation and eruption is followed by the development, calcification, and eruption of the *succedaneous* teeth apical to their roots. The eruption of these succedaneous teeth results in **resorption** of the roots of the primary teeth (that is, the gradual physiologic destruction or dissolution of the primary tooth root by the underlying erupting permanent tooth). When the secondary tooth is close to emergence, the primary tooth roots are resorbed so much that they can no longer support the remaining primary tooth crown. The primary tooth becomes loose and is eventually **exfoliated** (shed or lost). The exfoliation of the primary tooth is followed closely by the emergence of the succedaneous tooth just beneath the surface.

Now let us look at this entire process in more detail, discussing it step by step. All of the following information is derived from Table 9-1A.

1. CROWN CALCIFICATION OF PRIMARY TEETH

The crowns of all 20 primary teeth *begin* to calcify between *4 to 6 months in utero* (Fig. 9-4). *Crown completion* of all primary teeth occurs within the first year after birth, taking an average of 10 months from the beginning of tooth calcification. [The time from beginning hard tissue formation until complete enamel calcification ranges from a minimum of 9 months for incisors, to a maximum of 13 months for primary second molars.]

2. ROOT FORMATION AND EMERGENCE OF PRIMARY TEETH

Root formation for primary (and permanent) teeth begins immediately after the enamel on the crown is completely formed, and at this time the tooth starts its occlusal movement toward the oral cavity. This tooth movement is called **eruption**. In the process of eruption, the primary tooth crowns finally **emerge** into the oral cavity from age 6 months to 2 years (24 months). [The emergence of primary teeth ranges from about 3 months after crown calcification is complete for mandibular central incisors, to about 13 months after calcification for maxillary second molars.] The eruptive movement continues after emergence, until eventually the tooth comes into occlusion with teeth in the opposite arch. Even then these teeth continue to erupt to compensate for wear (attrition) on the incisal or occlusal surface, and/or when there are no opposing teeth.

3. ORDER OF EMERGENCE OF PRIMARY TEETH (FROM 6 MONTHS TO ABOUT 2 YEARS OLD)

The sequence of emergence for primary teeth presented in Table 9-2 shows that the first primary teeth to emerge are the mandibular central incisors, at about 6 months of age, followed by the mandibular laterals and then the maxillary incisors (centrals before laterals). (Note the difference in eruption patterns in Table 9-1B, where data showed that mandibular central incisors emerge first, but are followed by maxillary central incisors, maxillary lateral incisors, and finally mandibular lateral

FIGURE 9-4. Developing human primary molars. A. Occlusal view of a 19-week in utero maxillary right first molar. Note the large, well-developed, mesiobuccal cusp, which is covered with a mineralized enamel cap and is the first formed and largest cusp of the trigon, the early molar form that has three cusps. Original magnification x36. B. Buccal view of a 20-week in utero mandibular right first molar. Note the strongly elevated mesiobuccal cusp that dominates the mesial portion of the tooth. The mesiolingual cusp is the second to differentiate and shows incipient mineralization. Original magnification x36. These two examples illustrate that the mesiobuccal cusps of both the maxillary and mandibular molars are the first to form and mineralize.

incisors.) Next to emerge are the first molars, canines, then second molars. Thus, the last primary teeth to emerge, thereby completing the primary dentition, are the maxillary second molars, at about 2 years (24 months) of age.

4. ROOT COMPLETION OF PRIMARY TEETH

The primary tooth roots are completed between the ages of 1½ to 3 years. [The time from tooth emergence until the completion of the root ranges from about 10.5 months for maxillary central incisors to about 21 months for upper canines.] The *complete* primary dentition is in the mouth from about 2 years of age to 5¾ or 6 years, during which no permanent teeth are present. Shortly after the 4th birthday, as the maxillae and the mandible bones grow larger, spaces (called **primate spaces**) devel-

Table 9-2					

CHART REPRESENTING ORDER OF PRIMARY TOOTH EMERGENCE. (1 = FIRST TOOTH TO ERUPT, 2 = SECOND, ETC.) BASED ON DATA IN TABLE 9-1A.

	CENTRAL INCISOR	LATERAL INCISOR	CANINE	FIRST MOLAR	SECOND MOLAR
Maxillary	3rd (7½ mo.)	4th (9 mo.)	8th (18 mo.)	6th (14 mo.)	10th (24 mo.)
Mandibular	1st (6 mo.)	2nd (7 mo.)	7th (16 mo.)	5th (12 mo.)	9th (20 mo.)

op between the primary teeth. These frequently concern parents, but are perfectly natural and even beneficial since the spaces provide room for the secondary incisors and canines, which are considerably wider than their predecessors. Refer to Table 9-3 for differences in sizes between primary and adult teeth.

5. EXFOLIATION (SHEDDING) OF PRIMARY TEETH WITH THE SIMULTANEOUS ERUPTION AND EVENTUAL EMERGENCE OF THE SECONDARY (ADULT) TEETH

The roots of primary teeth are complete for a short period of time (Fig. 9-5). Only about 3 years after completion, primary tooth roots begin to **resorb**, usually at the apex, or on one side near the apex. Resorption of the primary tooth root occurs as the crown of the succedaneous tooth that is to replace it begins its occlusal migration, thus infringing upon the primary root. Increasing loss of root attachment from root resorption results in the eventual loosening of the deciduous teeth, so they "fall off" the jaw. This process of shedding is called **exfoliation**. As the primary teeth are shed, the crowns of the succedaneous teeth are close to the surface, ready to emerge shortly (Fig. 9-6).

6. MIXED DENTITION (PRESENT FROM 5 3/4 OR 6 YEARS TO 12 YEARS OLD)

During the time when *both* primary and secondary teeth are present in the mouth, the dentition is known as a **mixed dentition**. The mixed dentition begins at age 5 ¾ or 6 years old when the first (six-year) molars emerge. Next, the first primary incisors are gradually replaced by their larger successors. The mixed dentition ends at about age 12 when all primary teeth have been replaced. Usually 24 teeth are seen in the mouth throughout the mixed dentition (all 20 primary teeth OR their successors, *plus* the four six-year first molars). At 12 years old, all succedaneous teeth have replaced their primary predecessors (marking the end of mixed dentition). When the 12-year second molars erupt, 28 teeth are present. The full complement of 32 permanent teeth is not reached until the third molars erupt during the late teenage years or early twenties.

Soon after the 6-year first molars emerge, their eruptive forces, along with their tendency to drift toward the mesial, push the primary teeth forward. If this were to continue, there would be insufficient space for the premolars to come in. The flared roots of the primary molars, however, resist the mesial displacement (seen in Fig. 9-5). This, coupled with the fact that the primary molars are wider mesiodistally than their premolar successors, helps to preserve sufficient space for the premolars and secondary canines.[2]

7. CROWN FORMATION OF SECONDARY TEETH

The first *secondary* tooth crowns to begin forming (*at birth*) are the first molars. Crowns of the secondary dentition continue to form up to age 16 when crowns of third molars are completed. On average for the adult dentition, there is a *3- to 4-year span* from completion of crown calcification until the tooth emerges into the mouth [with a range of from 2.7 years for the lower anterior teeth to 4.7 years for the lower posterior teeth].

Table 9-3

DECIDUOUS TOOTH SIZE COMPARED TO THEIR SUCCESSORS

		CROWN LENGTH		ROOT LENGTH		OVERALL LENGTH		MESIO DISTAL CROWN		FACIO LINGUAL CROWN		MESIO DISTAL CERVIX		FACIO LINGUAL CERVIX		AVERAGE OF ALL MEASUREMENTS
		mm	%*	mm	%*	mm	%*	mm	%*	mm	%*	mm	%*	mm	%*	%*
Maxillary teeth	Central incisor	6.4	57	11.3	82	17.2	73	7.4	86	5.0	70	5.7	89	4.4	70	75.3
	Lateral incisor	7.4	76	10.9	81	16.8	75	5.8	88	4.9	79	4.0	85	4.5	78	80.3
	Canine	7.6	72	13.5	78	20.2	80	7.4	97	5.4	67	5.3	95	5.0	66	78.8
	First molar	6.0	70	12.5	93	17.1	80	8.1	114	9.5	103	5.9	123	8.9	108	98.7
	Second molar	6.4	83	10.4	74	15.9	75	9.7	147	10.3	114	7.1	151	9.6	118	108.8
Mandibular teeth	Central incisor	6.1	69	10.5	83	16.0	77	4.5	85	4.5	79	3.5	100	4.2	78	81.6
	Lateral incisor	7.3	78	10.6	78	16.5	75	4.9	86	4.8	79	3.7	94	4.5	78	81.4
	Canine	8.2	74	11.7	74	18.7	72	6.1	90	5.7	74	4.2	81	5.0	67	76.0
	First molar	7.1	81	9.7	67	15.9	71	8.7	124	7.4	96	7.2	150	5.3	78	95.3
	Second molar	6.6	80	10.8	68	15.5	70	10.3	145	9.2	112	7.6	152	7.1	97	103.4

Measurements are derived from 2392 maxillary and 2180 mandibular secondary tooth specimens compared to plastic model replicas of primary teeth made by the Shofu Dental Manufacturing Company reflecting the size of Japanese primary teeth. In most instances, these measurements on the plastic model teeth were 0.5–1 mm larger than measurements made by G.V. Black at the turn of the century (deciduous teeth).

* Percentage is based on the average size for the secondary dentition successor as equaling 100%. In instances in which the deciduous tooth dimension is greater than its successor, the percentage is over 100, even as high as 152% on the mandibular second molar mesiodistal cervix dimension, indicating that this part of the deciduous molar is 1.5 times larger than the corresponding region on its successor, the mandibular second premolar.

FIGURE 9-5. Models depicting the stage of development of the dentitions of a 3-year-old child. All primary teeth have emerged into the oral cavity, and they have full roots, prior to resorption. Notice the various amounts of crown development and locations of the partially formed crowns of the secondary dentition. (Models courtesy of 3M Unitek, Monrovia, CA.)

8. ORDER OF EMERGENCE FOR SECONDARY TEETH

Table 9-4 includes the sequence of emergence for secondary teeth. After the 6-year molars erupt just prior to the child's 6th birthday, the order of emergence for the succedaneous teeth is essentially the same as for the order of exfoliation of the primary teeth they replace. If you know the time *range* (for emergence of incisors, or for canines and premolars) and sequence of eruption within that time range, you can estimate the emergence time for any succedaneous tooth.

Recall that, very quickly after the 6-year molars emerge, the secondary incisors emerge between 6–9 years of age. The specific sequence within this range is: secondary incisors begin to replace primary incisors (centrals preceding laterals), and mandibular incisors precede maxillary incisors. Since the mandibular central incisors erupt first in this time range, they emerge closer to 6 years old, whereas maxillary lateral incisors erupt closer to the end of that time range, that is closer to 8 or 9 years old.

Next, the adult canines and premolars erupt from 9 to 12 years old. The eruption sequence during this range is as follows: *mandibular* canines replace primary mandibular canines, then premolars replace primary molars. Note in Table 9-4 that in the adult dentition, most teeth in the lower arch usually emerge slightly earlier than their maxillary counterparts; the ONLY maxillary tooth to emerge before its mandibular counterpart is the *maxillary* second premolar which precedes the *mandibular* second premolar. Finally *maxillary canines are the last primary teeth to be replaced.* Knowing the range and sequence, you can estimate the emergence time of the *mandibular* canine as close to 9 years, while the *maxillary* canine emerges last within this range, or at about 11½ to 12½ years of age.

Roots of secondary teeth are completed *about 3 years after their emergence* into the oral cavity.

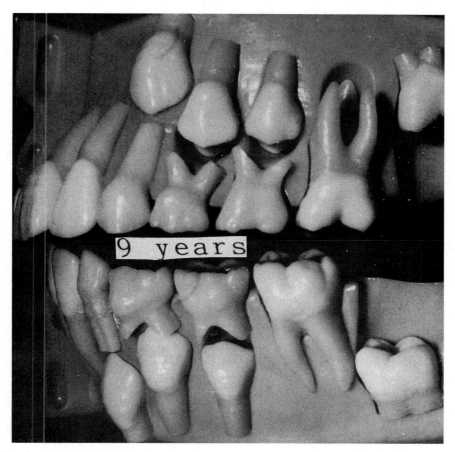

FIGURE 9-6. Tooth development of a 9-year-old child with mixed dentition. The secondary central and lateral incisors and first molars have emerged into a functional level. The deciduous canines and molars are still functioning although much of their roots have resorbed. You can see at this time why the maxillary canine is often the last permanent tooth to erupt except for the third molars (not shown). (Models courtesy of 3M Unitek, Monrovia, CA.)

Table 9-4

CHART REPRESENTING THE USUAL ORDER OF SECONDARY DENTITION TOOTH EMERGENCE BASED ON DATA FROM TABLE 9-1A. (1st = FIRST TOOTH TO ERUPT, 2nd = SECOND, ETC. SAME NUMBER WITH A "(t)" DENOTES ESSENTIALLY A TIE IN ERUPTION TIME.) Mandibular teeth often precede their maxillary counterpart within the time ranges given except for second premolars

	CENT INC	LAT INC	CANINE	1st PM	2nd PM	1st MOLAR	2nd MOLAR	3rd MOLAR
age range:	6 to 9 years old		9 to 12 years old			6 years	12 years	
Maxillary	2nd – t	3rd	6th (t)	5th (t)	5th (t)	1st (t)	7th (t)	8th (t)
	(7–8 yr.)	(8–9 yr.)	(11–12 yr.)	(10–11 yr.)	(10–12 yr.)	(6–7 yr.)	(12–15 yr.)	(17–21 yr.)
Mandibular	1st – t	2nd – t	4th	5th (t)	6th (t)	1st (t)	7th (t)	8th (t)
	(6–7 yr.)	(7–8 yr.)	(9–10 yr.)	(10–12 yr.)	(11–12 yr.)	(6–7 yr.)	(11–13 yr.)	(17–21 yr.)

SECTION III. Dentition Traits of All Primary Teeth

Your best specimens for the study of crown morphology of primary teeth can be found in the mouth of a 2- to 6-year-old who is willing to open his or her mouth wide, long, and often enough to permit your examination. Extracted or exfoliated primary teeth with complete roots and crowns are difficult to find since most of these have resorbed roots and severe attrition (occlusal wear). Plastic tooth models, if available, are most helpful and have the added advantage of complete roots.

First, consider the general traits of *all* primary teeth that set them apart from the secondary teeth:

- Primary teeth are smaller in size than the analogous secondary teeth (seen in the mandibular radiograph in Figure 9-7.
- Primary teeth are whiter in color.

FIGURE 9-7. Radiographs made of an 8-year-old child showing the first and second deciduous molars and first adult molars in the mouth. Notice the premolar crowns between the partially resorbed roots of the deciduous molars. Part of the 12-year second molar crown is seen on the far right. The lesser size, lesser enamel thickness, and larger pulp cavities are evident in the deciduous molars compared to the larger secondary molars just distal to them. (Courtesy of Professor Donald Bowers, Ohio State University.)

- The crowns and roots of primary teeth have a marked constriction at the cervix, appearing as if they are being squeezed with a rubber band. Thus, the enamel, rather than gradually tapering toward the occlusal surface as in secondary teeth, seems to bulge close to the cervical line forming labial cervical ridges and lingual cingula.[3] This is seen best from the proximal view in Appendix 9a and Appendix 10e.
- Primary teeth have longer roots relative to their crowns.
- The layers of enamel and dentin of primary teeth are thinner than on secondary teeth, but the pulp cavities are proportionally larger and are therefore *closer to the surface* (seen in the radiographs in Figure 9-7 where the outer layer of enamel is whiter, dentin is more gray, and the pulp, in the center of the tooth, is nearly black).
- Primary teeth are less mineralized so become very worn.[3,4] These teeth are prone to considerable **attrition**[at TRISH en] (tooth wear from tooth-to-tooth contact) which is made worse by the shifting relationship of the upper and lower teeth due to expanding growth of the jaws in young children. Attrition, therefore, is not really a dentition trait, but a fact of life or normal occurrence.[4]
- Primary teeth have more consistent shapes than the secondary dentition (fewer anomalies).[3]

Next, consider the unique traits of the **primary anterior teeth** (refer to Appendix page 9 while studying these traits):

- The cervical ridges on facial surfaces are prominent (running mesiodistally in the cervical third) (Appendix 9a, facial surfaces).
- The lingual cingula are prominent or seem to bulge and occupy about one-third of the cervicoincisal length (Appendix 9a, lingual surfaces).
- The roots of primary anterior teeth are long in proportion to crown length (Appendix 9f), and are relatively narrow mesiodistally (Appendix 9b).
- The roots of primary anterior teeth bend labially in their apical one-third to one-half by as much as 10° (Appendix 9c).
- Usually there are no depressions, mamelons, or perikymata on the labial surface of the crowns of the primary incisors. These surfaces are smoother than their successors.

Now consider the unique traits of the **primary posterior teeth** (refer to Appendix page 10 while studying these traits):

- The mesial cervical ridge on the buccal surface is prominent (it is easy to distinguish rights from lefts) (Appendix 10e).
- The roots are thin and slender, and spread beyond the outlines of the crown, more widely on primary second molars than the first molars (the opposite of the adult molars)[5] (Appendix 10g). This root divergence makes room for the development of the succedaneous premolars. Extraction of a deciduous molar when roots are complete and before they have started to resorb may cause the developing portion of the premolar to be removed along with the deciduous molar.[7]
- The root furcations are near the crown, with little or no root trunk (Appendix 10f).
- Due to the taper of the crown from the cervical bulges toward the occlusal surface, the molar crowns have a narrow **occlusal table** (Appendix 10c). (The occlusal table is the chewing surface inside the line formed by the continuous mesial and distal cusp ridges for all cusps, and the mesial and distal marginal ridges). In other words, the occlusal table is considerably smaller that the entire outline of the tooth from the occlusal view.
- From the buccal view, the molar crowns are wide mesiodistally relative to the height cervico-occlusally (Appendix 10a).
- The primary molar occlusal anatomy is shallow. In other words, the cusps are short (not pointed or sharp, almost flat) (Appendix 10d), the occlusal ridges are not pronounced, and the fossae and sulci are correspondingly not as deep as on secondary molars.
- There are few grooves or depressions in the crowns.
- Primary second molars are decidedly larger than primary first molars, different than in the secondary dentition (Appendix page 10, compare firsts to seconds).
- Microscopically, the enamel rods at the cervix slope occlusally, unlike in permanent teeth where these rods slope cervically.

SECTION IV. Class and Type Traits of Primary Teeth

A. PRIMARY INCISOR TRAITS

1. PRIMARY INCISORS FROM THE LABIAL VIEW

a. Outline Shape of Primary Incisor Crowns from the Labial View

Incisal edges of primary **maxillary central incisors** are relatively straight except for some rounding at the distoincisal angle. Mesial sides of maxillary central incisor crowns are fairly flat, whereas the distal sides are more convex. The crowns of **primary maxillary central incisors** are the ONLY incisor crowns (primary or secondary) which are wider mesiodistally than they are long incisocervically (Appendix 9e).

The **maxillary lateral incisor** crowns are similar in shape to the central incisor, but are longer incisocervically than wide mesiodistally, and are less symmetrical. Distoincisal angles of lateral incisors are even more rounded. Note this difference in Figures 9-8 and 9-9. Laterals are smaller than central incisors in the same dentition.

The crowns of the **mandibular incisors** resemble their replacement incisor crowns, but are much smaller. As with secondary mandibular incisors, primary **mandibular lateral incisor** crowns are a little larger than the crowns of central incisors and less symmetrical (with more rounded distoincisal angles) than the central incisors of the same dentition (Fig. 9-8).

The locations of proximal contact areas on primary incisors are comparable to those of their successors.

b. Surface Morphology of Primary Incisors From the Labial View

Labial surfaces of maxillary central incisors are smooth; usually there are no depressions. Mandibular incisors are also relatively smooth, but may have shallow depressions on their labial surfaces in the incisal third.

c. Root to Crown Proportion of Primary Incisors from the Labial View

Prior to root resorption, primary incisor roots are much longer relative to the crown length than on secondary incisors (Appendix 9f). Primary incisor roots are about twice the length of the crown. The roots of **maxillary lateral incisors** appear proportionally even longer. On primary extracted or shed teeth, there is usually some root resorption (Fig. 9-9). Often the entire root is gone.

FIGURE 9-8. Deciduous dentition, **facial views.**

D   M   D   M

Primary maxillary
lateral incisor (right)

Primary maxillary central
incisor (right)

FIGURE 9-9. Primary maxillary right lateral incisor (at left) and maxillary right central incisor. The central incisor crown is short and wide. There has been some resorption of the root tips on both teeth (moreso on the central incisor), but even so, the roots are twice as long as the crowns. The lateral incisor is less symmetrical and is longer than it is wide.

2. PRIMARY INCISORS FROM THE LINGUAL VIEW

Refer to Figure 9-10.

a. Cingula of Primary Incisors from the Lingual View

The cingula of primary **maxillary central incisors** are often proportionally large, so that lingual fossae are in only the incisal and middle thirds of the lingual surface. The lingual surface of **mandibular incisors** also has a cingulum and a slight lingual fossa.

b. Marginal Ridges of Primary Incisors from the Lingual View

On maxillary central incisors, marginal ridges are often distinct and prominent (like shovel-shaped incisors). On mandibular incisors, marginal ridges are more faint (Fig. 9-10).

DECIDUOUS DENTITION (Lingual)

LEFTS — RIGHTS

MAXILLARY

MANDIBULAR

DISTAL

FIGURE 9-10. Deciduous dentition, **lingual views**. Notice on molars that the lingual cusps are not as long as the mesiobuccal cusps.

3. **PRIMARY INCISORS FROM THE PROXIMAL VIEWS (MESIAL AND DISTAL)**

    a. **Primary Incisor Crown Outlines from the Proximal Views**

    Although the faciolingual dimension of these crowns appears small from these aspects, crowns are wide labiolingually in their cervical one third because of prominent, convex labial cervical ridges and lingual cingula.

    Similar to their successors, incisal ridges of primary maxillary central incisors are located labial to the root-axis line, whereas incisal ridges of mandibular incisors are located on the root axis line (Fig. 9-11).

    b. **Cervical Line of Primary Incisors from the Proximal Views**

    As on secondary incisors, the curve of the cervical line toward the incisal is greater on the mesial than on the distal. The cervical line is positioned more apically on the lingual than on the labial side.

    c. **Root Shape of Primary Incisors from the Proximal Views**

    The roots of **maxillary incisors** are curved from this view, bending lingually in the cervical third to half (Appendix 9d), and labially by as much as 10° in the apical half (Appendix 9c).[5] Roots of the **mandibular incisors**, in contrast, are straight in their cervical half, but then bend labially about 10° in their apical half (Appendix 9c).[5] This bend helps make space for the developing succedaneous incisors, which should be in a *lingual and apical position*.

4. **PRIMARY INCISORS FROM THE INCISAL VIEW**

    Incisor crowns have a smoothly convex labial outline. The 1-mm thick incisal ridge is slightly curved mesiodistally. The crowns have lingual surfaces that become narrower toward the lingual, at the cingulum.

FIGURE 9-11. Deciduous dentition, **proximal views**. Notice on the molars that more of the occlusal surfaces are visible from the distal view than from the mesial view. Also notice that the apical third of roots of anterior teeth bend labially, especially in the maxillary dentition.

Crowns of primary **maxillary central incisors** are much wider mesiodistally than faciolingually [by 2.4 mm] compared to maxillary lateral incisors which are only 0.9 mm wider mesiodistally. These proportions are evident in Figure 9-12. Both **mandibular incisor crowns** have mesiodistal and faciolingual dimensions that are essentially equal.

B. PRIMARY CANINE TRAITS

1. PRIMARY CANINES FROM THE LABIAL VIEW

a. Outline Shape of Primary Canines from the Labial View

Maxillary canine crowns may be as wide as they are long. They are constricted at the cervix. They have convex mesial and distal outlines, with distal contours more broadly rounded than mesial contours which are somewhat angular (Fig. 9-13). **Mandibular canine crowns** are longer incisocervically than wide mesiodistally [by 2.1 mm] and are 1.3 mm narrower mesiodistally than maxillary canine crowns (Appendix 9g).

1) Cusp Ridge Outlines

Maxillary canine cusps are often very sharp (pointed) with two cusp ridges meeting at an acute angle. The mesial cusp ridges of these maxillary canines are longer than the distal cusp ridges (similar to secondary maxillary first premolars, but just the *opposite* of all other premolars and canines, secondary and primary) (Appendix 9h, maxillary canine, and Fig. 9-13). These mesial cusp ridges are flat to concave and less steeply inclined[6] than the shorter

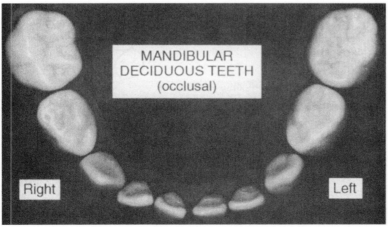

FIGURE 9-12. Deciduous dentition, **incisal and occlusal views**. Notice the striking resemblance of the second deciduous molar to a 6-year first molar.

Primary mandibular canine
A (right)

Primary maxillary canine (right)
B

FIGURE 9-13. Primary canines, labial views. A: Primary *mandibular* right canine. The root tip has begun to resorb. B: Primary *maxillary* right canine. Notice the longer mesial cusp ridge, the more cervically positioned mesial contact area, and the rounded distal contour compared to the more angular mesial contour.

distal ridges, which are more convex. **Mandibular canines** have sharp cusp tips pointed like an arrow (Fig. 9-13). As on the secondary mandibular canines, the mesial cusp slope is shorter than the distal cusp slope (Appendix 9h, mandibular canine).

2) Contact Areas

Distal contact areas of primary canines rest against the mesial surfaces of primary first molars since there are no primary premolars. Mesial and distal contact areas of **primary maxillary canines** are near the center of the crown cervicoincisally, with *the mesial contact more cervically located* (a condition UNIQUE to this tooth and the mandibular first premolar) (Appendix 9i).

b. Cervical Lines of Primary Canines from the Labial View

Cervical lines on maxillary canines are nearly flat on the labial surface.

c. Roots of Primary Canines from the Labial View

Maxillary canine roots prior to resorption are the longest of the primary teeth [13.5 mm] tapering to a blunt apex. The roots of mandibular canines are more tapered and pointed, and shorter than maxillary canine roots [by 1.8 mm].

2. PRIMARY CANINES FROM THE LINGUAL VIEW

The cingulum on a maxillary canine crown is bulky with well-developed mesial and distal marginal ridges which are, however, less prominent than on the secondary canines (Fig. 9-10).

A lingual ridge, with an adjacent mesial and distal fossa, is located on a maxillary canine crown somewhat distal to the middle of the crown. Distal fossae on these teeth are narrower and deeper than mesial fossae, which are broader and shallower.[5,6] In contrast, lingual ridges are barely discernible on mandibular canines, with faint marginal ridges and usually a single concavity or fossa (Fig. 9-10).[7]

3. **PRIMARY CANINES FROM THE PROXIMAL (MESIAL AND DISTAL) VIEWS**

   a. **Outline of Primary Canines from the Proximal Views**

   The cervical third of a primary canine is much thicker than on an incisor. On **maxillary** canines, cusp tips are positioned considerably labial to the root axis line (Fig. 9-11), whereas the cusp tip of **mandibular** canines is most often located slightly lingual to the root axis line. Labial cervical ridges are prominent on *both* maxillary and mandibular canines, bulging similar to lingual cingula. The S-shaped lingual crown outline of **maxillary** canines is more concave than on permanent canines.

   b. **Cervical Lines of Primary Canines from the Proximal Views**

   Cervical lines of both maxillary and mandibular canines curve incisally more on the mesial side than on the distal side, just like all other anterior teeth. They are positioned more apical on the lingual than on the labial.

   c. **Roots of Primary Canines from the Proximal Views**

   The roots of *both* maxillary and mandibular canines are bulky in the cervical and middle thirds, tapering mostly in the apical third where the apex is bent labially, similar to primary central and lateral incisors (Appendix 9c and 9d and Fig. 9-11).

4. **PRIMARY CANINES FROM THE INCISAL VIEW**

   a. **Crown Outline of Primary Canines from the Incisal View**

   The crown outline of **maxillary canines** taper noticeably toward the cingulum which is centered mesiodistally. The *mesial* half of these crowns is thicker faciolingually than the distal half (similar to secondary maxillary canines). From the incisal aspect, **mandibular canine** crowns have a *diamond shape* and are nearly symmetrical, except for the mesial position of the cusp tips and they appear to have slightly more bulk in the distal half (Fig 9-12). Cingula are centered or just distal to the center.

   b. **Crown Proportions and Size of Primary Canines from the Incisal View**

   Primary **maxillary canine** crowns are broader faciolingually than incisor crowns, but are still wider mesiodistally than faciolingually [by 2 mm]. The 1.5-mm thick mesial and distal cusp ridges curve toward the lingual at both ends. **Mandibular canine** crowns are only slightly wider mesiodistally than faciolingually [by 0.4 mm]. The smallness of these teeth, compared to their replacement counterparts, is quite noticeable.

C. PRIMARY MOLAR TRAITS

As stated earlier, primary molar roots are thin and widely spread to make room for the developing premolars crowns which are forming beneath them (Appendix 10g). Recall that primary *first molars* form over the crowns of developing *first premolars* and erupt just distal to primary canines and just mesial to primary second molars. Primary *second molars* form over the crowns of developing *second premolars*, just distal to primary first molars and, after age 6, just mesial to 6-year first molars. It could be said that these primary molars are saving a place in the arch for the teeth that will succeed them, namely the first and second premolars, respectively.

Primary second molars have considerable similarities to *secondary first molars* in their respective arches. Since these teeth are adjacent to one another during the time of mixed dentition (or longer in the case of retained primary teeth), it is important to distinguish between the primary second molars and the

6-year first molars which erupt just distal to them. One obvious difference between primary and secondary molar crowns is the presence of a prominent mesial cervical ridge on the buccal surface of primary molars. This bulge is sometimes called a buccal cingulum.[4] Also, primary second molars are smaller than 6-year first molars in the same dentition. Tooth position from the midline is also a clue. Primary second molars are normally the fifth tooth from the midline, whereas secondary first molars are sixth from the midline. The differences in size and position between the primary maxillary second molar and the secondary maxillary first molar are evident in Fig. 9-14.

FIGURE 9-14. Mixed dentition. **A.** In the maxillary arch, the fifth tooth from the midline on the left side of the photograph is a second premolar, but the fifth tooth on the right side is a primary second molar. Notice the similarity of the primary molar with the larger 6-year molar just distal to it. Also notice the position of the secondary maxillary canine which is normally the last succedaneous tooth to erupt (positioned just labial to the primary canine which is still present). **B.** In the mandibular arch, the fifth tooth from the midline on both the right and left sides is the primary second molar. Notice the similarity in morphology with the larger 6-year molar just distal to it (sixth from the midline). (Models courtesy of Dr. Brad Woodford, Ohio State University.)

Primary first molars are more unique in their shape. One author feels that primary *maxillary* first molars are the most atypical of human molars,[8] while another author feels they somewhat resemble the premolars (from the occlusal view).[9] It is agreed that primary *mandibular* first molars resemble no other tooth in either dentition.

When considering **arch traits** of primary molars, consider the number of roots. **Primary maxillary molars** generally have three roots (mesiobuccal, distobuccal and, palatal, as in the secondary dentition), whereas **mandibular molars** have only two roots (mesial and distal). Also, like secondary molars, *maxillary* primary molars tend to be wider buccolingually than mesiodistally, whereas *mandibular* molars tend to be wider mesiodistally than buccolingually.

Each type of primary molar will be discussed in detail at this time, emphasizing the traits that further differentiate each type. Discussion begins with primary *second* molars since they are similar to the 6-year first molars discussed previously in Chapter 7.

1.   TYPE TRAITS OF THE PRIMARY MAXILLARY SECOND MOLAR

Primary maxillary second molars *resemble the 6-year (adult) maxillary first molars* which erupt just distal to them (Fig. 9-14), but are smaller [by 13.2% when all dimensions are averaged]. They are similar in most respects, with the cusp ridges and fossae corresponding to those of permanent first molars. Maxillary primary second molars may even have a cusp of Carabelli (Fig. 9-15).

a.   Accentuated Crown Taper

Due to the prominent mesiobuccal cervical ridge and small occlusal table, these primary molars, when viewed from the proximal aspect, appear to taper narrower much more toward the occlusal (Appendix 10c and e).[5] From the occlusal aspect, the crown also tapers considerably from mesial to distal, accentuated by the prominent mesiobuccal bulge (seen in the Appendix page 10, occlusal view).

Further, the mesiolingual corner of the occlusal surface is flattened as though it were compressed toward the distal[5] (Appendix 10h), displacing the mesiolingual cusp more distally than on the permanent first molars. This results in more taper from buccal to lingual, an oblique ridge which is straighter in its course buccolingually,[5] and a smaller, oblong distal fossa buccolingually.

| A | Buccal Surface | B | Mesial surface | C | Occlusal Surface |

FIGURE 9-15. Primary maxillary right second molar. A. Buccal surface. B. Mesial surface. Notice the spread of the roots. The crown of the maxillary second premolar develops in the space bounded by these roots. Some root resorption has occurred (especially on the lingual root). C. Occlusal surface. From this aspect the primary maxillary second molar resembles a miniature 6-year first molar (even with a Carabelli cusp).

b. Relative Cusp Size

The mesiobuccal cusp is almost equal in size or slightly larger than the mesiolingual cusp (Appendix 10i). (Recall that the mesiolingual cusp is largest on permanent maxillary first molars.)

2. TYPE TRAITS OF THE PRIMARY MANDIBULAR SECOND MOLAR

The primary mandibular second molars *resemble the 6-year (adult) mandibular first molars* which erupt just distal to them (Fig. 9-14), but are smaller [by 17.3% when all dimensions are averaged]. They are similar in most respects, with the cusp ridges and fossae corresponding to those of secondary first molars (Fig. 9-16).

Compared to *secondary* mandibular *first* molars, *primary* mandibular *second* molars have a more prominent mesial cervical ridge, the roots are more slender and more widely spread, and the three buccal cusps (mesiobuccal, distobuccal, and distal) are of *nearly equal size* (Appendix 10j). The middle buccal cusp (called the distobuccal) is the widest (largest). As on the 6-year mandibular molars, these cusps are separated by mesiobuccal and distobuccal grooves. The mesiolingual and distolingual cusps are about the same size and height, slightly shorter than the buccal cusps.[5] A lingual groove separates these two lingual cusps.

From the proximal views, the mesial marginal ridge of the primary mandibular second molar is high and is crossed by a groove that may extend about one-third of the way down the mesial surface.[9] This mesial surface is generally convex but flattens cervically. The contact area with the primary first molar is in the shape of an inverted crescent just below the notch of the marginal ridge.[9]

Since the crown is shorter on the distal side, and the distal marginal ridge is lower (more cervical) than the mesial marginal ridge, all five cusps can be seen from the distal aspect. The distal contact with the mesial side of the 6-year first molar is round in shape and is located just buccal and cervical to the distal marginal groove (furrow) (Fig. 9-16).[9] The cervical line is almost flat on both the mesial and distal sides of the crown but slopes occlusally toward the lingual.

Roots of Primary Mandibular Second Molar

The roots are about twice as long as the crowns and are thin mesiodistally. The *mesial* root is broad and flat with a blunt apex, and has a shallow longitudinal depression. The *distal* root is broad and flat, and is narrower and less blunt at the apex than the mesial root. The root furcation is very close to the cervical line with very little root trunk.

| A | Buccal surface | B | Distal surface | C | Occlusal surface |

FIGURE 9-16. Primary mandibular right second molar. A. Buccal surface. The short root trunk and the wide-spread roots, as well as the small size, distinguish this tooth from the secondary mandibular first molar. The mesiobuccal, distobuccal, and distal cusps are often about the same size. B. Distal surface. C. Occlusal surface.

3. TYPE TRAITS OF THE PRIMARY MAXILLARY FIRST MOLAR

Primary maxillary first molars are quite unique in appearance (Fig. 9-17). According to one author, they do not resemble any other molars.[8] According to another author, they resemble maxillary first premolars that replace them (Appendix page 10, occlusal view).[9] The crowns are slightly wider than the premolars which will replace them [mesiodistally by 14%].

From the buccal aspect, these crowns appear very wide relative to their height, and are noticeably shorter occlusocervically toward the distal. The mesiobuccal cusp has a buccal ridge (running occlusocervically) that extends to the cervical line.

When the buccal surface is viewed from the proximal, the prominent mesial buccal cervical ridge and adjacent flat buccal outline from cervical ridge toward the occlusal surface results in a considerable taper from the wide cervical third to the narrow occlusal third (Appendix 10c and e, proximal views). The *lingual* outline from the proximal view is more gradually convex in the cervical and middle third and flat in the occlusal third.

Occlusal Shape and Anatomy (Cusps and Ridges) of Primary Maxillary First Molars

The occlusal outline is basically rectangular (wider faciolingually than mesiodistally [by 1.4 mm]) (Appendix 10m). Further, the prominent mesiobuccal cervical ridge (running mesiodistally in the cervical third) results in a wider dimension buccolingually in the mesial half, and a taper toward the distal. This tooth also tapers toward the lingual due to the mesial marginal ridge, which does not run straight toward the lingual, but rather runs obliquely in a distolingual direction. This taper is similar to that on the mesiolingual corner in the primary maxillary second molar (Appendix 10n). In contrast, the *distal* marginal ridge runs in a straight direction buccolingually, joining both the buccal and lingual borders at right angles,[7] best seen in Figure 9-17, occlusal views.

The mesial contact is flat where it contacts the canine in the occlusal third. The distal crown outline is decidedly more convex than the mesial, and contacts the primary second molar in the middle third.

Primary maxillary first molars, like secondary maxillary molars, usually have four cusps, but they may appear somewhat like maxillary premolars from the occlusal view since they have only *two prominent* cusps (a wide mesiobuccal cusp and a narrow, slightly more distinct, mesiolingual cusp). The other two cusps, the distobuccal and distolingual, are relatively indistinct and may blend into the distal marginal ridge. When a distolingual cusp is present (four-cusp type) it is

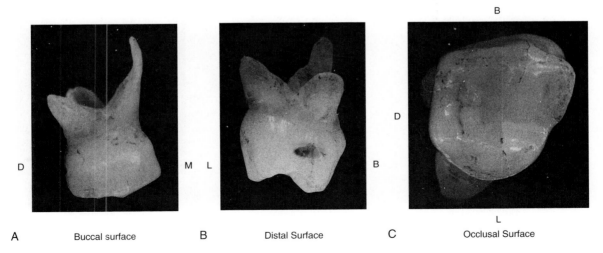

A   Buccal surface   B   Distal Surface   C   Occlusal Surface

FIGURE 9-17. **Primary maxillary right first molar.** A. Buccal surface. The mesiobuccal root is less resorbed than the distobuccal and lingual roots. The lingual root is barely discernible. B. Distal surface. C. Occlusal surface. The prominent cervical ridge below the mesiobuccal cusp gives the tooth an angular appearance. Notice the "H" shaped groove pattern.

inconspicuous, and it is often only a small nodule on the lingual half of the distal marginal ridge. Sometimes, the distolingual cusp is absent (three-cusp type), and the triangular ridge of the narrow distobuccal cusp actually becomes the distal marginal ridge.

The mesiobuccal cusp is the longest (but second sharpest) cusp.[5] The mesiolingual cusp is the second longest, but sharpest, cusp. In the four-cusp type, the triangular ridges of the distobuccal cusp joins the more distal of the two triangular ridges from the mesiolingual cusp as a barely discernible transverse ridge.[9] There is no buccal groove on the buccal surface, just a slight notch which divides the large mesiobuccal cusp from the indistinct distobuccal cusp (Appendix 10-l). This notch is distal to center. A groove between the two lingual cusps is present only when the distolingual cusp is definite.

There are three fossae on these maxillary first molars: a medium-size central fossa, a large and deep mesial triangular fossa, and a minute distal triangular fossa, each with a pit: central, mesial, and distal, respectively (Appendix 10o).

The occlusal grooves of the four-cusp type primary maxillary first molar teeth usually form an "H" pattern (seen in Fig. 9-17). The crossbar of the "H" is the central groove that connects the central and mesial triangular fossae. [Some textbooks say there is no central groove and that the crossbar is made up of a mesial and distal groove instead.[9]] Supplemental grooves running buccolingually just inside of the mesial marginal ridge form the mesial side of the "H," and the buccal groove (dividing the buccal cusps) combined with the distolingual groove (between the large mesiolingual and minute distolingual cusps on four-cusp type molars only) form the distal side of the "H." The mesial marginal ridge may be crossed by a marginal groove.

4. TYPE TRAITS OF THE PRIMARY MANDIBULAR FIRST MOLARS

These mandibular first molars do *not* resemble any other primary or secondary tooth (Fig. 9-18). According to one author, the chief differentiating characteristic may be an overdeveloped mesial marginal ridge (Appendix 10q).[9] The mesial marginal ridge is so well developed that it resembles a cusp[2] (Appendix 10q). This longer, prominent mesial marginal ridge is positioned more occlusally than the short (buccolingual), less prominent distal marginal ridge. (Compare mesial and distal views in Fig. 9-11 for marginal ridge heights and lengths.)

From the *facial* and *lingual* views, the crowns of these first molars are wider mesiodistally than high cervico-occlusally [by 1.6 mm] (Appendix 10a). Facially, they are longer (occlusocervically) on

| A | Buccal surface | B | Mesial surface | C | Occlusal surface |

FIGURE 9-18. Primary mandibular right first molar. A. Buccal surface. The distal root has been considerably shortened by resorption. Notice that the crown is longer mesially (right side) than distally. B. Mesial surface. Again the buccal cervical ridge is outstanding. Notice the very narrow occlusal surface and how the crown appears to tilt lingually. If the root apex was not partially resorbed, the root would appear to taper to a more blunt end. C. Occlusal surface. The buccal cervical ridge on the mesiobuccal cusp is conspicuous.

the mesial, due in part to the slope of the cervical line gingivally toward the mesial, separating the very prominent mesiobuccal cervical ridge from the root, and also due to the cervical slope of the occlusal border from mesial to distal. The mesial contact area with the canine is located more cervically than the distal contact area, which is in the middle of the crown.

The cervical line on the mesial, although it arcs toward the occlusal, also slopes gingivally toward the buccal (once again separating the mesiobuccal cervical ridge from the root, Fig. 9-18, proximal view). On the distal or lingual surface, the cervical line is practically flat or horizontal from buccal to lingual or from mesial to distal, respectively.

Recall that the crowns of all mandibular posterior teeth, primary and secondary, appear to lean lingually, even more so with primary teeth. This primary mandibular first molar crown appears to lean decidedly toward the lingual (accentuated by the prominent mesiobuccal cervical ridge), placing the buccal cusp tips well over the root base.[6] The lingual cusp tip may even be outside the lingual margin of the root (Fig. 9-18). From the proximal views, the buccal crown contour is nearly (but not quite) flat from the buccal crest of curvature to the occlusal surface and cervico-occlusally. The lingual surface is more convex cervico-occlusally.

a. Occlusal Shape and Anatomy of the Primary Mandibular First Molar

The general shape of the entire occlusal outline is somewhat oval or rectangular (wider mesiodistally than buccolingually). As with the primary maxillary molars, these teeth taper narrower toward the lingual, but do so primarily due to the taper of the mesial surface (Appendix 10s), and not of the distal side.[2] Subsequently, the mesiobuccal angle is acute, whereas the distobuccal angle is obtuse. The mesial crown contour is nearly flat buccolingually, whereas the distal surface is convex; the lingual surface is convex mesiodistally.

The shape of the occlusal table is that of a rhomboid, wider mesiodistally than buccolingually (Appendix 10r).[9] There is a *prominent transverse ridge* between the mesiobuccal and mesiolingual cusps (Appendix 10u). Even though the *entire tooth outline* from the occlusal view appears to be wider on the mesial half due to the prominent mesial cervical ridge, the occlusal table distal to the transverse ridge is larger than that portion mesial to the transverse ridge (Appendix 10v). Subsequently, the *mesial* triangular fossa and pit are relatively small, and the *distal* fossa is larger, extending almost into the center of the occlusal surfaces (Appendix 10v). In the large distal fossa, there is a central pit and a small distal pit near the distal marginal ridge. There is *no central fossa.*

This tooth has *four cusps*. The cusps are often difficult to distinguish, but careful examination of an unworn tooth will reveal (in order of diminishing size) a mesiobuccal , mesiolingual, distobuccal, and the smallest (also shortest) distolingual cusp. The *mesiobuccal cusp* of the mandibular first molar is always the largest and longest cusp, occupying nearly two-thirds of the buccal surface (Appendix 10t; Fig. 9-18A). This cusp is characteristically *compressed buccolingually*, and its two long cusp ridges extend mesially and distally serving as a blade when occluding with the maxillary canine.[5] The smaller *distobuccal cusp* is separated from the mesiobuccal cusp by a depression rather than a distinct groove. The *mesiolingual cusp* is larger, longer, and sharper than the distolingual cusp, and there is a slight groove between these two lingual cusps which ends in a depression near the cervix of the crown. The distal spur of the *distolingual cusp* forms the lingual third of the distal marginal ridge ending in a furrow.[5]

A central groove separates the mesiobuccal and mesiolingual cusps and connects with a mesial marginal groove (furrow). There is a short buccal groove and a short lingual groove on the occlusal surface. The buccal groove does not extend onto the buccal surface, and the lingual groove becomes a shallow depression on the lingual surface. Both marginal ridges have furrows or grooves between them and cusp ridges of lingual cusps[6] similar to the supplemental grooves in the triangular fossae of other posterior teeth. These grooves serve as escapeways during mastication.

b. Roots of Primary Mandibular First Molars

There are two roots—mesial and distal—with the mesial root wider (square and flat) and longer than the distal root. The distal root is more rounded, less broad, thinner, and shorter than the mesial root.

FIGURE 9-19. Primary *mandibular* right second molar, **cross-section** (buccal side ground off to expose pulp cavity). An interesting feature is the long narrow shape of the pulp horns, which often extend more into the crown, even higher or closer to the occlusal surface than seen in this cross-section.

FIGURE 9-20. Primary *maxillary* first molar, **cross-section** (mesial side removed). The root canals of the mesiobuccal root and of the lingual root (right side of picture) are exposed. An extensive area of decay beneath the enamel of the lingual cusp has reached the prominent pulp horn.

SECTION V. Pulp Cavities of Primary Teeth

Primary anterior teeth have pulp cavities that are similar in shape to the pulp cavities of the secondary teeth, but are much larger in proportion because of the thinner, more uniform enamel covering, and the thinner portion of dentin in the deciduous teeth. On anterior primary teeth, there are slight projections on the incisal border corresponding to the lobes, and there is usually no demarcation or constriction between the single canal and pulp chamber except on the mandibular central incisor.[9]

Primary molar teeth, when compared with secondary molars, have pulp chambers much less elongated vertically relative to the size of the tooth. In primary molars there is little or almost no root trunk, so the pulp chambers are mostly in the tooth crown (Fig. 9-19). Compare this to secondary molars where much of the pulp chamber is located in the root trunk. The pulp chambers of primary molars have long and often very narrow pulp horns extending beneath the cusps. Great care must be taken when preparing these teeth for restorations to avoid exposing the pulp horn to the oral cavity (Fig. 9.20).

LEARNING EXERCISE

1. If you are fortunate to have a collection of primary teeth, study the morphology for variations. Observe differences in the amount of root resorption, examine the occlusal surface for wear facets due to attrition, and evaluate the interior pulp chamber (after sectioning) for size, pulp horns, and thickness of enamel and dentin. Use the distinguishing characteristics in Table 9-5 and 9-6 to identify each tooth within your collection of deciduous teeth. If you don't have any teeth to study, try to recognize these traits as seen in the figures in this chapter.

2. Identify each tooth in a mixed dentition, and estimate "expected dental age" based on average eruption dates as follows: If you have learned the important range of dates for tooth eruption, and the sequence of eruption within those ranges, you should be able to estimate the "expected dental age" of a child based on what teeth are present in the mouth.

CASE 1: For example, look at Figure 9-21 and estimate the expected age of the child based on the

---

LEARNING EXERCISES, cont.

teeth visible in the mouth and those developing within the bone and still not erupted. Let us look at the facts. First, all primary teeth have erupted (which can be deduced based on their relatively small size, thin roots, and the fact that all permanent succedaneous teeth are forming apical to their primary tooth predecessors). Therefore the child is at least 2 years old. Next, the first permanent molars are not even close to emerging, so the child must be considerably younger than 6 years old. Finally, no resorption has begun on the primary tooth roots, so we can conclude that the child is closer to 3 or 4 years old, rather than to 5 or 6, since primary teeth roots begin to resorb about 3 years after eruption, which for the mandibular central incisors would be about $3^1/_2$ years old.

CASE 2: Next, estimate the dental age of the child based on the shapes of teeth in the radiographs in Figure 9-22. We see two mandibular premolar shaped crowns (with no roots) forming under the roots of two primary molars (evidenced by their divergent roots). Distal to the primary second

---

Table 9-5

ARCH TRAITS THAT DISTINGUISH PRIMARY MAXILLARY FROM MANDIBULAR TEETH

Maxillary Central Incisor	Mandibular Central Incisor
Short, wide, symmetrical crown	Long, narrow, symmetrical, very small
Root bends facially in apical $1/_3$	Root straighter but still bend facially in apical $1/_3$
Root long and bulky	Root long and thin
Large elevated cingulum	Smaller less prominent cingulum
Maxillary Lateral Incisor	Mandibular Lateral Incisor
Crown narrow and oblong	Smaller cingulum
Roots bend facially in apical $1/_3$	Root bends facially in apical $1/_3$
Maxillary Canine	Mandibular Canine
Wide crown mesiodistally	Crown longer, narrower, less symmetrical
Cusp tip sharp and centered	Cusp tip toward mesial
Mesial cusp ridge longer, steeper than D	Mesial cusp ridge shorter than D
Cingulum centered	Cingulum distally located
Mesial contact more cervical than distal	Distal contact more cervical than M
Root bends facially in apical $1/_3$	Root with less facial bend in apical $1/_3$
Flat labial cervical line	
Maxillary First Molar	Mandibular First Molar
3 roots (if intact): MB, DB, and L	2 roots (if intact): mesial and distal
3–4 cusps: MB largest, DB, ML, and DL may be absent	4 cusps: MB, DB, ML, and DL
Crown wider F-L than M-D; tapers to lingual	Crown much wider M-D than F-L
Crown wider F-L on mesial than distal; tapers to distal	Occlusal table has small mesial triangular fossa; large distal fossa
H-shape occlusal grooves	Well-developed mesial marginal ridge
Unique crown shape (or premolar-like)	Unique crown shape
Maxillary Second Molar	Mandibular Second Molar
3 roots (if intact): MB, DB, and L	2 roots (if intact): mesial and distal
Crown resembles small secondary maxillary first molar	Crown resembles small secondary mandibular first molar

---

LEARNING EXERCISES, cont.

---

molars are the larger, erupted 6-year molars with incomplete roots. The secondary maxillary canine and maxillary second molar crowns are still within the bone. By deduction, the child should be over 6 but not yet 12. Since the primary molars' roots are partially resorbed, the succedaneous premolars are close to emerging making the child closer to 8 or 9 years old. If you could confirm that the succedaneous incisors were all erupted, you could estimate the age at just over 9 years old.

CASE 3: Using the logic of deduction, look at the cut-away model in Figure 9-23 and see if you can estimate the expected dental age before reading the answer here.

ANSWER: The secondary first molars have emerged into the mouth making the child at least 6 years old. The relatively large size of the anterior incisor crowns, and lack of succedaneous teeth apical to the roots, indicate that the erupted incisors are succedaneous which places the age at 9 years old or older. The 12-year molar has not emerged, so the child is between 9–12. Since none of the succedaneous canines or premolars have yet emerged, the dental age is around 9.

Table 9-6

HOW TO TELL RIGHT FROM LEFT PRIMARY TEETH

Maxillary Central Incisor	Mandibular Central Incisor
90° mesioincisal angle	Difficult to discern
Distal contact more cervical than M	
Distoincisal angle more rounded	
Crown outline flat on mesial	
More cervical line curvature on mesial	
Maxillary Lateral Incisor	Mandibular Lateral Incisor
Flat mesial and rounded distal outline	More rounded distoincisal angle and distal crown bulge
Distal contact more cervical than mesial	Distal contact more cervical than mesial
More rounded distoincisal angle	More rounded distoincisal angle
More cervical line curvature on mesial	
Maxillary Canine	Mandibular Canine
Longer mesial cusp ridge:	Shorter mesial cusp ridge
Deeper and narrower D than M fossa	
Mesial contact more cervical than D	Distal contact more cervical than M
	Flat mesial crown outline
More cervical line curvature on mesial	More cervical line curvature on mesial
Maxillary First Molar	Mandibular First Molar
Crown longer on M than D (facial)	Crown longer on M than D (facial)
Crown wider (F-L) on mesial than distal	Occlusal table has small mesial triangular fossa; large distal fossa
Mesial cervical crown bulge	Mesial cervical crown bulge
D marginal ridge more cervical than M	D marginal ridge more cervical than M
DB root (if intact) is smallest; shortest	Mesial root (if intact) longer and wider (F-L)
	ML cusp pointed
Maxillary Second Molar	Mandibular Second Molar
Mesial cervical crown bulge	Mesial cervical crown bulge
Crown longer on M than D (facial view)	Crown longer on M than D (facial view)
Large ML cusp	Has fifth (distal) cusp
D marginal ridge more cervical than M	D marginal ridge more cervical than M
DB root shortest and smallest	Mesial root (if intact) longer and wider (F-L)

FIGURE 9-21. Case 1: Using the guidelines presented in this chapter, estimate the expected dental age of the child with this mixed dentition.

FIGURE 9-22. Case 2: Based on these radiographs of mixed dentition, estimate the expected dental age of this child. (Radiographs courtesy of Professor Donald Bowers, The Ohio State University)

FIGURE 9-23. Case 3: Estimate the expected dental age of the child with this mixed dentition.

Expected Teeth Based On Normal Position From The Midline	
Position from midline:	**Teeth expected in that position** **(if there are no missing or extra teeth):**
1st tooth from midline	Primary Central Incisor OR Secondary Central Incisor
2nd tooth from midline	Primary Lateral Incisor OR Secondary Lateral Incisor
3rd tooth from midline	Primary Canine OR Secondary Canine
4th tooth from midline	Primary First Molar OR First Premolar (adult)
5th tooth from midline	Primary Second Molar OR Second Premolar (adult)
6th tooth from midline	Secondary (Six-Year) First Molar
7th tooth from midline	Secondary (Twelve-Year) Second Molar
8th tooth from midline	Secondary Third Molar

FIGURE 9-24. Case 4: Identify each visible tooth in the unique dentition of this 15-year-old. Use the chart to guide your decision, but notice that some teeth are missing with the spaces filled in by adjacent teeth.

LEARNING EXERCISES, cont.

CASE 4: Finally, examine the unique dentition in Figure 9-24 to determine which teeth are present and which teeth are absent. Use the position from the midline as a guide to look for each tooth you expect to occupy that position, but always remember that the space could be occupied by the primary tooth OR its succedaneous tooth. Also realize that spaces are not always present when a tooth is missing. The teeth on either side of the space may move together and close the space either through orthodontic treatment, or due to a common tendency for teeth distal to a space to move (drift) into, and close, the space. Therefore, if a space is not occupied by the expected primary or secondary tooth, it may be because the tooth has been extracted or is missing, and you will have to adjust your positioning from the midline accordingly.

In this case, beginning at the midline, the large incisors appear to be adult central incisors, but the next teeth from the midline do not resemble lateral incisors. Instead, these teeth look like secondary canines, followed distally by first premolars. We therefore need to suspect that the lateral incisors are missing or still unerupted (impacted) within the maxillae. The teeth distal to the first premolars, which in an adult dentition should be the second premolars, instead resemble small maxillary first molars, followed by larger maxillary first molars. This leads us to conclude that the smaller molars, in the place of the maxillary second premolars, could be primary second molars (resembling the larger emerged 6-year first molars just distal to them). Since the 12-year second molars are also present (though partially cut off in the photo), the patient would be at least 12 years old. If that is true, we need to ask why there are no secondary lateral incisors or second premolars, and why the primary second molars are still present. A good history (which teeth have been extracted or have been confirmed as missing) along with excellent radiographs are needed to see whether the secondary lateral incisors or second premolars are still unerupted within the bone (impacted). If the lateral incisors are not present and never formed, they would be considered congenitally absent (that is, as a result of factors existing at birth). If the primary second molars were maintained into the adult dentition (usually because the second premolars were congenitally absent), the primary teeth in an adult would be called retained deciduous teeth. More on the topic of missing teeth will be presented in the chapter on dental anomalies.

LEARNING QUESTIONS

Learning questions on primary and mixed dentition and tooth morphology:

Circle the correct answer(s). More than one answer may be correct. Unless otherwise stated, teeth are identified using the Universal Identification System.

1.   Which primary teeth have crowns that are wider mesiodistally than they are long inciso- or occluso-cervically?
     a.   maxillary central incisor
     b.   maxillary first molar
     c.   mandibular lateral incisor
     d.   mandibular first molar
     e.   mandibular canine

2. Which one tooth is adjacent and distal to the primary maxillary second molar in a 7-year-old?
    a. maxillary first premolar
    b. maxillary second premolar
    c. secondary maxillary first molar
    d. secondary maxillary second molar
    e. primary maxillary first molar

3. How many teeth should be visible in the mouth of a 3-year-old?
    a. none
    b. 10
    c. 20
    d. 24
    e. 28

4. How many teeth should be present in the mouth of a 13-year-old?
    a. 10
    b. 20
    c. 24
    d. 28
    e. 32

5. Which primary molar most resembles a secondary maxillary right first molar?
    a. tooth A
    b. tooth E
    c. tooth F
    d. tooth T
    e. tooth B

6. What would you estimate to be the dental age of a child with the following teeth: all *primary* maxillary incisors, canines, and molars; *secondary* mandibular incisors and first molars.
    a. 2 to 4 years
    b. 5 to 7 years
    c. 8 to 9 years
    d. 10 to 11 years
    e. over 12 years

7. Which teeth (primary or secondary) have the mesial proximal contact positioned more cervically than the distal proximal contact?
    a. mandibular first premolar
    b. maxillary first premolar
    c. primary maxillary canine
    d. primary mandibular canine
    e. mandibular second premolar

8. Which teeth (secondary or primary) have the mesial cusp ridge of the facial cusp longer than the distal cusp ridge of the facial cusp?
    a. mandibular first premolar
    b. maxillary first premolar

    c. primary maxillary canine

    d. primary mandibular canine

    e. mandibular second premolar

9. Which succedaneous tooth erupts beneath tooth J?

    a. #1

    b. #5

    c. #10

    d. #13

    e. #16

10. Which of the following traits can be used to differentiate primary teeth from secondary teeth?

    a. Primary teeth have greater facial cervical bulges.

    b. Primary teeth have relatively thinner and longer roots.

    c. Primary teeth are whiter.

    d. Primary anterior teeth are larger than their successors.

    e. Primary teeth have relatively larger pulps.

11. Which of the following secondary teeth would you expect to be erupted in the average 9- to 10-year-old?

    a. maxillary lateral incisor

    b. maxillary central incisor

    c. mandibular canine

    d. maxillary canine

    e. mandibular second molar

12. Which traits apply to a primary mandibular first molar?

    a. Its roots are resorbed by the eruption of the 6-year mandibular first molar.

    b. It resembles a mandibular 6-year first molar.

    c. It has a prominent buccal cervical bulge.

    d. It has a prominent mesial marginal ridge.

    e. It has a prominent transverse ridge.

    f. It has an occlusal table larger in the mesial half than in the distal half.

ANSWERS: 1–a, b, d; 2–c ; 3. c; 4–d ; 5–a; 6–b; 7–a,c; 8–b,c; 9–d; 10–a, b, c, e; 11–a, b, c; 12–c, d, e.

REFERENCES

1. Hellman M. Nutrition, growth and dentition. Dental Cosmos Dec. 1923.
2. Brand RW, Isselhard DE. Anatomy of orofacial structures. St. Louis: C.V. Mosby, 1998:462–490.
3. Osborn JW, ed. Dental anatomy and embryology. Oxford: Blackwell Scientific Publications, 1981:144–151.
4. Huang L, Machida Y. A longitudinal study of clinical crowns on deciduous anterior teeth. Bull Tokyo Med Dent Univ 1987;28:75–81.
5. Jorgensen KD. The deciduous dentition—a descriptive and comparative anatomical study. Acta Odontologica Scandinavia 1956;14(Suppl 20):1–192.
6. Pagano JL. Anatomia dentaria. Buenos Aires: Editorial Mundi S.A., 1965:471–540.
7. DuBrul EL. Sicher's oral anatomy. 7th ed. St. Louis: C.V. Mosby, 1980:238–244.
8. Kraus B, Jordan R, Abrams L. Dental anatomy and occlusion. Baltimore: Williams & Wilkins, 1969:115–131.
9. Finn S. Clinical pedodontics. Philadelphia: W.B. Saunders, 1957:54–80.
10. Paulson RB, Gottlieb LJ, Sciulli PW, et al. Double-rooted maxillary primary canines. ASDC J Dent Child 1985; 52:195–198.

10 Functional Occlusion and Malocclusion

I. Jaw relationships of the mandible and maxillae
   A. Maximum intercuspal position (centric occlusion)
   B. Centric jaw relation (retruded contact position)
   C. Occlusal vertical dimension
   D. Jaw relations during horizontal movements of the mandible
II. Normal movements within the temporomandibular joint
   A. Movements within the lower joint space
   B. Movements within the upper joint space
   C. Total joint movement
III. The act of eating
   A. Incising
   B. Masticating (chewing)
   C. Swallowing (deglutition)
IV. Dislocation of the mandible (luxation or condylar subluxation)
V. Ideal occlusion versus malocclusion
   A. Ideal class I occlusion
   B. Dental malocclusions (including class I)
   C. Class II malocclusion (including division 1 and division 2)
   D. Class III malocclusion
VI. Parafunctional movements and contacts
VII. Treatment modalities
VIII. Accurate recording of the centric relation jaw position

An introduction to ideal *static* occlusion was discussed earlier in Chapter 3, Section VI. In this chapter, the more advanced aspects of tooth and jaw relationships *during function* are discussed, as well as the terminology and concepts associated with malocclusion (which literally means "bad" occlusion). The topics include the following:

OBJECTIVES

- Describe and recognize the following jaw relationships: maximum intercuspal position, centric jaw relation, and occlusal vertical dimension.
- Describe and recognize the following horizontal eccentric movements: protrusive (including the effect of horizontal and vertical overlap on incisal guidance) and lateral translation (including the effect of canine overlap on canine-protected occlusion).
- Define and recognize tooth relationships during lateral movements on the working and balancing sides.
- Describe and demonstrate mandibular movement within the lower joint space (rotation) and within the upper joint space (translation).

- Describe the relationship of teeth and adjacent oral structures during eating.
- Describe (and sketch) an ideal envelope of motion from the facial and sagittal views and label mandibular tooth positions or movements for each segment of the envelope.
- Describe mandibular dislocation (luxation) and demonstrate how to alleviate this problem with appropriate mandibular manipulation.
- Define Angle's Class I, II, and III relationships.
- List and describe types of tooth and jaw malocclusions.
- List and describe signs or symptoms of malocclusion (including the possible effects of premature contacts and parafunctional movements).
- List and describe possible methods of treatment for bruxing, myofunctional pain, and TMJ problems including the steps for construction of an occlusal device (bite guard).
- Describe a method for accurately recording a centric jaw relation position.

SECTION I. Jaw Relationships of the Mandible to the Maxillae

The maxillae (right and left) are firmly and immovably attached at suture lines to each other and to other bones of the facial skeleton. The maxillae move only as the head moves, not independently as does the mandible. The mandible articulates with the skull at the temporomandibular joints; it moves and changes its position in relation to the relatively stable maxillae and cranium. **Jaw relation** refers to the position of the mandible relative to the maxillae and could be thought of as a tooth-to-tooth relationship between maxillary and mandibular teeth, as well as a bone-to-bone (mandible to maxillae) relationship between the maxillae and mandible.

A. MAXIMUM INTERCUSPAL POSITION (CENTRIC OCCLUSION)

Maximum intercuspal position is a relationship between teeth. It is the tightest or best fit between maxillary and mandibular posterior teeth. (Fig. 10-1B). Other names for this are: maximum intercuspation, most occlusal position, acquired or habitual occlusion, centric occlusion, and natural bite. One can fit two casts of a person's upper and lower teeth together in the maximum intercuspal position without looking into the mouth (Fig. 10-2B).

B. CENTRIC JAW RELATION (RETRUDED CONTACT POSITION)

The most posterior position of the mandible relative to the maxillae with the mandible retruded maximally is called the **centric jaw relation**. It is a bone to bone relationship between the upper and lower jaws *without tooth contact* (or with one or only a few teeth *initially* contacting prior to closing teeth more tightly together into maximum intercuspal position).[1-3] It is most often behind (distal to) the maximum intercuspal position by 1–2 mm.[1,4,5] (In Figs. 10-1 and 10-2, compare the short vertical pencil lines connecting on each lateral view that line up between teeth in the maximum intercuspal position, but show the mandible distally positioned in centric jaw relation.) [Posselt found the distance to average 1.25 ± 1 mm with a range of 0.25–2.55 mm.[4]] Centric jaw relation also includes the *range of positions* with the mandible *retruded maximally* while rotating open *without bodily moving forward*. This relation can be obtained by tipping the head back with the mandible retruded, or by using an upward sloping gauge of variable thickness inserted between overlapping incisors to help guide a retracted closure of the mandible (a technique discussed later in this chapter and seen in Figs. 10-15 and 10-16).

In centric jaw relation, the condyles articulate with the thinnest avascular portion of their respective discs, and the condyle/disc complex is in an anterior-superior position against the posterior slopes of the articular eminence (recall Fig. 1-14). The presence or absence of teeth, or the type of occlusion or malocclusion, does not change this relationship.

It is a relatively rare but ideal occurrence when centric relation coincides with the maximum intercuspal position. This occurs when there is simultaneous, even contact between maxillary and mandibular teeth in maximum interdigitation as the mandible closes in its most retruded centric relation position.[2-4,6,7] This type of ideal occlusal relationship results from a balance between the guidance afforded by jaw muscles, condyle position, and fitting together of the teeth. This condition does not occur in most people unless they have just had a well-executed occlusal equilibration where small amounts of

CENTRIC JAW RELATION WITH TEETH
BARELY CONTACTING SOMEPLACE

A   VERTICAL
                     RELATIONSHIP

MAXIMUM INTERCUSPAL POSITION

B   RELATIONSHIP
                     OF MIDLINES

CENTRIC JAW RELATION WITH TEETH
BARELY CONTACTING SOMEPLACE

HORIZONTAL
OVERLAP   mm. DISTANCE

MAXIMUM INTERCUSPAL POSITION

LEFT SIDE

FIGURE 10-1. Maximum intercuspal position compared to centric jaw relation. A. Mandible has closed in the most retruded arc or **centric jaw relation** until the first tooth contact between any upper and lower teeth (indicating a prematurity or deflective contact). **B.** The mandible has continued to close from the first tooth contact into **maximum intercuspal position** and, as a result, the mandible has deviated (deflected) forward (as seen in the shift of the relationship of the vertical lines placed on the maxillary and mandibular first premolars) and laterally to the left (as seen in the shift of the alignment of the midlines of the maxillary and mandibular dentition). The deviation of the mandible was caused by deflective tooth interferences which guided the terminal (most upward) portion of jaw closure.

FIGURE 10-2. Maximum intercuspal position compared to centric jaw relation on a patient with severe deflective tooth contacts. A. Patient's casts (left side and right side) mounted in **centric jaw relation**. An articulator mounting of these casts in centric jaw relation using a leaf gauge revealed the *severe* deflective left second molar contact that is impossible to correct by an equilibration. This person's mandible would deflect forward 2 mm and to the right 1 mm as the teeth closed into maximum intercuspal position. **B.** Same patient's casts (left side and right side) mounted in **maximum intercuspal position**.

interfering occlusal enamel are removed by the dentist,[6] had a well-made removable denture, or had a complete dental arch rehabilitation replacing or reorienting all occlusal surfaces (seen later in Fig. 10-14).

When centric relation does *not* coincide with maximum intercuspal position, premature or deflective tooth contacts exist. **Premature or deflective occlusal contacts** refer to the teeth that contact first as the jaw closes in centric relation (most retruded position). Deflective occlusal contacts of opposing teeth are those which guide or direct the mandible away from centric relation, either forward or to one side or both, as the teeth slide together into maximum intercuspal position.

Mandibular deviation refers to the direction and movement of the mandible from the first slight premature tooth contact with the jaw in centric relation to the maximum intercuspal position. The direction of the deviation of the mandible is usually forward and upward with or without simultaneous lateral movement.[3,5,8] This is illustrated in Figure 10-1, where premature contacts deflect the mandible forward and to the left as the teeth move from centric jaw relation into maximum intercuspal position (from A to B), and in Figure 10-2, where the mandible is deflected forward 2 mm and to the right 1 mm (from A to B).

Most people have deflective malocclusion to some degree. (See Table 10-1, which gives information on deflective contacts for 811 dental hygienists).[6] Less than 1% of this group had maximum intercuspal position coincide with centric relation, yet most were asymptomatic. **Fremitus** is the palpable or visible movement of a tooth when subjected to occlusal forces. Fremitus is not necessarily an unhealthy condition, but may be an indication of a premature centric relation tooth contact or an interference during lateral excursions.

Edentulous people (with no teeth) who wear complete dentures or false teeth are provided with centric relation that coincides with maximum intercuspal position because they can learn to pull the mandible back and close into a *stable and repeatable position* of centric relation during jaw closure. This enables the tight occlusion of denture teeth to coincide with the repeatable closed-jaw position so the dentures will remain tightly secured against the mucosa and not rock loose when functioning. Dentists who make dentures attempt to duplicate and improve upon the patient's jaw relationships when teeth were present.

An **articulator** is a mechanical device that holds casts of the two arches, permitting a close duplication of the patient's open and closing centric jaw relations (Fig. 10-3). It is easier to study these relationships with the patient's dental arches (dental stone casts) on the articulator in your hands, rather than with your hands in the patient's mouth. What better way to determine whether or not the maxillary and mandibular lingual cusps fit together tightly or properly in the maximal intercuspal relationship?

Table 10-1

DEFLECTIVE CENTRIC RELATION TOOTH CONTACT DATA FROM 811 DENTAL HYGIENISTS

LOCATION OF FIRST CENTRIC RELATION TOOTH CONTACT	NUMBER OF HYGIENISTS	PERCENT
Premolars one side	232	28.6
Premolars both sides	90	11.1
Molars one side	328	40.5
Molars both sides	113	13.9
Molar one side; premolar one side	38	4.7
Canine	4	0.5
Maximum intercuspal position = centric jaw relation (no prematurities)	6[#]	0.7

TYPE AND PLACE OF DEFLECTIVE CONTACT	PERCENT
Premolars only	39.7
Molars only	54.4
Unilateral prematurity	69.2
Bilateral prematurity: same tooth	25.8
Bilateral prematurity: premolar-molar	4.7

[#]Three of the six recently had an equilibration by their dentists
Research conducted by Dr. Woelfel at The Ohio State University, 1974–1986

FIGURE 10-3. Casts mounted on an articulator. This articulator (Denar) can be used to mount casts of the patient's dentition in order to reproduce the position and movements of mandibular teeth relative to maxillary teeth. Notice the fit of the ball of the lower (mandibular) part fitting into a concavity on the upper part. This design somewhat simulates the head of the condyle fitting into the articular fossa. This mounting was used to design the tooth anatomy and occlusion for a fixed partial denture (bridge) from tooth 18 to 20 (replacing tooth 19) and a removable partial denture replacing teeth 12 through 15. (Mounting courtesy of Dr. Lisa Knobloch, The Ohio State University)

LEARNING EXERCISE

Tip your head way back with the teeth slightly apart, consciously retrude (pull back) your mandible, and close very slowly in a hinge motion (without sliding the jaw forward) until the first teeth initially touch gently. The relationship of your jaws prior to your first gentle tooth contact or contacts with the mandible retruded is your centric jaw relation. The relation of this retracted, pure hinge opening is a most important one to record when making extensive dental restorations for a patient. If your mandible is guided (hits and slides) forward as you continue to close your teeth together into their maximal intercuspal position where they fit together most tightly, you are experiencing deflective or premature occlusal contacts, and you are among the majority of people whose centric relation does not coincide with the maximal intercuspal position. The mandible will almost always slide forward from centric relation into maximum intercuspal position, either straight forward or to one side. More than likely, your own deflective tooth contacts will not be as severe as that shown in Figure 10-2. Can you determine which direction your premature tooth contacts deflect your mandible? Compare the location of your first (premature) tooth contact in centric relation with those in Table 10-1.

C. OCCLUSAL VERTICAL DIMENSION

Occlusal vertical dimension refers to the distance between a selected point on the mandible and a selected point on the maxillae. This dimension can be measured with the jaws positioned in centric relation or in maximum intercuspal position. **Vertical dimension of rest position** (or the **physiologic rest position**) is the position of the mandible when all of its supporting muscles (eight muscles of mastication plus the supra- and infrahyoids) are in their resting posture.[9] Physiologic rest position is further defined as the mandibular position when the person's head is upright, the muscles of mandibular movement are in equilibrium, and the condyles are in an unstrained position. Unless we are nervous, eating, talking, yawning, or using our muscles to perform other less natural functions, such as playing a clarinet, the mandible is in this comfortable resting position most of the time (over 23 hours each day).

FIGURE 10-4. Physiological rest position: effects of posture. A. This man assumes a normal posture with his mandible in physiologic rest position (r.p.). Posterior teeth, though not visible, are separated by an interocclusal distance. **B.** Now, the man is looking up and his mandible is again in physiologic rest position with his posterior teeth separated, but more so than in A, because of the stretch of fascia, skin, and the supra and infrahyoid muscles. The resting position of the mandible varies with such factors as body posture, fatigue, and stress.

When a person with an erect posture makes no conscious effort to open or close the mouth and the mandible is in its physiological rest position, there is a space between the occlusal surfaces of the maxillary and mandibular teeth called the **interocclusal distance** or **freeway space**. This space is normally 2 to 6 mm between the incisal and the occlusal surfaces of the maxillary and mandibular teeth. Of course, when the teeth are missing (in an edentulous person) there would be a 1 cm or more distance between the residual toothless ridges when the mandible is resting.[10]

A simple change in posture, such as looking up at the sky, or stretching the neck back in the reclined dental chair, will change the resting position of the jaw, separating the teeth farther than when in a comfortable upright position (Fig. 10-4). This change is due to the pull on the mandible by stretching skin and underlying fascia. Therefore, when a dentist places a restoration (filling) for a patient who is reclined in the dental chair, a final assessment and possible adjustment of the occlusion on this new restoration should take place with the patient in a relaxed *upright* position.

D. JAW RELATIONSHIPS DURING HORIZONTAL MOVEMENTS OF THE MANDIBLE

Relationships of the mandible relative to the maxillae can be documented as the mandible moves *horizontally* out of the centric relationship into other positions. **Eccentric** jaw relationships are any deviation of the mandible from the centric relation position. These relationships occur when the lower jaw moves anteriorly (**protrusion**), laterally (**mandibular lateral translation** or excursion), or any combination thereof.

1. PROTRUSIVE JAW RELATION

When pulled forward simultaneously by the lateral pterygoid muscles, the mandibular condyles and discs can slide forward down under the articular eminences in a movement known as **protrusion**. When pulled simultaneously by the posterior fibers of the temporalis muscles and assisted by the infra and suprahyoid muscles, the mandible can move backwards in a movement known as **retrusion** (**retraction**). As protrusion occurs, the movement of the mandible is influenced by the amount of overlap of the anterior teeth. When teeth are positioned in normal maximum intercuspal position, upper incisors and canines overlap lower incisors and canines (Fig. 10-5). This overlap can be described in terms of a **horizontal overlap** where maxillary incisal edges are labial to the mandibular incisal edges, and a **vertical overlap** where maxillary incisal edges overlap (and facially hide from view) part

MAXIMUM INTERCUSPATION

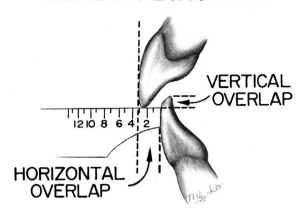

VERTICAL OVERLAP

HORIZONTAL OVERLAP

12 10 8 6 4 2

INCISAL AND CANINE GUIDANCE ANGLE ON 1114 STUDENTS

	Incisal Angle (Central Incisors)	Canine Rise Angle	
		Right Side	Left Side
Average	50°	56°	57°
Low	minus 26° (open bite)	0°	0°
High	86°	84.2°	83°

FIGURE 10-5. **Incisor and canine relationship and guidance.** Lateral view of maxillary and mandibular incisors showing the normal vertical and horizontal overlap of incisors when the posterior teeth are in maximum intercuspation. The incisal guidance angle is the angle formed between the occlusal plane (horizontal numbered line on illustration) and a line connecting the upper and lower incisal edges. It is only 37° in this illustration, which is less steep than in many dentitions. A canine guidance (rise) angle of 60° or more is necessary to provide canine guided disocclusion. **Chart:** Incisal and canine guidance angles of 1114 students.

of the mandibular incisor crowns. See Table 10-2 for the average and range of variations for these relationships.

Protrusive jaw relation is that position when the mandible moves anteriorly (as when incising food between the anterior teeth) so that both mandibular condyles *and* discs are forward in their glenoid or articular fossae, functioning against and beneath the articular eminences whose sloping morphology guides the mandible downward as it moves forward. Also, when a person with an *ideal* occlusal relationship moves the mandible forward, the incisal edges of the mandibular anterior teeth glide against the lingual surfaces of the maxillary anterior teeth, also guiding the mandible downward when protruding (recall Fig. 4-2). This is known as **incisal guidance.** It is influenced by the amount of movement and the angle at which the lower incisor and mandible must move downward and forward from the normally overlapping position of anterior teeth in maximal intercuspal position, to reach the edge-to-edge relationship of the mandibular and maxillary incisors. **Anterior guidance**

Table 10-2

INCISOR AND CANINE OVERLAP OF 1114 STUDENTS

NO. AND TYPE OF STUDENTS	INCISOR OVERLAP		CANINE OVERLAP			
			Horizontal		Vertical	
	Horizontal (mm)	Vertical (mm)	Right (mm)	Left (mm)	Right (mm)	Left (mm)
796 Dental Hygiene Students						
Average	2.78	3.27	2.01	2.02	3.23	3.19
Low	minus 2.5	minus 1.0	minus 1.0	minus 1.0	minus 1.0	minus 1.0
High	9.0	13.0	6.2	6.2	11.0	9.0
318 Dental Students						
Average	2.88	3.60	4.05	4.25	—	—
Low	minus 6.5 (prognathic)	minus 2.0 (open-bite)	0.0	0.0	—	—
High	10.0	8.0	8.5	9.0	—	—

Research conducted by Dr. Woelfel at The Ohio State University, 1974–1986

MAXIMUM PROTRUSION

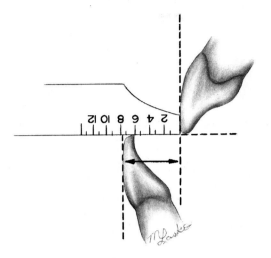

FIGURE 10-6. Maximum protrusive jaw relationship. This is the relationship of mandibular to maxillary central incisors when the mandible is maximally protruded. The mandible has protruded 11 mm because the mandibular central incisor was 3 mm lingual to the maxillary incisor in centric occlusion (see Figure 10-5).

(coupling) is a tightly overlapping relationship of the opposing maxillary and mandibular incisors and canines which produces disocclusion (separation) of the posterior teeth when the mandible protrudes or moves to either side from 1 to 4 mm.[11,12] [The average incisal guidance angle for 1,114 dental hygiene and dental students was 50° as shown in the chart is Figure 10-5. Many of these people did not have ideal Class I occlusion.]

When the mandible is *fully* protruded, the incisal edges of the mandibular incisors are in front of the maxillary anterior teeth. (Fig. 10-6) [The average maximum forward protrusion for 1,114 young men and women was 8.3 mm with a range from 2.5 to 16.0 mm (Table 10-3). These extremes included a very tight temporomandibular joint compartment that exhibited the smallest protrusion, and a very large jaw with loose ligament attachments which exhibited 16 mm protrusion.]

2. MANDIBULAR LATERAL TRANSLATION

During **mandibular lateral translation**, the mandible is moved to the right or left side and slightly downward as when masticating (chewing) food. When the mandible moves to one side, both condyles do not move equally toward that side. Rather, when the mandible moves to the *right side*, the *right condyle* rotates but remains relatively stationary, while the *left condyle and disc* move forward, downward, and medially within the articular fossa. Table 10-3 on maximum jaw movement reminds us that

Table 10-3

CAPABILITY OF MANDIBULAR MOVEMENT OF 1114 STUDENTS

NUMBER AND TYPE OF STUDENT	MAXIMUM JAW OPENING (MM)	MAXIMUM LATERAL JAW MOVEMENT		MAXIMUM JAW PROTRUSION (MM)	ENTIRE LATERAL JAW MOVEMENT (MM)
		Right (mm)	Left (mm)		
796 Dental Hygiene Students					
Average	51.01	7.68	7.71	8.44	15.39
Low	27.0	2.5	2.0	3.0	7.0
High	68.5	14.0	15.2	16.0	28.4
318 Dental Students					
Average	50.99	9.12	9.32	7.95	18.44
Low	35.5	2.0	3.0	2.5	6.0
High	71.0	14.0	15.4	13.5	32.0
Total Average of 1114 Students	50.29	8.09	8.17	8.30	16.26

Research conducted by Dr. Woelfel at The Ohio State University, 1974–1986

the mandible can move almost twice as far from side to side as it can directly forward. [The maximum average movement to either the right *or* left side was about 8.1 mm. Therefore, the *entire* lateral movement from right to left averaged 16.2 mm compared to an average forward protrusion of only 8.3 mm.]

Canine protected occlusion is an occlusal relationship in which the vertical overlap of the maxillary and mandibular canines produces a disocclusion (separation) of all the posterior teeth when the mandible moves to either side. **Disocclusion** refers to the separation of opposing teeth during eccentric movements of the mandible.[11,12] For example, in Figure 10-13I, note the separation of the right posterior teeth resulting from steep canine guidance on the left side as the mandible moves to the left. Many dentists consider this to be a desirable or healthy relationship to have. One study of 500 persons indicated that there was a lesser tendency toward bruxism (grinding the teeth together) with canine protected occlusion.[13] Another study found posterior tooth mobility to be higher in dentitions with canine protection than those with group function.[14] As seen in the chart in Figure 10-5, the average **canine guidance angle** was a little steeper (at 56° and 57°) than the anterior guidance (at 50°). To have a so-called **canine protected articulation** where the overlap of the canine teeth disengages the posterior teeth during excursive movements of the mandible, it is usually necessary to have a canine angle of over 60°. [Dr. Woelfel found canine protected articulation with posterior disocclusion in 37.7% of the natural dentitions of dental hygiene students (Table 10-4)]. When not present, it may be achieved through orthodontic treatment or by adding length or lingual thickness to the maxillary canines (by placing restorations).

Group function (or unilateral balanced occlusion) is an occlusal relationship in which *all* posterior teeth on a side contact evenly as the jaw is moved toward that side. This is much different from disocclusion, because multiple posterior teeth contact along with the canines on the working side.[7,15]

When the mandible moves to the right or to the left, the side where chewing (or work) occurs is called the working side, while the opposite side is called the nonworking side. In other words, the **working side** is the side toward which the mandible moves during lateral excursion. The **nonworking side** (previously known as the balancing side) is the side opposite the working side, or the side

---

Table 10-4

ECCENTRIC OCCLUSAL CONTACTS OF 342 HYGIENE STUDENTS

CONDITION	RIGHT QUADRANT	LEFT QUADRANT	TOTAL	PERCENT
Working Side Tooth Relationships:				
Canine Protected Articulation	207	205	412	60.2%
Group Function	135	137	272	39.8%
Nonworking Side Tooth Relationships:				
No contact	250	251	501	73.2%
Interference	92	91	183	26.8%

CONDITION	STUDENTS	PERCENT
Bilateral Canine Protected Articulation without nonworking side interference*	129	37.7%
Bilateral Canine Protected Articulation with nonworking side interference	29	8.5%
Bilateral Group Function without nonworking side interference	58	17.0%
Bilateral Group Function Articulation with nonworking side interference	34	9.9%
Different relationships on each side	92	26.9%

* Considered to be the best type of relationship

Survey conducted by Dr. Woelfel and his carefully trained staff. Doubtful recordings were personally reexamined by him for their validity (1980–1986). More than 30% of these 342 dental hygiene students had undergone orthodontic treatment.

which, during lateral movements, moves toward the median line. These terms are dependent upon which way the mandible is moved. For example, when the mandible moves to the right, the right side is the working side and the left is the nonworking, whereas when the mandible moves to the left, the left side is the working side, and the right is nonworking side.

The working side is the side where the "work" of chewing is occurring. As a person with an ideal occlusal relationship moves the mandible laterally, the posterior upper and lower teeth *on the working side* are aligned with the *upper buccal* cusps directly over the *lower buccal* cusps and with the *upper lingual* cusps directly over the *lower lingual* cusps. The condyle on the working side does not move much; it rotates on its vertical axis and moves laterally about 1 to 2 mm (called laterotrusion or Bennett's movement).

On the nonworking side, the *upper lingual* cusps are aligned over the *lower buccal* cusps, but ideally should *not* contact during the opposite side working tooth contacts. **Nonworking side** (mediotrusive or balancing) **interferences** refer to *any* tooth contacts on the nonworking side. The nonworking side mandibular condyle moves medially, downward, and forward perhaps 5 to 12 mm. If nonworking side interferences are heavy and frequent, they may actually be destructive to the supportive structures of the involved teeth, and can possibly cause temporomandibular joint pain on the opposite side because of the pivoting of the mandible and the stretching of opposite side ligaments and muscles. Poor occlusal relationships of any type can produce a variety of joint problems.[15-20] Canine protected dentitions generally do not have balancing side interferences . [As seen in Table 10-4, of 342 dental hygiene students examined, 26.8% had nonworking side interferences in at least one quadrant.]

The desirable type of relationship in a patient who has no teeth and must wear a set of complete dentures is **bilateral balanced occlusion**. This occurs when all of the posterior teeth contact on the working side *and* one or more teeth on the balancing side contact simultaneously. With complete dentures, the bilateral balancing contacts help to prevent the dentures from tipping and coming loose. It is considered potentially bad for a patient with natural teeth, however, to have any tooth contact on the nonworking side.

LEARNING EXERCISE

Feel the function of the temporomandibular joint by placing a finger on either side of your face just in front of your ears and opening and closing your mouth and moving the mandible from side-to-side. Then put your fingers in your ears and move the mandible sideways. Do you feel more movement when the jaw moves toward that side or when it moves away from that side? How do you account for this difference? (See reference 21 for interesting information on this subject.)

SECTION II. Normal Movements within the Temporomandibular Joint

The articular disc divides the articular space into two joint spaces (synovial spaces): an upper and a lower compartment.[22] (Recall Fig. 1-13). [In a healthy joint, with no clinical manifestations of joint disorder, the actual space (determined from radiographs) from the top of the mandibular condyles to the top of the temporal fossae measured 2.5 mm; to the anterior inferior surface of the eminence was 1.5 mm; and to the center of the external auditory meatus was 7.5 mm. This is based on averages from 50 subjects with teeth in centric occlusion, or 100 joints].[23]

The temporomandibular joint is a ginglymoarthrodial [[JIN gli mo ar THRO de al] joint, permitting both *hinge-like rotation* and *sliding* movements. Ginglymus [JIN gli mus] means rotation, and arthrodial [ar THRO de al] means freely moving. The *rotational* movements of condyles beneath the discs during centric relation occur in the *lower* joint space, whereas the *gliding* movements of the condyle *and* disc moving together over the articular eminence occur in the *upper* joint space.

A.   MOVEMENTS WITHIN THE LOWER JOINT SPACE

In the lower joint space, only a hinge-type or rotary motion can occur around a single terminal hinge axis, that is, the transverse horizontal axis that connects the condyles. The rotation of the mandible around a terminal hinge axis is possible only when the mandible is retruded in centric jaw relation, and only with a conscious effort or by the dentist's guidance. The purely rotational movement of the two rami around a horizontal axis connecting the two condyles can be compared to a playground swing with two supporting chains (similar to the supporting rami) that rotate front to back around a supporting pole (the swing's transverse horizontal axis). This purely rotational movement is only possible during the first part of mandibular opening while the jaws maintain a centric relation. [The maximum separation of the incisors for this pure-hinge opening (maximum hinge opening in Fig. 10-7) averages only 22.4 mm or 44% of maximum opening on 352 subjects (Table 10-5).]

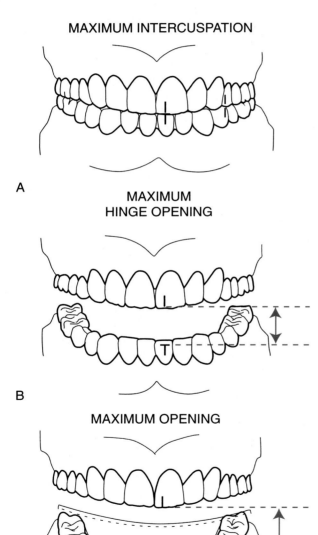

MAXIMUM INTERCUSPATION

A

MAXIMUM
HINGE OPENING

B

MAXIMUM OPENING

C

FIGURE 10-7. Range of opening for hinge and translation movements. **A.** Maximum intercuspal position. **B.** Maximum opening for hinge movement. **C.** Maximum normal total opening. Note: Movement from B to C would include both hinge *and* translatory movement. The curved horizontal line in C denotes the **mediolateral curve** (of Wilson) of the occlusal surface from side to side.

Table 10-5

TERMINAL HINGE (ROTARY) OPENING CAPABILITY OF 352 DENTAL HYGIENE STUDENTS

TYPE OF JAW OPENING	AVERAGE	RANGE	CONDYLAR ROTATION (AVERAGE IN DEGREES)	RANGE OF CONDYLAR ROTATION (IN DEGREES)
Maximum Opening at Incisors	51.0 ± 6.3 mm	27.0–68.5 mm	NA#	NA#
Hinge Opening at Incisors	22.4 ± 5.7 mm	9.5–40.5 mm	12.7*	4.4–24.2*
Percentage of Maximum Incisor Opening	44.0%	18.9–50.6%	—	—

#Unknown because translation has taken place in upper compartment.
*Results obtained by Dr. Woelfel (1980–1986).

B. MOVEMENTS WITHIN THE UPPER JOINT SPACE

Translation is the *bodily movement* of the mandible downward *and* forward, and occurs only within the upper joint spaces. When opening and closing the mouth wide, the discs *and* mandibular condyles together translate forward (upon opening) and backwards (retrude) upon closing. During translation, the horizontal axis between the condyles actually moves forward as the condyles and discs slide around within the articular fossa and adjacent eminence. Think of this translatory movement as taking the entire playground swing set with its horizontal axis in the previous example, and moving it forward, which moves the swing (mandible) bodily forward. If the swing is still swinging, a hinge movement is now combined with translation, similar to most movements within the jaw. Both translatory and rotational opening movement occur when a person continues opening beyond about halfway, beginning at the maximum hinge opening limit (Fig. 10-7B) continuing through the maximum possible opening (Fig. 10-7C).

The combined hinge and translatory motion follows a curved path primarily dictated by the movement of the condyle against the posterior inferior slope of the articular eminence, which is on the anterior portion of the articular (glenoid) fossa. Most functional movements of the mandible involve translatory motions with curved components because of the shape of the articular fossae and eminences, and because no conscious effort is made to open in a retruded manner.[24,25]

When the condyles and discs do not move forward simultaneously, the result may be crepitation. **Crepitation** (crepitus) is the crackling or snapping sound or noise emitted from the temporomandibular joints because of a disharmonious movement of the articular disc and the mandibular condyle, sometimes erroneously thought to be caused by the rubbing together of the dry synovial surfaces of joints. When the crackling noise is heard, the articular disc is snapping in or out of position too quickly or it becomes locked in the wrong position.[7,15,16,19,20,26] The frequency of crepitation among 1,099 dental hygiene and dental students was presented in Chapter 1 in Table 1-2. Over one-third of these students had some crepitus while opening widely; it was slightly more prevalent on the right side than on the left side, and was more common in women than in men. As you can see, crepitation is *not* a rare occurrence.

Usually, unless crepitation is accompanied by pain, limited jaw opening, or **trismus** [TRIZ mus] (a spasm of masticatory muscles associated with difficulty opening or locking of the jaw), treatment is not indicated.[19,27] The noise may disappear with time, or it may persist for many years being no more than a noisy annoyance. With practice, a person who has crepitus on one or both sides can learn to open the jaw like a hinge in a retruded position without any clicking noise, because the discs remain in position as the retruded condyles rotate beneath them.

LEARNING EXERCISE

Place your fingers in front of your ears and open and close your jaw to palpate the lateral heads of the mandibular condyles. When you open widely (as in yawning), you will now be rotating and translating your mandible. You may feel a bump, or hear a click or popping sound, or hear a grating noise (called crepitation) as the condyles move (translate) forward and slide down under the articular eminences. These sounds may be signs of pathology within the joint such as a disc that does not follow the movements of the condyle. How far are you able to open in the incisor region before you feel the condyles slide or slip forward (translation in the upper part of the joints)? Compare this limited amount of opening with your maximum opening in the incisor region and compare with Dr. Woelfel's measurements shown in Table 10-5.

C. TOTAL JOINT MOVEMENT

During the normal day-to-day activities and functioning of the masticatory complex, a *pure* hinge type rotation of the mandible does *not* occur since all functional mandibular movements involve both translation with some rotation, but not around a stationary, single axis as described earlier. Normal functional motion such as eating, swallowing, yawning, relaxing the jaw, and talking, occurs simultaneously in both the upper and lower spaces of the temporomandibular joints, resulting in combined translatory and rotary movement. This combination of both hinge and sliding movement is a specific characteristic of human jaw opening. Even in the highest order of apes (chimpanzee), the mandible drops open in a simple hinge movement.

An exhaustive study on the temporomandibular joint by Turell includes color pictures of many human temporomandibular joints—some healthy, some with displaced discs, and others diseased with osteoarthritis.[20] This project involved dissection and analysis of joints from 100 cadavers (dead for less than 12 hours). Joint conditions were found to be directly related to existing occlusal relationships. Older people with their teeth and natural occlusion had normal joints. Internal joint changes were determined to be more common in the elderly only because of occlusal interferences, loss of teeth, heavy attrition, and uncorrected malpositions of teeth. It was concluded that many of the alterations seen in osteoarthritic temporomandibular joints had been caused by abnormal, heavy forces within the joints from poor occlusion.[20]

Try to find a copy of reference 27 in your library. It has a glossary, a review of significant research on the temporomandibular joint, 488 references, and contains original research on the joints of 318 oral rehabilitation patients compared to those of 61 other patients. It is a fascinating treatise.

SECTION III. The Act of Eating

Eating involves the intake of food by placing it in the mouth, **incising** to obtain a manageable size morsel, chewing (also called **mastication** [mas ti KA shun]), and swallowing (also called **deglutition** [deg loo TISH un]).

A. INCISING

Incising is the articulation of the anterior teeth performed to cut food into chewable morsels. Eating begins as the mandible drops downward to open the mouth, food is placed between the opposing anterior teeth, and the mandible is protruded (by the lateral pterygoid muscles). The mandible then closes in this protrusive position until the incisal edges of the anterior teeth meet the morsel. The mandible is then moved up and posteriorly with the mandibular incisors against lingual surfaces of the maxillary incisors, thus cutting a portion of the food free.

B. MASTICATING (CHEWING)

Next, food is transferred by the tongue to the posterior teeth; it is held in position on the teeth of the working side by the buccinator muscles in the cheeks and the action of the tongue. The teeth are brought together, engaging the food with the mandible in a slightly lateral position toward the working side. The upper buccal cusps are directly over the lower buccal cusps with the mandible in this lateral position. The closing motion slows as the mandible is forcibly closed[28] (by the masseter and medial pterygoid muscles), and the canine overlap and inclines of posterior tooth cusps guide the mandible into maximum intercuspation of the posterior teeth. As this happens, the crushed food squirts out into the buccal and lingual embrasures and grooves, and down over the tooth curvatures toward the cheek and onto the tongue where it can be tasted, mixed with saliva, placed back over the teeth, and chewed some more. Once the posterior teeth contact in maximum intercuspal position, there is a pause of about 0.16 second (silent period). Next, the mandible opens and moves laterally to commence the next chewing stroke. The duration of each chewing stroke varies from 0.7 to 1.2 seconds in most people.[28] We usually chew like this on one side for several strokes and then switch the food over to the opposite side where a similar chewing cycle occurs.

Tooth cusp slopes and triangular ridges act as cutting blades, whereas major and supplemental grooves serve as escape pathways (escapeways or sluiceways) for crushed food to squirt out buccally and lingually. This mechanism significantly reduces lateral forces applied to the teeth which could be damaging to the teeth and their supporting bone.

A helpful method for analyzing a patient's mandibular movement is to attach a stylus to the mandibular teeth that can trace (on paper) the movements of the mandible as viewed from the front (a frontal view), or from the side (a sagittal view). Figure 10-8 shows these two tracings, both reproducing the outer maximum border movements of the mandible, each called an **envelope of motion**. Trace the *frontal* envelope in order to appreciate what it reveals. Begin in the maximum intercuspal position (MIP) at the top and fol-

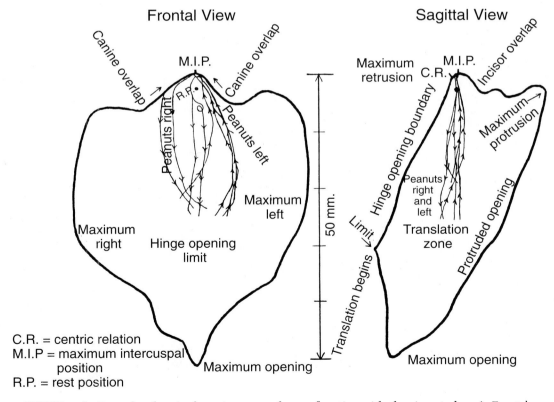

FIGURE 10-8. Frontal and sagittal maximum envelopes of motion with chewing strokes. A. Frontal view: Four chewing strokes are shown within the large envelope of motion as the patient chewed on 3 gram portions of peanuts, first on the left and then on the right sides (arrows denote direction of chewing strokes). **B.** Sagittal view of same patient during chewing.

lowing clockwise. The mandible with the teeth in contact first slides laterally to the patient's left (our right) as far as possible. The canine overlap results in the mandible initially moving down as it moves to the side. Next, the jaw opens downward in its most left lateral position until open about 30 mm, then begins veering toward the center to a maximum opening of 51 mm. From this point, the jaw moves to the patient's right (our left) as far as possible as it begins to close. Finally, from the closed maximum right side position, the teeth slide into maximum intercuspal position as the jaw slowly moves back and upward (due to the canine overlap) into the starting point (MIP).

To trace the *sagittal* envelope of motion, begin at the most retruded posterior position (centric relation or CR). Due to a slight deflective (premature) contact, the mandible is directed forward and slightly upward into maximum intercuspal position (MIP). With the teeth held together lightly as the mandible continues to protrude maximally, the initial downward movement is due to incisal overlap, followed by an upward and forward movement beyond the edge-to edge position into the most protruded position. With the mandible protruded, it moves down to the maximum opening of 51 mm. From this point, the jaw closes while firmly retruded which develops the curved *translation* portion of closure, followed by the straighter hinge opening boundary (with rotary motion only), and finally back to the starting point (MIP). We can tell from this envelope of motion that upon opening, this man can *rotate* his retruded mandible open 30 mm at the incisors with a hinge movement before it begins to translate forward.

Now focus on the smaller pattern (enclosed within the larger frontal envelope of motion) of that person chewing peanuts on the right and left sides. The line traced during the *opening* stroke (denoted by opening arrows pointing downward) is somewhat straight, whereas the *closing* stroke is considerably convex or bulges as the mandible moves toward the working side to obtain working side tooth contacts. The chewing cycles occupy only 25 of the maximum 51 mm opening range for this man. The chewing strokes on peanuts in a lateral direction utilize only 12 mm of the total side-to-side range of mandibular movement.

Frontal envelopes of motion for three young men

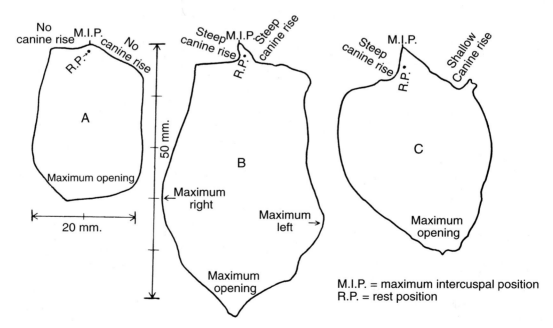

FIGURE 10-9. Variations in movement and canine guidance: The frontal envelopes of motion of three men, demonstrating the wide range of variability between the movement capabilities and their canine guidances.

On the *sagittal* view, note that the chewing stroke begins at the maximum intercuspal position (MIP), and the opening stroke is more posterior than the closing stroke. [The opening stroke is only 7 mm anterior to the hinge opening boundary, whereas the closing stroke is 10 mm anterior to that boundary.] However, as the jaws are closed to crush the food bolus, the mandible is slightly more retruded than the maximum intercuspal position. Crushing of the food bolus occurs at this maximal intercuspal position.

Now, study Figure 10-9 to compare the uppermost portions of the frontal envelopes of motion of three subjects in order to visualize differences in the superior portion related to the amount of canine guidance (overlap). Subject A has the smallest and narrowest range of movement for his mandible (32 mm vertically, 21 mm sideways). No lowering of the mandible on either side of the MIP indicates he did not have canine protection (deeply overlapping canines) to lower the mandible and disocclude the posterior teeth. Subject B can open his mandible 53 mm and move it laterally 31 mm. He has a canine protected occlusion as indicated by the steep portion where the mandible drops on either side of the MIP. Patient C had a medium-sized envelope of motion with canine protection on the patient's right side and group function occlusion with shallow canine rise on the patient's left. This patient preferred to chew mostly on the left side where his envelope is lopsided.

LEARNING EXERCISE

Look in a mirror and move your jaw as far as possible in all directions (wide open, and from right to left) as far as possible to discover exactly how wide and long your total envelope (range) of motion is. Then chew some sugarless gum and notice that you use perhaps only half of this overall range of motion. Observe the pattern of movement of your mandible from the facial view during chewing to see if you move your mandible in a tear drop or circle shape similar to the envelope of motion seen on the left in Figure 10-8. Your side or sagittal view could also be viewed using a second mirror placed at 45°.

C. SWALLOWING (DEGLUTITION)

Swallowing begins as a voluntary muscular act (when we decide to) but is completed involuntarily by reflex action. The mechanics are as follows:

- The anterior part of the mouth is sealed (lips closed).
- The teeth are closed into their maximum intercuspal position.
- The soft palate is raised.
- The hyoid bone is raised as we close off the trachea (windpipe). This prevents food from passing into the lungs.
- The posterior part of the tongue is engaged in a piston-like thrust causing the small mass of chewed food (**bolus**) to be pushed into the oral pharynx [FAR inks] (throat).
- The act of swallowing takes place.
- Once the bolus is in the pharynx, the superior portion of the posterior wall presses forward to seal the pharynx, and then the esophageal phase of swallowing commences. This is accomplished by involuntary **peristalsis** (waves of contraction), which moves the food bolus through the entire length of the digestive tract.
- Then the mandible usually drops open, assuming its physiological resting posture. Several swallows are necessary to empty the mouth of a given food mass. However, even without food or drink, we swallow a number of times every hour without thinking about it.

Bite off a piece of firm food and analyze your jaw movements by looking in a mirror as you prepare the food for swallowing. This process is called mastication, to be followed by deglutition (swallowing). Observe and feel the hyoid bone above the voice box move as you swallow. Also, notice how difficult it is to swallow with your lips and teeth apart. Dental professionals must remember this fact as they keep patients' mouths open for extended periods of time without providing an opportunity for them to close their teeth together and swallow.

SECTION IV. Dislocation of the Mandible (Luxation or Condylar Subluxation)

During an extreme opening of the mandible, the disc and head of the condyle may move forward so far that they slip out of the articular fossa and forward beyond the articular eminence. Thus, the mandible will be partially dislocated or **subluxed**. This dislocation occurs in the upper joint compartment where translation occurs. If the closing muscles suddenly contract, the mandible could become painfully locked open. The patient's jaw opening muscles are not nearly as powerful as the closing muscles and, therefore, are unable to unlock a mandibular dislocation. [Perhaps you have seen an alligator trainer hold the alligator's jaws closed with only one hand (comparatively weak lateral pterygoid muscles)].

A subluxed position could be released only by another person who must depress the mandible with heavy force by pushing downward and backward with the thumbs on the buccal shelf next to the first molars. Recall that the disc is loosely attached to the condyle and normally travels with it. The loose capsular tissue surrounding the joint does not usually tear when dislocation occurs, but there would be a lot of pain until the contracted muscles relax after the mandible is depressed and repositioned by the thumbs of the rescuer.

SECTION V. Ideal Occlusion versus Malocclusion

Ideal occlusion is the relationship of teeth and jaws that dentists and dental specialists would like to reproduce when restoring a patient's entire mouth to form and function. **Malocclusion**, on the other hand, is literally a "bad" occlusion with poor tooth alignment or interferences that result from abnormalities in the size or arrangement of teeth, in the relative sizes of the dental arches and their alignments, or in the types of poor occlusal relationships acquired naturally or from incomplete orthodontic treatment. Malocclusions include tooth or *dental* malocclusions, *skeletal* relationships that adversely affect the occlusion, or a combination of both.

Malocclusion can be detrimental to oral health if it adversely affects appearance, comfort, or function. It could even cause ringing in the ears, sinus pain, dizziness, and migraine-type headaches, and could contribute to tooth wear (facets), and/or bone loss, loose teeth, or joint pain.[10] Myofascial [my o FASH i el] pain dysfunction syndrome (MPD) is a common disorder and it originates in the jaw muscles.[16,17] (Muscle fascia is the thin connective tissue covering that connects muscles.) The pain from this condition can often be alleviated simply when the patient wears a maxillary occlusal bite plane (occlusal device), as shown in Figure 10-13 and discussed later.

Three classes of *skeletal* relationships are recognized. They were first classified by Dr. Edward H. Angle in 1887. The ideal *skeletal occlusal* relationship is called Class I occlusion. In contrast, Class II and Class III relationships are considered to be *skeletal mal*occlusions because of the considerable difference in size, or the abnormal positional relationship, of the maxillae and the mandible (Fig. 10-12). Each class of skeletal relationship is defined by describing the occlusion of the first teeth to erupt in the adult dentition: namely, the maxillary and mandibular first molars.

A. *IDEAL* CLASS I (SKELETAL) OCCLUSION (ALSO CALLED NORMAL OCCLUSION OR NEUTROCCLUSION)

The profile of a person with Class I occlusion is called **orthognathic** [or thog NA thik], characterized by a lack of obvious protrusion *or* retrusion of the resting mandible relative to the maxillae. Recall from Chapter 3 that Class I occlusion is defined by the relationship of the first permanent molars: the tip of the mesiobuccal cusp of the maxillary first molar is aligned directly over the mesiobuccal groove on the mandibular first molar and the maxillary canine fits into the facial embrasure between the mandibular canine and first premolar (Fig. 10-12, column A).

The static *tooth* relationships considered to be normal or ideal include the following:

- The incisal edges of maxillary teeth are labial to the incisal edges of mandibular teeth (horizontal overlap in Fig. 10-5).
- The incisal edges of mandibular incisors are hidden from view by the overlapping maxillary incisors (vertical overlap in Fig. 10-5).
- Buccal cusps and buccal surfaces of the *maxillary* teeth are buccal to those in the mandibular arch whereas the lingual cusps and lingual surfaces of the *mandibular* teeth are lingual to those in the maxillary arch (Fig. 10-11A).
- Lingual cusps of *maxillary* teeth rest in occlusal fossae of the mandibular teeth whereas the buccal cusps of the *mandibular* teeth rest in the occlusal fossae of the maxillary teeth (Fig. 10-11A).
- The vertical (long) axis midline of each maxillary tooth is slightly distal to the vertical axis of the corresponding mandibular tooth (seen best in Fig. 10-2B).
- Normal occlusion is an absence of individual dental malocclusions, although they may occur even in Class I relationships.[15]

During function, *ideal* or normal occlusion exists when only the canines touch as the mandible moves laterally (without molar and premolar contacts) known as canine protected articulation; no nonworking side contacts exist; and the anterior teeth occlude (couple) together to disocclude the posterior teeth during protrusive movements (known as anterior guidance or anterior protected articulation).

B. *DENTAL* MALOCCLUSIONS (INCLUDING CLASS I)

Dental malocclusions can occur in mouths with a Class I, II, or III skeletal relationship. They include malalignments of teeth such as (a) crowded arch (Fig. 10-10), (b) a loss of arch continuity, (c) poor alignment of the anterior teeth (aesthetic malocclusion, Fig. 10-10), (d) abnormal buccolingual tooth relationships such as crossbite or buccoversion of the maxillary posterior teeth (Fig. 10-11B or C), and/or (e) heavy or premature occlusal contacts (Fig. 10-2A). Possible effects of dental malocclusion include tooth facets, bone loss, loose teeth, and joint pain.

C. CLASS II MALOCCLUSION (INCLUDING DIVISION 1 AND DIVISION 2)

This is a skeletal type of malocclusion with a *small mandible* relative to the maxillae (Fig. 10-12, column B). This could involve a very small mandible, or very large protruding maxillae, or both. The mandibular teeth are in a distal and sometimes lingual relationship to their normal maxillary opponents (buccoversion in Fig. 10-11B). The patient's curved **retrognathic** [ret ro NATH ik] convex facial profile appears to have a receded chin. Often there is an abnormally large horizontal overlap of anterior teeth with the maxillary incisors 5-10 mm labial to the mandibular incisors. Some evidence indicates that people with this type of malocclusion have more crepitus because of the frequent necessity to protrude the jaw consider-

FIGURE 10-10. **Esthetic malocclusion: crowding.** Extreme anterior crowding in a mandibular dentition. The mandibular lateral incisors emerged lingual to, rather than beneath, their deciduous predecessors, which were subsequently extracted with nearly half of their roots intact.

FIGURE 10-11. **Molar relationships in cross-section. A.** Views of the **normal** occlusion with the buccal surfaces of maxillary molars buccal to mandibular molars. **B.** Maxillary molars in **buccoversion** or more buccal than normal; common with Class II malocclusion where the mandible is small relative to the maxillae. **C. Posterior crossbite** (reverse articulation) with mandibular molars positioned buccally to maxillary molars; common with Class III malocclusion, where the mandible is large relative to the maxillae.

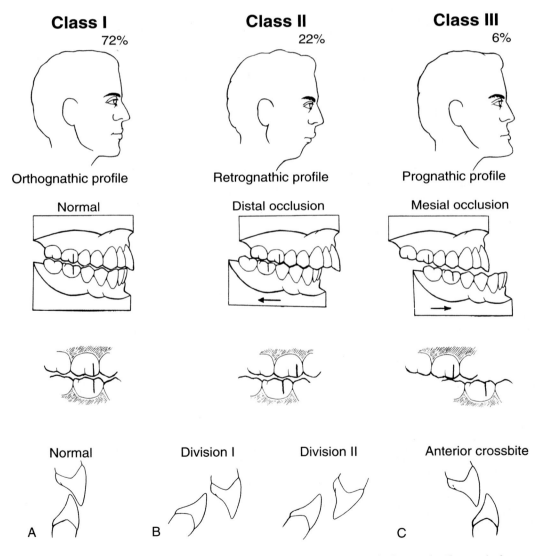

FIGURE 10-12. **Angle's classifications of occlusal relationships: Class I** (column A), **Class II** (column B), **and Class III** (column C). Top row: expected facial profile; second row: occlusal relationships of casts in maximum intercuspal position; third row: a close-up of the first molar relationships; fourth row, incisor relationships for each class.

ably forward in order to properly enunciate and to incise. There are two subdivisions of this type of skeletal malocclusion based on the inclination of the maxillary incisors. They are known as Division I and Division II (as seen in the lowest row in Fig. 10-12, column B).

- Class II, Division I is where the maxillary incisors have a labial inclination similar to that found in normal Class I occlusion. People with this subdivision of malocclusion have a long face, a tapered arch with high palate, a large horizontal overlap of maxillary incisors labial to mandibular incisors, super-eruption of mandibular incisors, diminished muscle tone in the upper lip, and an overactive lower lip.[26]
- Class II, Division II is where the maxillary incisors have a lingual inclination. Also these people have a short, wide face, square arch, less horizontal overlap than in Division I, a deep vertical overlap, severe anteroposterior curve (of Spee), anterior crowding, and well-developed chin musculature.[26]

D. CLASS III MALOCCLUSION (ALSO CALLED MESIAL OCCLUSION, MESIOOCCLUSION OR MANDIBULAR PROGNATHISM)

This is a skeletal type of malocclusion with a relatively *large mandible* compared to the maxillae, and with the mandibular teeth in a mesial, and often facial, relationship to their upper counterparts (Fig. 10-12, column C). In addition to a massive mandible, people with this class of malocclusion have a long narrow face, a tapered upper arch with a high vaulted palate, increased activity of their upper lip, and decreased activity of their lower lip. The anterior teeth may be in an edge-to-edge or crossbite relationship (lowers are facial to uppers) (seen anteriorly in Fig. 10-12, column C, lowest row, and seen posteriorly in Fig. 10-11C). The patient's facial profile will be concave with a very prominent chin (or **prognathic** [prog NATH ik]). Other terms for this anterior tooth relationship are underbite, anterior crossbite, or reverse articulation. Crepitus is not common with Class II malocclusion since little, if any, protrusion is required to clearly enunciate or to incise.

Treatment of Class II and Class III malocclusions using orthodontics (including braces) usually require much longer correction time and often involve surgical intervention compared to treatment of Class I malocclusions. This is due to the greater disparity from an ideal relationship of the corresponding teeth in the maxillae and mandible. A sliding **osteotomy** [ahs te OT o me] where the jaw bones are cut and reshaped may, in conjunction with orthodontics, be used to correct Class II and II skeletal malocclusions. This technique will dramatically and suddenly improve appearance, provide better tooth relationships and, eventually, better function as well.

From eight unrelated surveys of the prevalence of malocclusion done by orthodontists on 21,328 children, ages 6 to 18, in the United States between 1951 and 1971, Dr. Woelfel averaged the results and derived the following information:

- 71.7% had malocclusion (range: 31–95%)
- 28.3% had acceptable occlusion
- 72.3% had Angle's Class I malocclusion (range: 62–88%)
- 22.0% had Angle's Class II malocclusion (range: 8–32%)
- 5.7% had Angle's Class III malocclusion (range: 2–12%)

SECTION VI. Parafunctional Movement and Contacts

Functional tooth contacts (articulation) occur during the normal day-to-day processes of mastication and deglutition. **Parafunctional** contacts, on the other hand, are those which occur outside of these normal functions. Parafunctional movements that influence and contribute to these parafunctional tooth contacts include, for example, **clenching** (squeezing the teeth together without jaw movement), **bruxing** (grinding the teeth together in movements other than chewing), smoking a pipe (which involves chewing on the pipe stem), playing a reed instrument such as an oboe, and playing a violin (which affects jaw alignment and tooth contacts due to the tipping of the neck).

Parafunctional contacts can result in tired muscles, **trismus** (a disturbance of the trigeminal nerve resulting in spasms of the masticatory muscles and limited jaw opening), sore tooth or teeth, joint pain, loose tooth or **fremitus** [FREM i tus] (detectable as a vibration of the tooth upon tapping), **facets** (flattened areas of the tooth due to rubbing away of tooth structure, especially due to heavy or premature tooth contacts), and pain of the face, head and even the neck. The pain can sometimes be severe.[15-18, 29,30] It is not surprising, therefore, that parafunctional habits and contacts are undesirable and should be avoided. **Temporomandibular disorders (TMD)** from abnormal functions of the temporomandibular joints can result from loss of vertical dimension from tooth wear or tooth loss, loss of posterior tooth support, and/or other malocclusions. Symptoms of TMD can include headaches, ringing of the ears (**tinnitus** [ti NI tis]), ear pain, and impaired hearing.

Tooth contacts during parafunctional movements, especially if they involve considerable force and frequency, can be potentially damaging to teeth, to tooth supportive structures and to the temporomandibular joint. Unfortunately, when a person develops a bruxing habit, these heavy potentially damaging tooth contacts are exercised almost constantly under stressful situations. In a healthy person without occlusal problems, functional tooth contacts over a 24-hour period, including eating three meals, will total only 7–8 minutes. Parafunctional tooth contacts, in contrast, may amount to several hours per day.

Biting strength in bruxers or clenchers can be as much as six times higher than the in nonbruxers, so it takes little imagination to understand why bruxing can be a dangerous and damaging habit.[24] [Natural dentition chewing forces are well below maximum bite force on average foods, ranging from 0.5 to 33 pounds, seldom exceeding 100 pounds.[25] The human jaw muscles are very powerful, however. The largest maximum bite strength ever recorded was that of a 37-year-old man who maintained a force of 975 pounds for 2 seconds.[24] The average maximum biting force for 20 subjects was 192 pounds (range: 55–280 lbs.)].

Fortunately, we have a natural mechanism that protects teeth from heavy (or deflective) tooth contacts. Our fifth cranial nerve (trigeminal nerve) provides nerve branches to the periodontal ligaments of each tooth, and these nerve fibers send messages to the brain from sensory end organs (called **proprioceptors** [PRO pree o SEP ters]). These stimuli direct movements of the muscles that move the mandible in order to *avoid* heavy traumatic or deflective contacts. Several animal studies using cats have found that canines are more richly represented by neuron units (mechanoreceptors in the periodontal ligament) than any other teeth.[31-33] Another study reported that the periodontal ligament proprioceptors were directionally sensitive to forces of a few grams.[34] Such evidence lends credence to the canine protection theory.[7,11,12] By virtue of this complex protective mechanism, traumatic or deflective tooth contacts are most often avoided during normal function (chewing, talking, and swallowing).[1-3,6,7]

SECTION VII. Treatment Modalities

Treatment modalities for bruxing, myofascial pain, and temporomandibular joint disorders (TMD) may involve or include (a) conscious effort by the patient to avoid clenching, (b) biofeedback, (c) tranquilizers, (d) muscle relaxants (medication), (e) occlusal corrections including orthodontics, and tooth equilibration (selective recontouring of enamel), (f) jaw muscle exercise, (g) patient education, (h) nutritional guidance, (i) psychological counseling, and (j) occlusal bite guard (occlusal device) therapy.[29,30,35]

To succeed and to correct a patient's unfortunate parafunctional bruxing habit is not an easy task and takes time, skill, and patience at best. A basic principle of treating occlusal dysfunction is to get the teeth to come together evenly with the jaw in the most comfortable position. This can be accomplished through a combination of therapies that includes anterior deprogramming, use of an occlusal device, occlusal equilibration, orthodontics, a full mouth rehabilitation, and/or surgery to improve abnormal jaw alignment.

Anterior deprogramming[8,36-45] is the process of getting the temporomandibular joints into a relaxed or comfortable neuromuscular position (centric relation) by interrupting or negating the proprioceptors surrounding the teeth in the periodontal ligaments. These proprioceptors would otherwise automatically or subconsciously direct the mandible into the habitual or acquired intercuspal position. Anterior deprogramming is usually accomplished in 10–15 minutes by interposing something between the anterior teeth[3, 37-39,42,43] (such as a leaf gauge, Lucia jig, or sliding guide) while the patient retrudes the mandible and squeezes slightly on the centered anterior fulcrum (see Figs. 10-15C and 10.16B and C). The posterior teeth must remain separated several minutes for deprogramming to occur.[3,41] Once it has occurred, the posterior teeth seem to the patient to occlude (contact) improperly or in a strange way (with deflective contacts). In some instances, the deprogramming will not occur until the patient has worn an occlusal device for several weeks, and has maintained a stable and comfortable mandibular position for at least 1 week.[41]

An **occlusal device** (sometimes called a bite plane, bite guard, or night guard) is a removable artificial occlusal surface that can be used to stabilize occlusion, treat temporomandibular disorders, or prevent tooth wear. A detailed description of the method for constructing a maxillary occlusal device is presented in Figure 10-13. The occlusal device is constructed of a thin, horseshoe-shaped layer of transparent plastic, and is relatively easy

FIGURE 10-13. **Stages of construction and adjustment of a maxillary occlusal device. A.** A *template* from a thin plastic sheet (1.5–2.0 mm thick) has been heated and vacuum-molded (sucked down) onto a clean, dry, accurate cast of the maxillary teeth. The center palatal portion and excess on the sides and posteriorly has been removed leaving only a 3-mm overlap on the facial surfaces of the teeth. The occlusal surfaces are roughened with a carbide bur so additional acrylic resin will adhere securely. **B.** A triangular-shaped *anterior ramp* of cold-curing acrylic resin has been added lingually between the central incisors to maintain vertical dimension and to guide the mandible posteriorly (like a leaf gauge or sliding guide). **C.** Contact with the anterior ramp shows an excessive increase of the vertical dimension, so this is *adjusted* leaving only a point of contact with the mandibular incisors so they will contact at an incline of about 45° upward and posteriorly. **D.** The softened dough roll of orthodontic cold-curing clear acrylic *resin is adapted* over the roughened occlusal and incisal portion of the template with the anterior portion slightly longer and thinner than the posterior part. **E.** The template with the molded softened acrylic resin dough is *placed in the mouth* and the patient closes gently two or three times in the terminal hinge position and just far enough upward so that the mandibular incisors are stopped and the mandible is guided posteriorly by the previously adjusted narrow anterior hard resin ramp. The resin dough is permitted to harden. **F.** With the acrylic resin hardened, return the occlusal device or bite plane to the cast, mark the *cusp indentations* with a bright red felt marker, then *grind off all excess* acrylic except the imprints of only the tips of the cusps resulting in a flat plane. **G.** *Relieve the anterior portion* of all tooth imprints and slope it sharply upward toward the lingual to provide a ramp for disocclusion during lateral jaw movement. The posterior imprints are correct for initial placement of the device. While on the cast, the roughened acrylic resin is lightly buffed with a rag wheel and polishing compound. **H.** Place the maxillary occlusal device with the patient initially closing in centric relation. The mandibular posterior teeth contact *uniformly* (without deflections) on a flat smooth plane. The mandibular anterior teeth are just barely out of contact until the jaw moves forward or to either side. **I.** The patient slides the mandible to the left, and all teeth on the right side disocclude as the lower left canine slides up the lingual ramp. (Courtesy of Dr. Richard W. Huffman, Professor Emeritus, Ohio State University.)

to construct and use. It fits over the upper teeth to provide a smooth flat surface for the mandibular teeth to contact. A properly constructed occlusal device negates input to proprioceptive sensors in the teeth[1-3,6,7,15,31] providing a noninvasive, reversible therapy. Its use permits the mandible to seek its centric jaw relation, which is the most neuromuscularly comfortable and stable position (centric relation).

Patients are advised to wear the occlusal device 24 hours each day except when eating, and the devise should be periodically evaluated and adjusted as needed. After a few days, the patient may experience tremendous re-

FIGURE 10-14. **Stages of a full mouth rehabilitation. A and B.** Preparations of 15 teeth are ready for impressions (reversible hydrocolloid). **C and D.** Completed castings (crowns and inlays or onlays) are constructed on casts of the prepared teeth mounted on an articulator in the centric jaw relation such that the maximum intercuspal position of the newly formed occlusal surfaces is now simultaneous with the patient's centric jaw relation. The preparations and gold castings were as follows: one DO inlay-onlay (21), three $\frac{3}{4}$ crowns (6, 11, 15), three full cast crowns (28, 29, 30), eight MOD inlay-onlays (3, 4, 5, 12, 13, 18, 19, 20), and two pontics (14, 31). The pontic for tooth 31 is very small for a molar pontic because it has no posterior support, only the three splinted or soldered units anterior to it (28, 29, 30). Notice the ideal embrasure design and the multiple small ridges (cutting blades) and grooves or escapeways (gnathologic design) that provide for the highest possible masticatory effectiveness while directing all forces parallel to the long axes of the teeth. E. Mandibular gold castings in the mouth including the pontic replacing tooth 31. F. The patient in maximum intercuspal position, which is now simultaneous with centric jaw relation. The canines have been lengthened and thickened lingually to provide canine protection. (Courtesy of Dr. John Regenos, Cincinnati, Ohio.)

lief from severe facial muscle pain, headaches, or even some backaches that are related to an imbalance of the TMJ and tooth occlusion. For example, the patient in Figure 10-2 exhibited trismus and limited jaw opening over a 4-year period. He was only able to open 35 mm at the incisors, but after he wore a maxillary occlusal device for 18 months, his mandible stabilized into a comfortable centric relation position and he was able to open at the incisors 55 mm.

Definitive dental work (restorations, bridges, equilibration, orthodontics, etc.) should be postponed until the patient has remained comfortable for several weeks, and upon return visits requires little if any adjustment of the device.

Occlusal equilibration is the process by which a dentist modifies the occlusal or incisal form of the teeth by using revolving stones or burs in a dental handpiece to remove very small amounts of enamel at the sites of the tooth prematurities.[6] An occlusal equilibration should never be attempted without first having the patient wear a maxillary occlusal device for 1–6 weeks which assures natural and comfortable repositioning of the mandible and its temporomandibular joints. Thus, the equilibrated teeth will be in harmony with physiologically relaxed joints. The occlusal equilibration should be reevaluated at appropriate intervals to confirm the need for follow-up treatment.

Long centric articulation is actually a range of mandibular movement where a person can smoothly (without interferences) move the mandible from centric relation directly forward in a horizontal plane to the position of maximum intercuspation. There is no upward or lateral component. This range of movement is often the goal during an equilibration to provide the patient with a long centric relationship by relieving all deflective or premature tooth contacts that had previously caused the mandible to deviate either sideways or upward from centric relation to the maximum intercuspal position. The patient with a long centric articulation will have a small anteroposterior range (0.5 to 2.0 mm) of uniform posterior tooth contact occurring at the same vertical dimension of occlusion.

When teeth are so poorly aligned that too much tooth structure would have to be removed during an equilibration (and sensitive dentin or even pulpal tissue would be exposed), the dentist needs to consider other treatment options. **Orthodontic** treatment can be used to bodily move the teeth into an improved alignment. The results of a severe unilateral molar prematurity in the centric relation position is presented in Figure 10-2. This patient underwent 2 ½ years of orthodontic therapy to correct the enormous discrepancy between centric jaw relation and maximum intercuspal position. Other alternatives would have been surgery (intrusion of molars) or possibly root canal therapy on the molars followed by eight cast crowns (reducing molar cusp height). Ordinarily, the very common centric relation prematurities are not as severe as this, and often can be corrected when necessary with minimal occlusal equilibrations or minor orthodontic tooth movement.

Another technique that can be used to perfect the contours and occlusion of teeth that are not too badly out of alignment is to reconstruct the occluding surfaces of all or most teeth by constructing crowns, fixed partial dentures (bridges), or using large, stress-bearing restorations. This technique is a **full mouth rehabilitation**. An example of the stages of a full mouth rehabilitation is presented in Figure 10-14. Prior to having this extensive treatment, the patient in this figure wore a maxillary occlusal device for 4 months to ensure comfort, stability, and compatibility between his temporomandibular joints and the new occluding surfaces. Upon completion of treatment, his mandible could move freely to the right or left with all of the teeth disoccluding except the canines, which had been reshaped (lengthened and thickened lingually) to provide this canine protection or steeper guidance angle.

When the jaws are so poorly aligned or so different in size that it is impossible to perfect tooth contour using only restorations or orthodontics, **surgical techniques** can be used to reshape and realign jaw bones, usually followed by orthodontic treatment to perfect tooth alignment.

SECTION VIII. ACCURATE RECORDING OF THE CENTRIC RELATION JAW POSITION

The process of obtaining an accurate **centric relation jaw registration** or occlusal record is seen in Figure 10-15. First, a **leaf wafer**[2,8,39] is selected and deformed in the mouth as the patient bites into it. Then a **leaf gauge** or sliding guide (also known as an anterior deprogrammer)[1,6,8,36-39,41] is inserted at an upward angle between the incisors as the patient arcs the mandible open and then closes (hinge type or rotational opening) until the incisors engage the leaf gauge of sufficient thickness so all other teeth separate slightly (Fig. 10-15C). In this manner, the mandible is "tripodized" (stabilized by two condyles and the leaf gauge) by the patient's neuromusculature, and the patient is momentarily unable to aim the jaw into

FIGURE 10-15. Procedure for making a centric relation jaw registration. This jaw relation registration (interocclusal record) is used for mounting casts in centric jaw relation on an articulator for analysis and possible tooth alteration or orthodontic movement. **A.** A Woelfel Leaf Wafer used to carry a leaf gauge (in B) of predetermined thickness and the registration medium into the mouth. **B.** Paper leaf gauges above (color-coded for thickness) and below, a numbered plastic leaf gauge. **C.** Patient, with head tipped back, is arcing his mandible in the hinge position and closing on the leaf gauge of minimal but sufficient thickness to separate all teeth to negate any learned habitual closure. **D.** The recording material, polyether rubber, is applied to tooth indentations on the wafer. **E.** The patient closes firmly onto the leaf gauge as the recording material sets. **F.** The centric relation registration with leaf gauge. **G.** The leaf wafer registration is used to orient the lower to upper cast for assembly on an articulator. A brittle, strong sticky-wax (shaded areas on drawing) is used to maintain the relationship of the maxillary and mandibular casts until the mounting plaster attaching the casts to the articulator sets.

the acquired or habitual occlusion because no signals can be sent to the brain from the proprioceptors in the separated teeth.[31] Otherwise, the teeth could contact deflectively causing the mandible to move forward from the retruded position. Next, the leaf gauge is inserted in the wafer, and a recording medium (such as the impression material polyether or polyvinylsiloxane) is thinly spread over tooth indentations in the leaf wafer (Fig. 10-15D). Next, the entire assembly is carried to the mouth (Fig. 10-15E), and the patient retrudes and closes firmly, as previously, onto the leaf gauge until the recording medium sets.

    This centric relation registration (Fig. 10-15F) is used to relate models (casts) of each arch mounted on the articulator (Fig. 10-15G). This **diagnostic mounting** procedure should always be accomplished prior to attempting any type of tooth equilibration in the mouth.[1,2,6] These dental *stone* models, mounted in their neuromuscularly relaxed centric relation position, can be used to evaluate the extent of tooth malalignment in order to decide the best treatment. The dental stone teeth with interfering or premature contacts can be reshaped (reduced) in order to predict the amount of tooth reduction that will be required during the equilibration. If the amount of tooth structure that must be removed during the equilibration would likely expose dentin or pulp, then orthodontics or surgical procedures must be considered.

Another device used for anterior deprogramming of the mandible and for recording centric jaw relation is the *sliding guiding inclined gauge* or *sliding guide*[36-38,41,45] (Figs. 10-16 and 10.17). It comes in three maximum thicknesses, and the thickness used is dependent on the severity of the malocclusion (Fig. 10-16A). The thickness gradually increases from tip to handle, and the curvature of the sliding guide is critical so that it can be placed in the mouth between overlapping incisors at a relatively steep angle relative to the plane of occlusal without injuring the rugae or hard palate (Fig. 10-16B). The exact thickness between the incisors is read on the millimeter scale (Fig. 10-16C). Minimal incisal separation is the goal for deprogramming and jaw position registration, just so long as no posterior teeth touch, thus avoiding proprioceptive impulses. This is particularly important for the centric jaw relation registration to minimize errors between the articulator and the patient. The sliding guide is made of a non-brittle autoclavable plastic, and works well with a custom bite deformed Woelfel leaf wafer for centric relation jaw registrations (Figs. 10-16D and 10-17).[36-38,41]

FIGURE 10-16. **A. Three sliding guiding inclined gauges.** The millimeter scales denote the amount of incisal separation between overlapping incisors (left sliding guide 16 mm, center one 9 mm, right one a maximum thickness of 4 mm). **B.** A 4 mm sliding guide is held between the incisors at a steep angle to the occlusal plane separating them by 2.5 mm, just enough to keep all of the posterior teeth from touching. **C.** A 9 mm sliding guide is placed in the mouth so the incisors are separated by 6.5 mm during the muscular deprogramming period. **D.** A centric relation jaw registration made with a 4 mm sliding guide inserted into a previously constructed custom "bite deformed Woelfel leaf wafer." The minimal amount of incisal separation (2.5 mm) was determined prior to the centric relation registration that was used to mount diagnostic casts of the patient on an articulator in centric jaw relation.

FIGURE 10-17. **Three views of a registration made with a 4-mm sliding guide**. A sliding gauge may be used in conjunction with the previously bite-deformed leaf wafer and a semi-rigid impression material (polyvinylsiloxane) to obtain the centric relation (retruded) jaw registrations. **A.** The curvature of the sliding guide and its proper angle above the occlusal plane are seen. **B.** Maxillary side of the registration showing the tooth indentations and the 3.5 mm incisal separation. **C.** Inferior view with mandibular tooth imprints in the registration media and pertinent patient information written with a Sharpie fine point marker. This centric jaw relation registration is seen in the mouth in Figure 10-16D.

LEARNING EXERCISE

LEARNING EXERCISE ON YOUR OWN JAW MOBILITY OR MANDIBULAR MOVEMENT CAPABILITY

It should be an educational and interesting experience for you to complete this simple exercise in order to increase your awareness of your own jaw movements. During this exercise, as you move in each direction as indicated, think about which muscles bring about these jaw movements and which ligaments limit the amount of jaw movement. It will take about 20 minutes to do this exercise.

Obtain a clean, plastic millimeter ruler cut off even with the zero mark. Make the following measurements as described while observing your tooth relationship in a mirror.

1. Horizontal overlap (H) of incisors and canines
   Using a mirror, measure the Horizontal overlap (H in Fig. 10-18) in the following three locations while holding your teeth together in maximum intercuspal position (or on hand-held tooth models with teeth tightly closed).
   1a. ___ mm = horizontal overlap between the labial surfaces of central incisors at the midline
   1b. ___ mm = horizontal overlap between labial surfaces of left canines
   1c. ___ mm = horizontal overlap between labial surfaces of right canines

2. Protrusive overlap (P) = ___ mm
   Measure the Protrusive overlap (P in Fig. 10-18) with your lower jaw moved forward as far as possible (like a bulldog), between the labial surface of the maxillary central incisors and the labial surface of the mandibular incisors. (This movement requires contraction of both lateral pterygoid muscles simultaneously.)

3. Horizontal overlap of canines during lateral excursions (right and left sides)
   Measure the horizontal distance between the facial surfaces of the upper and lower canines during maximum movements in lateral excursions, first with the lower jaw moved to the left as far as possible as seen in Fig. 10-19A. This is just like the measurement P in Figure 10-18, only between the facial surfaces of the maxillary and mandibular left canines. This movement requires contraction of the right lateral pterygoid muscle.
   3a. ___ mm = left horizontal overlap of canines
   Next, measure the horizontal distance between the facial surfaces of the upper and lower canines during a maximum lateral movement of the jaw to the right side as far as possible, as seen in Figure 10-19B. This movement requires contraction of the left lateral pterygoid muscle.
   3b. ___ mm = right horizontal overlap of canines

4. Vertical overlap of central incisors (V) = ___ mm
   Measure the vertical overlap (V in Fig. 10-20) at the midline between the incisal edges of your central incisors while holding your back teeth tightly closed, or on your tooth models in maximum intercuspal position.

5. Opening movements (hinge opening and total opening)
   The hinge opening is the distance between incisal edges at the maximum hinge-only opening. Practice opening your jaw slowly as far as possible while firmly retruding it in centric relation. Hinge opening is usually only half or less than half of the maximal opening (first portion of O in Figure 10-20, and represented in Figure 10-8B as the limit of the hinge opening). If you open properly, there should not be any crepitation because the articular discs and condyles are fixed posteriorly.
   5a. ___ mm = Hinge opening
   Now open as widely as you can and measure the maximum opening (O in Fig. 10-20) between the incisal edges (usually you can fit four fingers between your incisors). If you noticed a noise near one or both ears when you opened widely, it is probably caused by a disharmony between the movement of the jaw and the movement of the disc that fits between the jaw condyle and the skull on either side. It is usually not a serious problem, and many people experience crepitation for a while during their lifetime.
   5b. ___ mm = Maximum opening (O in Fig. 10-20)

6. **Calculate maximum movements:**
    6a. Add measurements 4 plus 5b to obtain total incisor opening = ____ mm
    6b. Add 4 and 5a to obtain maximum hinge opening at incisors = ____ mm
    6c. Add measurements 1b and 3a to obtain maximum left lateral movement = ____ mm
    6d. Add measurements 1c and 3b to obtain maximum right lateral movement = ____ mm
    6e. Add measurements 1a and 2 to obtain maximum protrusion = ____ mm

    6f. Add totals 6c and 6d to obtain total lateral movement (from right to left) = ____ mm
    Are you surprised that you can move your mandible farther from side-to-side than you can move it directly forward? Usually your jaw can move about twice as far sideways (laterally) as it can protrude or move directly forward. Compare the results of your own jaw movement capability with that of 796 dental hygienists and 318 dental students in Tables 10-2 and 10-3.

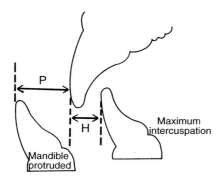

FIGURE 10-18. H is the horizontal overlap of central incisors with the teeth in maximum intercuspation, and **P** is the horizontal overlap with the mandible protruded as far as possible.

A   B

FIGURE 10-19. Lateral jaw movements of the mandibular moved as far as possible to the left (A) and to the right (B).

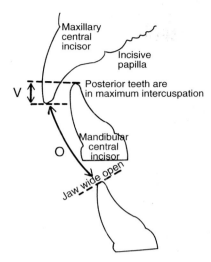

FIGURE 10-20. V is the vertical overlap of central incisors in maximum intercuspation. O denotes the maximum opening distance between incisors.

REFERENCES

1. Williamson EH, Steinke RM, Morse PK, Swift TR. Centric relation: a comparison of muscle determined position and operator guidance. Am J Orthod 1980;77:133–45.
2. Woelfel JB. New device for accurately recording centric relation. J Prosthet Dent 1986;56:716–27.
3. Carroll WJ, Woelfel JB, Huffman RW. Simple application of anterior jig or leaf gauge in routine clinical practice. J Prosthet Dent 1988;59:611–17.
4. Posselt U. The Physiology of Occlusion and Rehabilitation. Philadelphia: F.A. Davis, 1962.
5. Rosner D, Goldberg G. Condylar retruded contact position correlation in dentulous patients Part I: Three-dimensional analysis of condylar registrations. J Prosthet Dent 1986;56:230–37.
6. Huffman RW. A cusp-fossa equilibration technique using a numbered leaf gauge. J Gnathology 1987;6:23–36.
7. Williamson EH. Occlusion: understanding or misunderstanding. Angle Orthod 1976;46:86–93.
8. Fenlon, MR, Woelfel JB. Condylar position recorded using leaf gauges and specific closure forces. Intern J Prost 1993;6(4):402–8.
9. Williamson EH, Woelfel JB, Williams BH. A longitudinal study of rest position and centric occlusion. Angle Orthod 1975;45:130–36.
10. Winter CM, Woelfel JB, Igarashi T. Five-year changes in the edentulous mandible as determined on oblique cephalometric radiographs. J Dent Res 1974;53(6):1455–67.
11. Brose MO, Tanquist RA. The influence of anterior coupling on mandibular movement. J Prosthet Dent 1987;57:345–53.
12. Kohno S, Nakano M. The measurement and development of anterior guidance. J Prosthet Dent 1987;57:620–30.
13. Barghi N. Clinical evaluation of occlusion. Tex Dent J 1978;96(Mar):12–14.
14. O'Leary J, Shanley D, Drake R. Tooth mobility in cuspid-protected and group function occlusions. J Prosthet Dent 1972;27(Jan):21–25.
15. Ramjford SP, Ash MM Jr. Occlusion. Philadelphia: W.B. Saunders, 1966:142–59.
16. American Dental Association. Temporomandibular disorders. JADA Guide to Dental Health Special Issue 1988;45–6.
17. Locker D, Grushka M. The impact of dental and facial pain. J Dent Res 1987;66:1414–17.
18. Gross A, Gale EN. A prevalence study of the clinical signs associated with mandibular dysfunction. JADA 1983;107:932–6.
19. Seligman DA, Pullinger AG, Solberg WD. The prevalence of dental attrition and its association with factors of age, gender, occlusion, and TMJ symptomatology. J Dent Res 1988;67:1323–33.
20. Turrell J, Ruiz HG. Normal and abnormal findings in temporomandibular joints in autopsy specimens. J Craniomandibular Disorders: Facial & Oral Pain 1987;1:257–75.
21. Sicher H, DuBrul EL. Oral anatomy. 7th ed. St. Louis: C.V. Mosby, 1975:174–209.
22. Montgomery RL. Head and neck anatomy with clinical correlations. New York: McGraw-Hill, 1981:202–14.
23. Ricketts RM. Abnormal functions of the temporomandibular joint. Am J Orthod 1955;41:425, 435–41.
24. Gibbs CH, Mahan PE, Mauderli A, et al. Limits of human bite strength. J Prosthet Dent 1986;56:226–40.
25. Guernsey LH. Biting force measurement. Dent Clin North Am 1966;10:286–9.
26. Renner RP. An Introduction to Dental Anatomy and Esthetics. Chicago: Quintessence Publishing, 1985:162.

27. Lindblom G. On the anatomy and function of the temporomandibular joint. ACTA Odontol Scand 1960;17(Supp 28):1–287.

28. Woelfel J, Hickey JC, Allison ML. Effect of posterior tooth form on jaw and denture movement, J Prosthet Dent 1962;12:922–39.

29. Green CS. A critique of nonconventional treatment concepts and procedures for TMJ disorders. Comp Cont Educ 1984;5:848–51.

30. Pierce CJ, Gale EN. A comparison of different treatments for nocturnal bruxism. J Dent Res 1988;67:597–601.

31. Crum RJ, Loiselle RJ. Oral perception and proprioception. A review of the literature and its significance to prosthodontics. J Prosthet Dent 1972;28:215–30.

32. Kruger L, Michel F. A single neuron analysis of buccal cavity representation in the sensory trigeminal complex of the cat. Arch Oral Biol 1962;7:491–503.

33. Kawamura Y, Nishiyama T. Projection of dental afferent impulses to the trigeminal nuclei of the cat. Jpn J Physiol 1966;16:584–97.

34. Jerge CR. Comments on the innervation of the teeth. Dent Clin North Am 1965;117–27.

35. Young JL. Successful restorative dentistry for the internal derangement patient. Mo Dent J 1987;67:21–6.

36. Woelfel JB. New device for deprogramming and recording centric jaw relation: the sliding guiding inclined gauge. Advanced Prosthodontics Worldwide, Proceedings of the World Congress on Prosthodontics, Hiroshima, Japan, Sept 21–23, 1991:218–9.

37. Woelfel JB. A new device for mandibular deprogramming and recording centric relation: the sliding guiding inclined gauge. Protesi occlusionone ATM a cura di Giorgio Vogel FDI 1991. Milan, Italy: Monduzzi Editore III, 1991:35–40.

38. Woelfel JB. Sliding and guiding the mandible into the retruded arc without pushing. The Compendium of Continuing Education in Dentistry 1991(Sept);12(9):614–24.

39. Paltaleao JF, Silva-Netto CR, Nunes LJ, Woelfel JB. Determination of the centric relation. A comparison between the wax prepared method and the Leaf Gauge-Leaf Wafer System. RGO 1992;40(5):356–60.

40. Tsolka P, Woelfel JB, Man WK, Preiskel HW. A laboratory assessment of recording reliability and analysis of the K6 diagnostic system. J Craniomandibular Disorders: Facial & Oral Pain 1992;6:273–80.

41. Woelfel JB., An easy practical method for centric registration. Jpn J Gnathology 1994;15(3):125–31.

42. Donegan SJ, Carr AB, Christensen LV, et al. An electromyographic study of aspects of "deprogramming" of human jaw muscles. J Oral Rehabil 1990;17:509–18.

43. Carr AB, Donegan SJ, Christensen LV, et al. An electrognathographic study of aspects of "deprogramming" human jaw muscles. J Oral Rehabil 1991;18:143–8.

44. Christensen IV, et al. Observation on the motor control of brief teeth clenching in man. J Oral Rehabil 1991.

45. Yaegashi Y, Tanaka H. An electromyographic study of the effect on masticatory muscle activity applying the leaf gauge. J Prosthet Dent 1994.

General References

The glossary of prosthodontic terms. J Prosthet Dent 1999;81(1):48-106.

Dental Anomalies

Acknowledgments:
This chapter was originally contributed by Connie Sylvester, R.D.H., B.A., M.S. former faculty of the Ohio State University and the University of Texas Schools of Dental Hygiene. Special thanks to Drs. C.C. Dollens, Rudy Melfi, and Donald Bowers for their gracious assistance in obtaining several of the photographs and radiographs used in this chapter. Also, special thanks to the first-year dental hygiene students at Ohio State University, who brought in numerous anomalies and casts depicting such unusual teeth.

Topics
I. Anodontia: absence of teeth
   A. Total anodontia
   B. Partial anodontia
II. Extra or supernumerary teeth
   A. Maxillary incisor area
   B. Third molar area
   C. Mandibular premolar area
III. Abnormal tooth morphology
   A. Abnormal crown morphology
   B. Abnormal root morphology
   C. Additional anomalies

OBJECTIVES

This chapter is designed to help the learner perform the following:
- Identify variations from the normal (anomalies) for the number of teeth in an arch.
- Identify anomalies in crown morphology and, when applicable, identify the anomaly by name and give a possible cause (etiology).
- Identify anomalies in root morphology and, when applicable, identify the anomaly by name and give a possible cause (etiology).
- Identify anomalies in the alignment of teeth within an arch.

Definition: An **anomaly** [a NAH mah lee] is a deviation from normal, usually related to embryonic development that may result in the absence, excess, or deformity of body parts.[1] Dental anomalies are abnormalities of teeth that range from such "common" occurrences as malformed permanent maxillary lateral incisors that are peg-shaped, to such rare occurrences as complete anodontia (no teeth at all). Dental anomalies are most often caused by hereditary factors (gene related) or by developmental or metabolic disturbances. While more anomalies occur in the permanent than primary dentition, and in the maxilla than the mandible, it is important to remember that their occurrence is rare. For example, only 1–2% of the population have some form of anodontia (one or more missing teeth), while another 1–2% have supernumerary (extra) teeth.[2-4] When specific deformities or abnormal formations of teeth occur with greater frequency, it is difficult to determine whether the deviation is a "true" anomaly or simply an extreme variation in tooth morphology.

Familiarity with dental anomalies is essential to the clinical practice of dentistry and dental hygiene. Recognition and correct labeling of anomalies is important for your communication with other dental team members, especially in the case of referral to or from another dentist. Additionally, your communication with the patient (or, in the case of a child, the parent) should reflect knowledge of abnormal oral conditions. Your assurance that the fused front tooth of a 4-year-old child occurs with 0.5% frequency and rarely affects the number of teeth in the permanent dentition, will go a long way to promote the patient's confidence in you and the office. Likewise, the informed patient who understands why the accessory cusp on the buccal of his maxillary or mandibular molar is more prone to decay than normal, will likely be more receptive to home care instructions that are specific to his mouth and his needs. Finally, understanding the etiology (cause) of the anomaly is important in determining the course of treatment, if any. Additional information related to the etiology of the following anomalies is found in the study of both oral histology/embryology and oral pathology.

SECTION I. Anodontia: Absence of Teeth

A. TOTAL ANODONTIA

True anodontia is the total *congenital* absence of a set of teeth. **Total anodontia** is characterized by the absence of the entire primary and secondary dentitions, and is extremely rare. It is most often associated with a generalized congenital deformation (a sex-linked genetic trait) such as the abnormal development of the ectoderm or outer embryonic cell layer. Faulty ectodermal development further affects such structures as hair, nails, sebaceous and sweat glands, and salivary glands.

B. PARTIAL ANODONTIA

Partial anodontia, also referred to as congenitally missing teeth, involves one or more missing teeth from a dentition. Though not proven to be a hereditary trait, tendencies toward missing the same tooth do run in families.

1. MOST COMMONLY MISSING PERMANENT TEETH

The *most commonly missing* permanent teeth are third molars, with the maxillary thirds absent from the dentition more often than the mandibular thirds.

2. SECOND MOST COMMONLY MISSING TEETH

The permanent maxillary lateral incisors are the next most commonly missing teeth (Fig. 11-1). Approximately 1–2% of the population is missing one or both of these maxillary incisors.[4,5]

FIGURE 11-1. Partial anodontia. Congenitally missing maxillary lateral incisors.

FIGURE 11-2. Partial anodontia. Missing second premolar. Routine radiographic examination of a 10-year-old female revealed both mandibular right and left second premolars to be missing. The first premolar can be seen situated under the deciduous first molar crown between its roots. Notice the fully erupted secondary first molar and the unerupted second molar (extreme left). The deciduous second molar is functional and its roots have not begun to resorb.

3. THIRD MOST COMMONLY MISSING TEETH

The mandibular second premolars are the third most frequently missing permanent teeth (Fig. 11-2), with 1% of the population missing one or both.[4] [Some studies indicate the order of most commonly missing teeth to be: third molars, maxillary and mandibular premolars, and maxillary lateral incisors.[6]]

Some observers state that missing teeth follow evolutionary trends in that the teeth most commonly missing from the dentition (third molars) are those that are most expendable in terms of their role in oral function.[4] Conversely, the most stable teeth in the permanent dentition, the canines, are the least likely to be absent from the dentition.[6]

Other congenitally missing permanent and deciduous teeth are evident in Figure 11-3.

FIGURE 11-3. Partial anodontia. A. Congenitally missing deciduous mandibular central incisor. **B.** Both deciduous mandibular central incisors congenitally missing. **C.** Congenitally missing secondary mandibular central incisor.

SECTION II. Extra or Supernumerary Teeth

Supernumerary teeth are teeth that form in excess of the normal dental formulas for each quadrant (deciduous quadrant: I-2, C-1, M-2; permanent quadrant: I-2, C-1, P-2, M-3). They occur in 0.3–3.8% of the population.[22] They are found in both permanent and deciduous dentitions, with 90% of all occurrences in the maxilla.[7] Specifically, the most frequent supernumerary specimens are found in one of two locations: maxillary incisor area (Fig. 11.4) or maxillary third molar region. One report states that supernumerary teeth occurred eight times more often in the maxillary than mandibular regions, and twice as frequently in men than in women.[29] Another study of 50 patients from 16 months to 17 years of age, found 20% of the supernumerary teeth to be inverted.[23] Fourteen percent of these patients had multiple supernumerary teeth, and 80% of the extra teeth were in a lingual position relative to the dental arch. These teeth can vary considerably in size and shape (Fig. 11-5).

A. MAXILLARY INCISOR AREA

A **mesiodens** is a small supernumerary tooth that forms between central incisors. It has a cone-shaped crown and short root (Fig. 11-6). It may be visible in the oral cavity or remain unerupted. If unerupted, a diastema (space) may be present.[8] One study of 375 children with mesiodens reports that they are often in an inverted position and rarely erupt into the oral cavity.[29] The prevalence of mesiodens in the permanent dentition in the Caucasian populations is 0.15–1.9%.[9]

Less frequently, supernumerary teeth may be positioned between central and lateral incisors or between lateral incisors and canines. The occurrence of supernumerary teeth in the deciduous dentition is low (approximately 0.5%).[9] The most common supernumerary teeth in the secondary dentition, however, are either midline mesiodens or supplemental lateral incisors.

B. THIRD MOLAR AREA

The presence of supernumerary teeth distal to the third molars is more common in the maxillary arch but does occur in the mandible. These supernumerary teeth are often called **distomolars, paramolars** or **fourth molars**. These extra teeth rarely erupt into the oral cavity and thus are usually discovered through radiographs (Fig. 11-7).

C. MANDIBULAR PREMOLAR AREA

The most common location for supernumerary teeth in the *mandible* is the second premolar region (Fig. 11-8). Supernumerary teeth appearing in this area generally resemble normal premolars in size and shape.[10]

FIGURE 11-4. Supernumerary tooth. Maxillary dentition with three incisors shaped like central incisors.

FIGURE 11-5. **Supernumerary teeth** of various sizes and shapes. Some resemble premolars, some appear like peg-shaped incisors, and others look like very small third molars.

FIGURE 11-6. **Supernumerary mesiodens.** A. Radiograph: notice the mesiodens next to the fully erupted maxillary permanent central incisor. B. Fully erupted mesiodens: one has a peg shape and one is shaped more like a small lateral incisor.

FIGURE 11-7. **Paramolars or fourth (supernumerary) molars. A.** Maxillary. **B.** Mandibular. The extra molars (arrow) are just distal to the secondary third molars.

FIGURE 11-8. **Supernumerary teeth** in mandibular premolar region. **A.** Extra first premolar fully emerged but crowded. (Courtesy of Dr. L. Claman.) **B.** Extra first premolars on each side of the mandibular arch are positioned lingually.

SECTION III. Abnormal Tooth Morphology

A. ABNORMAL CROWN MORPHOLOGY

Crown malformations may be seen clinically upon visual inspection of the oral cavity.

1. THIRD MOLAR MALFORMATIONS

Maxillary third molars have the *most variable* crown shape of all permanent teeth followed by mandibular thirds. These anomalies can range in shape from a small peg-shaped crown, to a multi-cusped, malformed version of either the first or second molar.

2. PEG-SHAPED LATERAL INCISORS

The most common anomaly in tooth shape in the anterior of the secondary dentition is the **peg-shaped** (or cone-shaped) **lateral incisor** (Fig. 11-9), occurring in 1–2% of the population.[4] The tooth is generally conical in shape, broadest cervically, and tapers toward the incisal to a blunt point. Several studies of identical twins seem to indicate that missing and peg-shaped lateral incisor teeth may be varied expressions of the same genetic trait.[11,12] A most unusual occurrence is that of peg-shaped maxillary central incisors (Fig. 11-10). Peg-shaped teeth develop from one facial lobe (instead of the three facial lobes normally present on anterior teeth).

3. GEMINATION OR TWINNING

Gemination or **twinning** results from the splitting or twinning of a single forming tooth (germ). Since the tooth division is incomplete, the twinned crown appears doubled in width compared to a single tooth and possibly notched (Fig. 11-11). The single root is not split and has a common pulp canal. Most commonly seen in the anterior area in the region of the maxillary incisors and canines,[3] this condition occurs in less than 1% of the population. It occurs more frequently in the primary dentition

FIGURE 11-9. Peg-shaped maxillary lateral incisors: A viewed from the facial. B viewed from the incisal.

FIGURE 11-10. Peg-shaped maxillary central incisors, a very rare occurrence. Above: Facial view. Below: Incisal view showing both canines and one lateral incisor.

FIGURE 11-11. Gemination. A. It appears that the left lateral incisor germ split or divided into two since, if that tooth is counted as two, there are five incisors, one more than expected. The geminated tooth will generally have a single root and common pulp canal. B. Deep labial grooves on all four maxillary central incisors and four canines (maxillary and mandibular) of a Native American. Notice the similarity in crown morphology of these wide, grooved teeth with geminated crowns.

FIGURE 11-12. **Fusion.** Two mandibular first premolars fused together. Buccal aspect (left) and lingual aspect (right). Some separation between the roots is visible. There would be two pulp canals.

than in the permanent dentition. If the doubled tooth is counted as *two* teeth, the dental arch containing the geminated tooth will generally have an *extra* tooth beyond the normal number of teeth. Note in Figure 11-11B that the wide crowns of the anterior teeth of Native Americans may exhibit deep labial grooves that resemble gemination.

4. **FUSION**

Fusion is the union of two adjacent tooth germs, always involving the dentin. Upon clinical examination, this condition appears similar to gemination since the fused teeth have one crown that appears doubled in width. However, unlike gemination, radiographs usually reveal two separate but fused roots with separate pulp chambers (Fig. 11-12). Another way to differentiate fusion from gemination is to count the teeth in the arch. If the fused teeth are counted as *two*, the total number of teeth will reflect the normal number of teeth in that arch (Fig. 11-13).

Like geminated teeth, fused teeth occur more commonly in the anterior portion of the mouth (in less than 1% of the population), and more often in the deciduous dentition than in the permanent dentition. The mandibular incisor area is affected more often than the maxilla.[2,3]

FIGURE 11-13. **Fusion. A.** If the double wide tooth is counted as two, the number of incisors is four: the expected number. Therefore we suspect that the maxillary right lateral and central incisor have fused. Another possibility is the fusion of the central incisor and a supernumerary mesiodens with the lateral incisor is congenitally absent. **B and C.** Fused mandibular central and lateral incisors from different individuals. In C, the fused teeth are seen from both lingual and facial aspects.

FIGURE 11-14. Fusion. Unusual maxillary third molar with a supernumerary paramolar fused to its distal surface.

Fusion is thought to be caused by pressure or force during development of adjacent roots. Many of the reports of fusion involve a supernumerary tooth joining with an adjacent tooth, such as the fusion of a mandibular third and fourth molar seen in Figure 11-14, and the fusion of a maxillary lateral incisor and anterior supernumerary tooth seen in Figure 11-15.[13-15]

5. HUTCHINSON'S TEETH

Unusual incisor and molar shapes may occur in both dentitions as the result of prenatal syphilis. Maxillary and mandibular incisors may be screwdriver shaped, broad cervically, and narrowing incisally, with a notched incisal edge. These teeth are often referred to as **Hutchinson's incisors**. Note in Figure 11-16 that the crowns of Hutchinson's incisors resemble somewhat the notched crowns of fused teeth seen in Figure 11-13A. Also, first molars in these dentitions may have occlusal anatomy made up of multiple tiny tubercles with poorly developed indistinguishable cusps. Because of the berry-like shape on the occlusal, these molars are called **mulberry molars**.

6. VARIATIONS IN THE NUMBER OF LINGUAL CUSPS ON MANDIBULAR SECOND PREMOLARS

Mandibular second premolars vary in the number of lingual cusps, ranging from one to three (recall Table 6-3). Occlusal morphology can vary greatly in terms of groove and fossa patterns established by the number of lingual cusps.[16]

FIGURE 11-15. Fusion. Extracted maxillary central incisor with a fused mesiodens.

FIGURE 11-16. Hutchinson's (notched) maxillary incisors of a nine-year-old female. (Model courtesy of Dmitri J. Harampopoulos, D.D.S.)

7. ACCESSORY CUSPS OR TUBERCLES

Any tooth may exhibit extra small enamel projections called **tubercles** (Fig. 11-17), or extra accessory cusps. These enamel projections may result from developmental localized hyperplasia (increase in volume of tissue caused by growth of new cells) or crowded conditions prior to eruption where fusion of a supernumerary tooth may be viewed as an extra cusp (Fig. 11-18).

a. Enamel Pearls

Enamel pearls are small, round nodules of enamel with a tiny core of dentin. They are found most frequently on the distal of third molars and the buccal root furcation of molars[17] (Fig. 11-19). Radiographically enamel pearls appear as small round radiopacities (that is, areas appearing light or white on the exposed film). Being covered with enamel, they prevent the normal connective tissue attachment and consequently may channel disease (periodontal problems) into this region.

FIGURE 11-17. Tubercles. A. Two elevations or tubercles or cusplets on the canine, three on the lateral incisor. **B.** Pronounced tubercles on the cingula of maxillary anterior teeth, most noticeable (due to lighting) on the patient's *left* central and lateral incisor and canine. **C.** Proximal views of contralateral first premolars from a young Native American showing tubercles emanating from the buccal triangular ridges just lingual to the buccal cusps.

FIGURE 11-18. **Extra cusp**, cusps, or paramolar fused to mandibular third molar in **A**, to the buccal surfaces of maxillary second molars in **B**, **C**, and **D**, and to the mesiobuccal cusp of a mandibular second molar in **E**.

b. Taurodontia

In **taurodontia**, or so-called bull or prism teeth, the pulp chamber is very long, without a constriction near the cementoenamel junction (Figure 11-20). This occurs only in permanent teeth, with a frequency of less than 1 in 1,000 among American Indians and Eskimos.[24] Taurodontia is caused by a disorganization of the calcified tissues and possibly occurs in dentitions subjected to heavy use.

c. Talon Cusp

A small enamel projection in the cingulum area of maxillary or mandibular anterior permanent teeth is a **talon** ("claw of an animal") **cusp** (Fig. 11-21A). Frequently, the cusp has a pulp horn so that radiographically it may be mistaken for a supernumerary tooth superimposed over an anterior tooth or dens in dente. Removal of this cusp is often necessary because of its interference in jaw closure in the maximum intercuspal position. Since the pulp horn is present, endodontic treatment is usually required when this cusp is removed.[2,18] Notice that the deep lingual grooves found on some anterior teeth may somewhat resemble the grooves of a talon cusp (Fig. 11-21B).

FIGURE 11-19. **Enamel pearls** of various sizes on maxillary third molars.

FIGURE 11-20. **Taurodontia.** Photograph of extracted tooth on left; radiograph on right. (Courtesy of Professor Rudy Melfi, D.D.S.)

8. VARIATIONS IN TOOTH SIZE

Microdontia (very small, but normally shaped teeth) and **macrodontia** (very large, but normally shaped teeth) may occur as a single tooth, several teeth, or an entire dentition.[36] Macrodontia most frequently involves incisors and canines whereas microdontia affects maxillary lateral incisors and third molars.[8,19,20] Some examples of variation in size of teeth are shown in Figure 11-22. One report shows a maxillary canine 39 mm long and a maxillary first molar 31 mm long (compared to average lengths of 26.3 mm and 20.1 mm , respectively), both removed from a pituitary giant.[36]

9. SHOVEL-SHAPED MAXILLARY INCISORS

Possibly not a true anomaly, **shovel-shaped incisors** are a frequently occurring trait that reflect biologic differences between races.[4] The lingual anatomy includes a pronounced cingulum and marginal ridges, thus the scoop or "shovel" appearance (Fig. 11-23A). These teeth are observed most frequently in the Asian, Mongoloid, Eskimo, and American Indian races. Double shoveling refers to the pro-

FIGURE 11-21. **Talon cusps. A.** Lingual view of two maxillary central incisors with talon cusps. **B.** Lingual view of a maxillary left lateral incisor shows a lingual groove at the junction of the prominent mesial and distal ridges which might, at first glance, be confused with a talon cusp.

FIGURE 11-22. Variation in tooth size from **microdontia** (very small) to **macrodontia** (very large). Microdontia of four very short central incisors with dwarfed roots (one tooth only 16 mm long) and macrodontia of two very long incisors (one 34 mm long).

nounced *lingual* marginal ridges as well as prominent ridges on the mesial and distal portions of the *labial* surface as seen in Figure 11-23B.

B. ABNORMAL ROOT MORPHOLOGY

Root malformations are not usually obvious without the aid of radiographs. Close examination of extracted specimens reveals wide variations.

1. DILACERATION OR FLEXION

Dilaceration is a severe bend or distortion of a tooth root and/or crown, often approximating an angle from 45° to more than 90° (Figure 11-24).[25] This unusual occurrence may be the result of a traumatic injury or of insufficient space for development, as is often the case with third molars (Figure 11-25). **Flexion** is another term used to describe a sharp curvature or bend (less than 90°) on a tooth root. Dilaceration and flexion are often observed in teeth with accessory roots.

2. DENS IN DENTE

Dens in dente (literally "tooth within a tooth") is a developmental anomaly resulting from the invagination of the enamel organ within the crown of a tooth. Clinically, it appears as a deep crevice primarily in the cingulum region of incisors. Most commonly found in maxillary lateral incisors, it can appear in upper central incisors and in mandibular incisors. Radiographically, dens in dente appears as a mass of elongated enamel within the dentin of a normal sized tooth (Fig. 11-26 A and B). Usually it appears in the coronal third of the tooth, but may extend the entire root length. Often peg-

FIGURE 11-23. **A. Shovel-shaped** permanent incisors from a young Native American dentition (incisal view). Note the prominent marginal ridges on the lingual surface. **B.** The range of prominent labial ridges on **double-shovel shaped incisors** varies from barely discernable labial ridges on the left to prominent labial ridges on the right.

FIGURE 11-24. **Dilaceration,** where the root and/or crown are severely twisted. Maxillary teeth crowns are down; mandibular teeth crowns are above the roots.

FIGURE 11-25. **Dilaceration** (severe) of the roots of mandibular molars.

FIGURE 11-26. **Dens in dente** ("tooth within a tooth"). **A.** Faciolingual cross-section of a maxillary lateral incisor with a dens in dente (tooth within a tooth). This tooth section is only 50 micrometers thick. **B.** Radiograph of dens in dente on maxillary right central incisor. It connects with the lingual pit as clearly seen in A. It is caused by an invagination of the epithelium of the enamel organ before the formation of hard tissue. (Courtesy of Professor Rudy Melfi, D.D.S.)

FIGURE 11-27. Concrescence. The junction or joining of cementum between adjacent maxillary first and second molars. Left: Lingual view. Right: Disto-occlusal aspect with the buccal toward the right.

shaped lateral incisors, with failure of mesial and distal lobes to develop, are found to have dens in dente upon radiographic examination. Their occurrence is from 1–5% of the population.[2]

3. CONCRESCENCE

Concrescence is a type of superficial fusion or growing together of two adjacent teeth at the root through the *cementum only* (Fig. 11-27). Unlike fusion, the teeth involved are originally separate but become joined, usually after eruption into the oral cavity, because of the close proximity of the roots and excessive cementum deposition.[6] This anomaly occurs most frequently in the maxillary molar region.

4. DWARFED ROOTS

Maxillary teeth often exhibit normal sized crowns with abnormally short (**dwarfed**) roots (Fig. 11-22). The incisal edge is usually displaced lingually as in the mandibular incisors. This condition is often hereditary, however, isolated or generalized dwarfing of roots may also result from orthodontic movement of the teeth (with braces) when the movement has occurred too rapidly.

5. HYPERCEMENTOSIS

Hypercementosis is the excessive formation of cementum around the root of a tooth after the tooth has erupted (Fig. 11-28). It may be caused by trauma, metabolic dysfunction, or periapical inflammation. The excess amount of cementum may cause webbing of the roots.

6. ACCESSORY (EXTRA) ROOTS

Usually occurring in teeth whose roots form after birth, accessory roots are probably caused by trauma, metabolic dysfunction, or pressure. Third molars are the multi-rooted teeth most likely to exhibit accessory roots (Fig. 11-29).[2] The single-rooted teeth most frequently affected are the mandibular canines and premolars. Two roots (one facial and one lingual) are found rarely enough on mandibular canines to be interesting, but frequently enough not to be amazing (Fig.11.30A). Mandibular first premolars may also exhibit a bifurcated root (one buccal and one lingual, a condi-

FIGURE 11-28. **Hypercementosis** or excess cementum thickness. Top row: Maxillary third molar, first premolar and two first molars. Lower row: Mandibular first molar, maxillary first molar, and second premolar.

tion less common for this tooth than for mandibular canines (Fig. 11-30B). A Japanese study of 500 mandibular first premolars found this type of bifurcation occurred in 1.6% of their teeth. These researchers also found one very rare specimen with two buccal and one lingual roots.[40] A somewhat rare occurrence of two roots on mandibular premolars (one mesial and one distal) is evident on the radiographs in Figure 11-30C.

Another unusual root formation includes maxillary first premolars with three roots (two buccal and one lingual) similar to the roots of a maxillary molar (Fig. 11-31). The somewhat rare occurrence of the primary maxillary canines with their root divided mesiodistally is shown in Figure 11-32.[30-36] There have been six reported cases of contralaterally bifurcated roots on primary maxillary canines: five discovered from routine radiographic examination, the sixth on a routine dental recall examination.[30-35]

FIGURE 11-29. Three examples of distolingual **extra (accessory) roots** in a young Native American; two permanent contralateral first mandibular molars and a deciduous second molar.

FIGURE 11-30. Unusual bifurcated roots.
A. Two mandibular canines with an uncommon furcated root (one facial and one lingual). B. Two mandibular right first premolars with bifurcated roots, a condition that is less common for this tooth than on mandibular canines. C. Radiograph showing both first and second mandibular premolars with mesial and distal roots. This mesiodistal split is quite rare. A more common occurrence is for mandibular first premolars to have their root divided buccolingually (as in B). (Root and pulp cavity images have been enhanced.)

MAXILLARY
RIGHT FIRST PREMOLAR

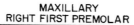

FIGURE 11-31. Unusual trifurcation of a maxillary premolar. Three views of a maxillary right first premolar with a normal looking crown, but with three roots: two buccal and one lingual root (mesiobuccal, distobuccal and lingual). Except for a lesser spread, these roots resemble those found on maxillary molars.

FIGURE 11-32. Unusual bifurcation of buccal views of primary maxillary canines.[41] The left one was extracted from a 9-year-old African-American child (mesial to the right). The middle and right tooth came from a 5-year-old Native American child in Woods County, Ohio, believed to be 2580 years old. Mesial sides face each other. (Courtesy of Dr. Ruth B. Paulson.)

C. ADDITIONAL ANOMALIES

Additional anomalies, including those that tend to affect the entire dentition rather than one or two specific teeth, and those related to mechanical retention and injury, should be noted.

1. ENAMEL DYSPLASIA

Enamel dysplasia is a broad term used to describe abnormal enamel development. Specifically, it is any disturbance in the ameloblasts during the enamel matrix formation, while enamel hypocalcification is a disturbance in the maturation of the enamel matrix. Enamel dysplasia may be hereditary (amelogenesis imperfecta), or could result from systemic causes (such as drugs, infection, and nutritional deficiencies) or local disturbances (such as trauma and periapical infection). Generally, variations in color (from white to yellow and brown) or morphology (pitted and roughened enamel) can result. Common occurrences include:

a. Amelogenesis Imperfecta

Amelogensis imperfecta is a hereditary disorder that affects the enamel formation of both dentitions (Fig. 11-33). The partial or complete lack of enamel results in rough yellow to brown crowns that are highly susceptible to decay. This condition is extremely rare, with an incidence in the United States of 1 in 15,000.[2]

FIGURE 11-33. **Amelogenesis imperfecta. A.** Deciduous maxillary dentition. **B.** Permanent mandibular dentition. This condition occurs only once in about 15,000 people. (Courtesy of Professors Donald Bowers and Rudy Melfi.)

FIGURE 11-34. Fluorosis. This example of mottled enamel is generalized in a 25-year-old female. It consists of a chalky white coloration in the cervical and/or middle third of all permanent teeth. Some pitting of the enamel surface is also visible.

b. Fluorosis

Fluorosis is a condition caused by the ingestion of a high concentration of fluorine in drinking water that greatly *exceeds* the concentration recommended for controlling decay. The fluorine content of some naturally occurring mineral water that causes this condition is *many times greater* than the one part per million that is added to drinking water in many cities to so effectively reduce the prevalence of decay. Clinically, all permanent teeth may be involved and can exhibit a color change from white to yellow/brown spots called mottled enamel (Fig 11-34), and/or a morphologic change of pitted enamel. These teeth are generally very resistant to decay.

c. Enamel Damage Due to High Fever

Pitted enamel on permanent teeth is often the result of early childhood fever from such diseases as measles.[4] Usually, the specific crowns that are developing at the time of the fever are affected (Fig. 11-35). Thus, there are identifiable patterns, such as the pitting of enamel in all permanent first molars, as well as the permanent incisors.

d. Focal Hypomaturation

Focal hypomaturation or hypoplasia is seen as a localized chalky white spot on a tooth. During enamel formation, this condition may result from trauma, a local infection of an adjacent abscessed primary tooth, or some other interference in enamel matrix maturation (Fig. 11-36). Un-

FIGURE 11-35. Dysplasia of the enamel due to high fever. A. Permanent dentition. Patient reported a history of high fever between the ages of 2 and 3 years. Notice that the teeth whose enamel matrix was forming at the time of the fever are affected: mandibular first and second premolars and second molar, and maxillary second premolar and second molar. B. Deciduous dentition. Patient had a high fever during the first 6 weeks after birth. (Courtesy of Professor Donald Bowers.)

FIGURE 11-40. **Misplaced** left maxillary lateral incisor and canine.

c. Tooth Rotation

Rotation is a rare anomaly, most common for the maxillary second premolar, sometimes the maxillary incisor, first premolar, or mandibular second premolar.[27] A tooth may be rotated on its axis by as much as 180° (see rotated maxillary second premolar in Fig. 6-17).

d. Ankylosis

Teeth that erupt into the oral cavity but fail to reach occlusion with the opposing arch appear submerged or ankylosed. **Ankylosis** may be initiated by an infection or trauma to the periodontal ligament. The ankylosed tooth has lost its periodontal ligament space and is truly fused to the alveolar process or bone. Deciduous mandibular second molars most often fail to continue erupting as the jaw grows. Many times, the ankylosis occurs when the permanent successor is missing. Consequently, the ankylosed tooth will be 2–4 mm short of contacting an opposing tooth.

4. REACTIONS TO INJURY

Reactions to injury are not really anomalies, but are unique changes in tooth morphology associated with a specific cause. It is important to recognize these conditions so that their etiology (causes) can be identified and modified, when possible, to avoid the causative factor(s) that could worsen the condition.

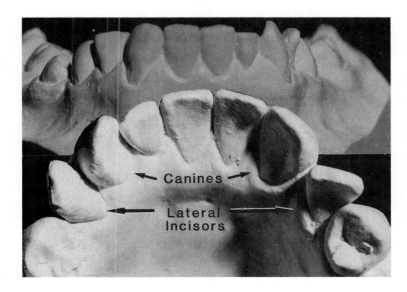

FIGURE 11-41. Bilaterally **misplaced** mandibular canines and lateral incisors, a rare occurrence. Also note the small retained left deciduous lateral incisor.

a. Attrition

Attrition is the wearing away of enamel and dentin from the movement of mandibular teeth against maxillary teeth during normal function, and is made worse by excessive grinding or gritting together of teeth known as **bruxism**. Two examples of severe attrition are shown in Figure 11-42. Stress greatly increases bruxism. This is not really an anomaly, but it must be recognized and distinguished from other forms of tooth wear such as abrasion and erosion.

b. Abrasion

The wearing away of tooth structure by *mechanical* means is called **abrasion**. Abrasion from improper tooth brushing most often results in worn enamel on the facial surfaces of premolars and canines at the cementoenamel junction (Fig. 11-43). It is caused by use of a hard toothbrush and/or a horizontal brushing stroke and/or a gritty dentifrice. Occlusal abrasion results from chewing or biting hard foods or objects, or from chewing tobacco, and results in flattened cusps on all posterior teeth and worn incisal edges. An unusual type of abrasion, caused by the use for many years of a toothpick between the maxillary central incisors, has been reported by Melfi.[39] The same type of proximal abrasion has been reported from the use of a straight pin for the same purpose over many years. A similar looking condition resulting from tooth flexure due to heavy occlused forces is called **abfraction**.

ATTRITION
Deciduous Dentition

Secondary Dentition

FIGURE 11-42. Attrition from prolonged bruxism or grinding of the teeth. The deciduous maxillary central incisors have been worn down almost to the gingival sulcus. The secondary mandibular incisors are worn down to a level where the pulp chamber was at one time many years previously (note the circular and oval regions on the incisal ridges).

ABRASION

Toothbrush

Tobacco

FIGURE 11-43. **Abrasion.** Above: From incorrect horizontal tooth brushing. Below: From chewing tobacco over a 30-year span. (Courtesy of Professor Rudy Melfi.)

c. Erosion

Erosion is the loss of tooth structure from *chemical* (non-mechanical) means and affects smooth and occlusal surfaces. Erosion can be the result of excessive intake or use of citric acid (lemons), carbonated beverages, industrial acids, or the result of regurgitated stomach acids (seen in bulimic individuals who habitually induce vomiting, as in the "binge and purge" syndrome).[2] Erosion can also occur from an unknown cause (idiopathic) (Fig. 11-44).

5. UNUSUAL DENTITIONS

During a routine check of a dental hygiene student's completed oral prophylaxis on a 23-year-old man, the instructor noticed what appeared to be an oblique ridge and cusp of Carabelli on the left mandibular first molar. Alginate impressions were made and casts poured (Fig. 11-45). Careful examination of the casts by both the instructor and Dr. Woelfel revealed not only that the mandibular left first molar closely resembled a maxillary first molar, but also that first and second mandibular premolars and first, second, and third mandibular molars on both sides were remarkably similar morphologically to maxillary posterior teeth. The mandibular six anterior teeth unquestionably belonged to the mandibular dentition. The occlusion of the young man's teeth was remarkably good considering the fact that maxillary posterior teeth were occluding against practically identical maxillary teeth on both sides!

FIGURE 11-44. **Erosion** from an unknown cause (idiopathic). Restorations have been placed in the cervical regions of the mandibular teeth, but the erosion process continues beyond the amalgam margins and is evidenced on the maxillary central incisors.

A MOST UNUSUAL MANDIBULAR DENTITION

FIGURE 11-45. *Mandibular* dentition of a 23-year-old man who has premolars and molars with crown morphology more similar to *maxillary* premolars and molars, particularly on the left side. Both dentitions are seen from the occlusal aspect and on the left as they fit together well into the maximum intercuspal position. The lower premolar crowns do not resemble mandibular premolars in any fashion. The six mandibular anterior teeth are truly mandibular, however. The mandibular right first molar has three buccal cusps, but otherwise seems to be a mixture of both maxillary and mandibular first molars, oblong mesiodistally like a lower, but with a much larger mesiolingual cusp and Carabelli cusp like an upper first molar. The mandibular left three molars seem to have only morphologic characteristics of maxillary molars. This man's maxillary dentition seems entirely normal. It is most interesting to note that the lower left posterior teeth (particularly the premolars) have the morphology of maxillary right side teeth. Likewise, the lower right teeth belong in the upper left quadrant.

A most unusual maxillary dentition with a total of 24 erupted or partially erupted teeth is seen in Figure 11-46. This was the maxillary dentition of a foreign exchange student from Africa. There are 4 incisors, 1 canine, 6 premolars, and 13 molars (5 of which somewhat resemble mandibular molars).

A mandibular dentition with five incisors is seen in a radiograph (Fig. 11-47).

FIGURE 11-46. Very unusual permanent maxillary dentition with 24 teeth, including 13 molars. This cast was furnished courtesy of J. Andrew Stevenson (D.T.L.) and Dr. Robert Stevenson, Columbus, Ohio.

FIGURE 11-47. Radiograph of the mandibular incisor region depicting three central incisors and two lateral incisors, all non-fused and with normal pulp cavities.

Learning questions on anomalies. Circle the correct answer(s).

1. What may result when a forming succedaneous tooth is located next to an abscess on an adjacent deciduous tooth?
    a. Turner's tooth
    b. Fluorosis
    c. Tetracycline staining
    d. Dentinogenesis imperfecta
    e. Amelogenesis imperfecta

2. When you observe only three maxillary incisors but one crown is doubled in width and notched, what do you suspect?
    a. fusion
    b. twinning
    c. gemination
    d. concrescence
    e. cementosis

3. Which condition may be caused by habitually sucking on lemons (which are quite acidic)?
    a. attrition
    b. erosion
    c. abrasion
    d. amelogenesis imperfecta
    e. hypoplasia

4. Which *three* of the following locations are most likely to have supernumerary teeth form?
    a. mandibular premolar area
    b. maxillary premolar area
    c. maxillary incisor area
    d. mandibular incisor area
    e. third molar area

5. Which *one* of the following teeth that are normally single-rooted are most likely to have a bifurcated root?
    a. maxillary central incisors
    b. maxillary lateral incisors
    c. mandibular canines
    d. mandibular first premolars
    e. mandibular second premolars

6. Which *two* of the following are most likely to exhibit anomalous crown morphology?
    a. maxillary central incisors
    b. maxillary lateral incisors
    c. mandibular canines
    d. maxillary third molars
    e. maxillary first molars

Answers: 1–a; 2–a; 3–b; 4–a, c, e; 5–c; 6–b,d.

REFERENCES

1. Dorland's Pocket Medical Dictionary. Philadelphia: W.B. Saunders, 1965.

2. Smith RM, Turner JE, Robbins ML. Atlas of Oral Pathology. St. Louis: C.V. Mosby, 1981

3. Croll TP, Rains JR, Chen E. Fusion and gemination in one dental arch: report of case. ASDC J Dent Child 1981;48:297.

4. Rowe AHR, Johns RB, eds. A Companion to Dental Studies: Dental Anatomy and Embryology. Vol. 1, Book 2. Boston: Blackwell Scientific Publications, 1981.

5. McDonald TP. An American Board of Orthodontics case report. Am J Orthod 1981;80:437–442.

6. Fuller JL, Denehy GE. Concise Dental Anatomy and Morphology. Chicago: Year Book Publishers, Inc, 1984:264–5.

7. Jones AW. Supernumerary mandibular premolars. Report of a case in a patient of mongoloid origins. Br J Oral Surg 1981;19:305–6.

8. Robinson HB, Miller AS. Colby, Kerr and Robinson's Color Atlas of Oral Pathology. Philadelphia: J.B. Lippincott Comp., 1983, p. 38.

9. Primosch RE. Anterior supernumerary teeth—assessment and surgical intervention in children. Pediatr Dentistry 1981;3:204–15.

10. Ranta R, Ylipaavalniemi P. Developmental course of supernumerary premolars in childhood: report of two cases. ASDC J Dent Child 1981;48:385–8.

11. Rubin MM, Nevins A, Berg M, Borden B. A comparison of identical twins in relation to three dental anomalies. Multiple supernumerary teeth, juvenile periodontosis, and zero caries incidence. Oral Surg 1981;52:391–94.

12. Zvolanek JW. Maxillary lateral incisor anomalies in identical twins. Dent Radiogr Photog, 1981;54:17–8.

13. Hemmig SB. Third and fourth molar fusion. Oral Surg 1979;48:572.

14. Good DL, Berson RB. A supernumerary tooth fused to a maxillary permanent central incisor. Pediatr Dentistry 1980;2:294–6.

15. Powell RE. Fusion of maxillary lateral incisor and supernumerary tooth. Oral Surg 1981; 51(3):331.

16. Speiser AM, Bikofsky VM. Premolars with double occlusal surfaces. JADA 1981;103:600–1.

17. Melfi, RC, Alley KE. Permar's Oral Embryology and Microscopic Anatomy: A Textbook for Students in Dental Hygiene. Philadelphia; Lippincott, Williams and Wilkins, 2000.

18. Myers CL. Treatment of a talon-cusp incisor: report of case. ASDC J Dent Child 1980;47:119–21.

19. Hayward JR. Cuspid gigantism. Oral Surg 1980;49:500–1.

20. Ruprecht A, Singer DL. Macrodontia of the mandibular left first premolar. Oral Surg 1979;48:573.

21. Becker A, Smith P, Behar, R. The incidence of anomalous maxillary lateral incisors in relation to palatally-displaced cuspids. Angle Orthod 1981;51:24–9.

22. McKibben DR, Brearley LJ. Radiographic determination of the prevalence of selected dental anomalies in children. J Dent Child 1971;28:390–8.

23. Nazif MM, Ruffalo RC, Zullo T. Impacted supernumerary teeth: a survey of fifty cases. JADA 1983;106:201–4.

24. Hamner JE, Witkop CJ, Metro PS. Taurodontism. Oral Surg 1964;18:409–18.

25. Pindborg JJ. Pathology of the Dental Hard Tissues. Philadelphia: W.B. Saunders, 1970:15–73.

26. Schachter H. A treated case of transposed upper canine. Dent Rec 1951;71:105–8.

27. DeJong TE. Rotatio dentis. Gegenbaurs Morphologisches Jahrbuch 1965;108:67–70.

28. Schulze C. Developmental abnormalities of the teeth and jaws. In: Gorlin RJ, Goldman HM, eds. Thoma's oral pathology. 6th ed. St. Louis: C.V. Mosby, 1970, 138–40.

29. Rothberg J, Kopel M. Early versus late removal of mesiodens: a clinical study of 375 children. Comp Cont Educ Pract 1984;5:115–20.

30. Paulson RB, Gottlieb LJ, Sciulli PW, et al. Double-rooted maxillary primary canines. ASDC J Dent Child 1985;52:195–8.

31. Bimstein E, Bystrom E. Birooted bilateral maxillary primary canines. ASDC J Dent Child 1982;49:217–8.

32. Kelly JR. Birooted primary canines. Oral Surg 1978;46:872.

33. Brown CK. Bilateral bifurcation of the maxillary deciduous cuspids. Oral Surg 1975;40:817.

34. Kroll SO. Double rooted maxillary primary canines. Oral Surg 1980;49:379.

35. Bryant RH Jr, Bowers DF. Four birooted primary canines: report of a case. ASDC J Dent Child 1982;49:441–2.

36. Goldman HM. Anomalies of Teeth (Part 1). Comp Cont Educ Pract 1981;2:358–67.

37. Jackson M, Leeds, LD. Upper canine in position of upper central. Brit. Dent. J 1951;90:243.

38. Curran JD, Baker CG. Roentgeno-oddities. Oral Surg 1973;41:906–7.

39. Dr. Rudy Melfi, Columbus, Ohio, personal communication.

40. Takeda Y. A rare occurrence of a three-rooted mandibular premolar. Ann Dent 1988; 44:43-4.

41. Paulson RB, Gottlieb LJ, Sciulli PW, et al. Double rooted maxillary primary canines. ASDC J Dent Child 1985; 52:195–8.

Operative Dentistry

Robert G. Rashid, D.D.S., M.A.S, contributed this chapter for this edition.

OBJECTIVES

After studying this chapter, readers should be able to:

- Define operative dentistry, dental caries, dental plaque, intra- and extracoronal restorations, and restorative dentistry.
- Classify dental caries according to pit and fissure versus smooth surface, and describe the pattern of spread of each within enamel and dentin.
- Define and identify root caries.
- Describe and identify each G.V. Black Class of dental caries clinically and radiographically.
- List and describe the principles of cavity preparation.

- Describe the indications for restoring a tooth for each class of caries.
- List and describe characteristics of commonly used restorative materials.
- For each class of caries, describe the unique application of the principles of cavity preparation dependent upon the material used.
- For each class of caries, define terms used to describe cavity walls, cavosurfaces, line angles, and point angles.
- Define and identify the types of restoration used to restore large tooth defects.
- Define and identify the restorations used to replace lost teeth.

SECTION I. Operative and Restorative Dentistry: Definitions

Tooth destruction can occur from dental caries (decay), attrition or abrasion, erosion, and fracture; and old restorations can break down. **Dental caries**, known more commonly as tooth decay, is the most common cause of tooth destruction. Caries (which literally means "rotten") results from the **demineralization** of mineralized tooth structures (that is, the loss of minerals or inorganic content from enamel, dentin, and cementum). This demineralization process occurs when specific bacteria firmly adhere to teeth (in a layer called **dental plaque**) *and* are exposed to certain carbohydrates over extended periods of *time* to form acids (such as lactic acid) which react with the hard tooth structure causing mineral loss. *Streptococcus mutans* and lactobacilli are bacteria known to contribute to the caries process. Sugar-containing food items, such as candy, honey, pastries, and especially non-diet soft drinks, contribute to acid formation that can destroy mineralized tooth structure.[1]

Demineralization can be reversed if plaque is removed frequently enough through good oral hygiene measures, if sweets in the diet are limited, and minerals (especially calcium in healthy saliva and fluoride) are available for uptake (remineralization) into the porous demineralized tooth. This tug-of-war between demineralization and remineralization is constant and is the basis for prevention methods that are applied and taught by dental professionals.

Patient education and preventive treatment are important aspects of dental patient care. Prevention and treatment should be based on personalized risk-based assessment of each patient's caries history, which includes their history of fluoride use, their salivary flow rate, and the frequency of sugar uptake (especially snacks).[2,3] **Fluoride** applied to teeth in appropriate concentrations has been shown to reduce dental caries incidence because it increases the tooth's resistance to breakdown by caries-forming acids. Therefore, caries prevention includes daily use of fluoride-containing paste and fluoride-containing mouthwashes (either prescription or over-the-counter), as well as office applied fluorides that contain higher concentrations. Further, when saliva flow is reduced (from damage to the salivary glands due to radiation therapy, or as a side effect to many medications), the teeth are more susceptible to tooth decay. Artificial saliva or sugarless chewing gum could be used to alleviate this problem. Finally, snacks provide the ingredients that, with certain bacteria found in dental plaque, form acids that contribute to demineralization. (Most soft drinks are quite acidic themselves as well as containing sugars that can produce even more acid during the caries-forming process.) Therefore, frequent snacking must be curtailed.

In a 1979–80 survey representing 45.3 million United States school children between the ages of 5 and 17 years, the estimated prevalence of breakdown in permanent dentition was 4.77 decayed, missing, or filled surfaces per child.[4] Comparing data from two studies conducted for the Centers for Disease Control and Prevention, the number of carious permanent teeth (both treated and untreated) in children from 6 to 18 years old decreased by 57% from 1971 to 1974 through 1988 to 1994 [decreasing from 4.44 to 1.9 carious teeth].[5] These studies also showed a 40% decline in the number of carious primary teeth in 2 to 10 year olds [from 2.29 to 1.38].

These and other reports have shown a worldwide decrease in the incidence of coronal caries, especially in children and adolescents, ranging from 10 to 60% depending on the article cited. However, the number of adults older than 65 is expected to double by 2025, and people are keeping their teeth longer (53% of persons older than 65 still have at least 20 natural teeth).[6] Further, the prevalence of root caries in the elderly is increasing,[7] with one study reporting 75% of elderly women with clinically detectable root caries.[8] Therefore, the restoration of damaged teeth (from caries and other reasons) will continue to be a part of the practice of general dentistry for some time to come.

Operative dentistry is the phase of dentistry involving the art and science of the diagnosis, treatment and prognosis of defects in teeth which do *not* require restorations that cover the entire tooth (full coverage). Restoring *conservative* tooth defects, such as those resulting from small carious lesions which are confined to enamel or have progressed just beyond the dentinoenamel junction, usually requires placement of **intracoronal** restorations whose preparations are cut *within* the tooth and, if located occlusally, are narrower buccolingually than the distance between the cusps.

As tooth destruction increases in size, **extracoronal** restorations may be a more appropriate restoration of choice. These larger extracoronal restorations surround and cover all or part of the exposed tooth, and include crowns (also known by many as "caps") or onlays (which have an intracoronal component but also include coverage of cusp tips). Treatment with extracoronal and intracoronal restorations should result in the restoration of proper tooth form, function and esthetics while maintaining the physiological integrity of the teeth in harmonious relationship with the adjacent hard and soft tissues, all of which enhances the general health and welfare of the patient.[9] **Restorative dentistry** is the phase of clinical dentistry that includes not only the prevention and treatment of defects of individual teeth, but also the replacement of teeth that were lost or never formed. Lost teeth can be replaced using a fixed partial denture (also known as a bridge), a removable partial denture, an implant (surgical insertion or placement of an artificial root over which a crown may be constructed), or complete dentures (also known as false teeth). Thus, restorative dentistry involves the restoration of lost tooth structure *and/or lost teeth* with the ultimate goal of reestablishing a healthy, functioning, and comfortable dentition.

SECTION II. Classification of Carious Lesions

There are two *broad* classifications of tooth decay based on the anatomy of the tooth surface involved: *pit and fissure*, and *smooth surface*. The pattern by which the spread of dental caries occurs as it enlarges and deepens differs in these two types.

Pit and fissure carious lesions begin in the depth of pits and fissures which form from incomplete fusion of enamel lobes during tooth development and are nearly impossible to keep clean. Note the deep occlusal fissure in cross-section of a tooth in Figure 12-1A and B. As you should recall, fissures and pits are commonly located on the occlusal surfaces of posterior teeth (molars and premolars), as well as on the lingual surface of maxillary molars, the buccal surface of mandibular molars, and in the lingual fossae of maxillary incisors, especially lateral incisors.

A small pit and fissure lesion can be almost undetectable externally but, as it progresses deeper, the caries widens within the fissure as it approaches and spreads beyond the dentinoenamel junction (DEJ) (occlusal surface in Fig. 12-1 A and B). This widening is due to the decreased mineral content at this junction and in dentin when compared to hard enamel.

In contrast to pit and fissure caries, **smooth surface** carious lesions occur on the smooth surfaces of the anatomic crown of a tooth in the areas which are least accessible to the natural cleansing action of the lips, cheeks, and tongue. These areas include the proximal surfaces of teeth just *cervical* to the proximal contact, and the facial and lingual surfaces just *cervical* to the crest of curvature of the crown (in the gingival one-third of the crown). The pattern of spread within enamel for smooth surface caries is different than for pit and fissure caries since it begins as a relatively broad area of destruction just beneath the outer layer of enamel, but it *narrows* as it progresses more deeply toward the dentinoenamel junction. Once it reaches dentin, however, it spreads out wider at the dentinoenamel junction, just like pit and fissure caries.

Root surface caries is another type of smooth surface caries that occurs on cementum, most frequently in patients with disease of the periodontium, patients with decreased saliva flow, or in older patients who have had gingival recession which increases the potential for accumulation of caries-forming plaque on the cementum of root surfaces. This type of caries is a softening, destructive process that may not require a restoration if there is only minimal involvement.[10] Treatment in these cases can include polishing the root, applying fluoride (topical or fluoride containing varnishes), and keeping the roots clean through good oral hygiene.

In 1908, Dr. G. V. Black developed a comprehensive method of classifying carious lesions that has been useful when describing specific principles of cavity preparation.[11] The original classifications were G.V.Black Class I, II, III, IV, and V. All pit and fissure type lesions are Class I, whereas Class II, III, IV, and V caries are all smooth surface type lesions.

FIGURE 12-1. **Pattern and location of pit and fissure and smooth surface caries.** A. Drawing of a cross-section of a mandibular molar showing the usual pattern of spreading decay. The occlusal lesion (Class I, pit and fissure) is small externally, widening toward the depth of the fissure as it approaches the dentinoenamel junction. Once within dentin, the caries spreads out laterally as well as progressing toward the pulp. The mesial lesion (Class II, smooth surface) is broad externally, narrowing toward the dentinoenamel junction. Once within dentin, this lesion spreads out laterally (like the Class I), as well as progressing toward the pulp. B. Cut section of a mandibular molar. Notice the very deep fissure beneath the central groove (top arrow), and the lateral spread of decay at the dentinoenamel junction (arrows). C. Cut section of a smooth surface Class II lesion. Note the width of the lesion near the surface of enamel, the narrowing as it progresses toward the DEJ, and then the spread of the decay once it reaches dentin.

A. IDENTIFICATION OF CLASS I CARIES

Class I lesions (Fig. 12-2A) form in enamel pits and fissures, and may form wherever deep inaccessible pits and fissures occur. In a 1979–80 survey of United States school children aged 5 to 17 years, 54% of all carious lesions were found on the occlusal surfaces,[4] which constitute one-fifth of the surfaces of any premolar or molar. More recently, studies of teeth at risk show that the occlusal surfaces of the first molars are

FIGURE 12-2. **Class I carious lesions**. On the left is a small lesion in the central pit on tooth number 18 at the depth of stained grooves, which must be detected with a sharp explorer by feeling for tugback. On the right is an enormous, clinically obvious lesion on tooth number 2 that has resulted in the collapse of most of the occlusal enamel by the undermining spread of the decay in dentin. Both teeth appear to be restorable, but the one with extensive decay would probably require endodontic therapy (root canal) and an inlay-onlay or crown.

FIGURE 12-3. **Radiograph of a Class I lesion** on tooth number 31. By the time it appears this deep on the radiograph, the caries has destroyed dentin to such a depth that a thermal-insulating base of some type of dental cement will be needed to protect the pulp from thermal conductivity through the metal filling. This pit and fissure caries should have been detected earlier with a good clinical examination. [There is also a large distal Class II lesion on tooth number 4, which appears to be rotated (top right)].

at greatest risk for *initial* caries, followed by the occlusal surfaces of lower, then upper second molars.[12] Detecting Class I lesions clinically requires visual inspection and tactile evaluation. Careful visual analysis of a clean, dry, well-lit occlusal surface will reveal this type of caries as a fissure or pit surrounded by enamel that is chalky or more opaque (less translucent) than the adjacent enamel. Some dentists prefer to confirm caries within these suspicious defects by probing with a very sharp explorer. After pressing the explorer into the defect with moderate to firm pressure, sensing a resistance to removing the explorer (known as **tugback**) helps to confirm the presence of softness and therefore caries within the defect or fissure wall. However, the firm use of the explorer for the detection of occlusal caries should be used with caution. One study suggests that the sensitivity and specificity of this technique is poor, and excessive force could actually damage fragile enamel rods on the tooth.[13] Even in the absence of obvious tug-back, loss of translucency of enamel around a pit or fissure may be considered to be reliable evidence of attack. It is especially important to avoid undue pressure with the explorer point in larger, frank lesions (as seen in Fig. 12-2, right tooth) because injudicious probing may cause pain or additional enamel rod destruction.

A Class I lesion is usually not detectable on a radiograph until it is quite deep into dentin because the lesion is superimposed between the thick buccal and lingual surfaces of enamel which show up whiter (radiopaque), thereby masking the darker caries. By the time the cavity is visible on the radiograph (Fig. 12-3), the size of the preparation required to remove all of the decay would be considerably deeper (toward the pulp) than if the decay had been detected during a good clinical examination when the lesion was smaller. Thus, early Class I decay can be best diagnosed during a thorough, systematic *clinical* examination of clean, dry teeth using good lighting and a sharp exploring point.

B. IDENTIFICATION OF CLASS II CARIES

A Class II lesion is one that forms on the smooth proximal surface of *posterior teeth* just cervical to proximal contact (Fig. 12-4A). It results from inadequate plaque removal in these hard to reach interproximal surfaces. Judicious use of dental floss is one method for preventing (or reversing) Class II (and Class III) caries.

Clinical detection of small Class II lesions in the mouth without the aid of radiographs is often difficult due to the inability to visualize or probe the areas where they form. A loss of translucency of the enamel

FIGURE 12-4. **Class II lesions. A.** Left: An incipient (beginning) lesion without cavitation on the mesial surface of tooth number 14, probably visible only on a radiograph if an adjacent tooth were present. Right: A larger Class II lesion with cavitation on the mesial surface of tooth number 15, with color changes to the enamel that would be evident beyond the proximal contact area in the mouth. **B.** A Class II lesion on the mesial surface of tooth number 30 which resulted in the collapse of the entire mesial marginal ridge of enamel.

seen when examining the overlying marginal ridge may be the first clinical evidence of Class II caries. As the carious lesion increases in size, it may appear as a dark, cavitated area (hole) that can be detected by a thin probe (explorer) in the buccal or lingual embrasure. A very large Class II lesion may actually undermine the entire marginal ridge, permitting the entire ridge of enamel to break off during mastication (Fig. 12-4B).

Radiographic detection of an incipient (beginning, small) Class II lesion is most predictably accomplished using bitewing radiographs because the Class II lesion is normally visible on the radiograph before it can be detected clinically (Fig. 12-5). A Class II lesion is seen as a narrow triangular shadow within the enamel *just cervical to the proximal contact* (Fig. 12-5A, arrow). The wide base of the triangle is located at the enamel surface, and it tapers to a point toward the dentinoenamel junction. When the lesion gets large enough to reach dentin, it can be seen spreading out beneath the dentinoenamel junction (seen in two large lesions in Fig. 12-5B).

FIGURE 12-5. **Radiographs of Class II lesions. A.** Radiographic evidence of a Class II lesion which has barely spread into dentin on the distal surface of tooth number 20 (arrow). Note the location of the lesions just cervical to the proximal contacts, and that the lesion is wider at the surface of enamel than at the DEJ. **B.** Several Class II lesions (arrows), some of which are confined to enamel, and two that have spread out in dentin. [Note the existing Class II amalgam on tooth number 13 with a deep base and large undesirable overhang (i.e., excess bulk of amalgam beyond the gingival cavosurface margin)].

C. IDENTIFICATION OF CLASS III CARIES

Class III lesions are smooth surface lesions located on the proximal surfaces of *anterior teeth*, just cervical to the proximal contact, but *not* involving the incisal angle (or corner) of the tooth (Fig. 12-6).

An incipient (small or beginning) Class III lesion can usually be detected clinically by carefully examining the enamel facially or lingually for changes in translucency *just cervical to the proximal contact*. The underlying lesion causes overlying enamel to appear slightly darker or more opaque than surrounding, sound enamel. These changes are most evident when a source of light (such as fiber optics) is placed lingually against the proximal enamel of the tooth, revealing the change in translucency facially. This method of clinical detection is called **transillumination**.

Periapical radiographs of the anterior teeth (and the bitewing radiographs for the distal of canines) may also be used to confirm a Class III lesion (Fig. 12-7, arrow). The location (just cervical to the proximal contact) and pattern of spread is typical of smooth surface lesions as described earlier for a Class II lesion.

D. IDENTIFICATION OF CLASS IV CARIES

A Class IV lesion involves the proximal surface of an anterior tooth (as does a Class III lesion), but, *in addition*, it involves the incisal angle (or corner) of the tooth (Fig. 12-8). The Class IV lesion is frequently the result of a Class III lesion that became so large that the undermined tooth angle broke off. A similar shaped defect occurs when the tooth corner fractures off due to a blow to the mouth. The loss of an incisal angle is plainly visible upon clinical examination. Radiographs are not needed to detect the Class IV lesion, but may be useful to determine the depth of the lesion relative to its proximity to the pulp chamber (Fig. 12-9).

E. IDENTIFICATION OF CLASS V CARIES

The Class V lesion is located in the cervical one-third of the facial or lingual surface of any (anterior or posterior) tooth crown (Fig. 12-10). It is a smooth surface lesion that results from poor hygiene in the area of the tooth just cervical to the buccal or lingual crest of curvature, adjacent to the gingiva, where the nat-

FIGURE 12-6. Class III lesion on the mesial of tooth number 6 with an area of obvious cavitation or hole in the enamel surface. If this lesion involved any more of the mesial incisal angle, it would become a Class IV, rather than a Class III, lesion.

FIGURE 12-7. Radiograph of a Class III lesion on the mesial of tooth number 8. Note the location of this decay just cervical to the proximal contact, and the characteristic spread or widening of the decay at the dentinoenamel junction.

FIGURE 12-8. An enormous **Class IV carious lesion** involving the mesioincisal angle of tooth number 26.

FIGURE 12-9. Radiograph of a Class IV lesion involving the distoincisal angle of tooth number 10.

ural cleansing action of the lips, tongue, and cheeks is ineffective. This area of the tooth is susceptible to plaque accumulation and resultant caries. Over the lifetime of a tooth, the gingiva and supporting bone may recede apically, exposing greater amounts of the root surface. With decreased salivary flow and/or poor oral hygiene, the incidence of caries increases in this area (Fig. 12-10, right tooth).

The Class V lesion is best detected by careful visual examination of the smooth gingival portion of the tooth crown with good lighting to determine a chalky white or stained appearance, often with a break (cavitation or hole) in the enamel surface. *Care should be taken with the explorer* not *to break through an area of beginning demineralization that has not yet cavitated*, since excellent oral hygiene and fluoride has been shown to reverse the caries process. These lesions may extend slightly apical to the level of inflamed gingiva, so that the use of the tactile sense obtained through the explorer is critical for detection of cavitation,[10] and to distinguish these lesions (which are cavitated) from a calcified buildup of calculus (which is felt as a bump attached to the surface of the tooth).

As with a Class I lesion, the Class V lesion is superimposed over buccal or lingual surfaces of enamel that show up whiter (radiopaque), thereby masking the darker caries. By the time a Class V lesion is evident on radiographs, it has progressed far beyond the incipient stage, and will require a much larger

FIGURE 12-10. Class V lesions. Left: Incipient (beginning) buccal lesion that is seen as chalky and discolored and is flaking away. **Right:** An obvious cavitated Class V facial lesion that has destroyed much of the enamel on the buccal surface of the crown and adjacent cementum and dentin of the root.

FIGURE 12-11. **Radiograph of a Class V lesion** on tooth number 22. It is impossible to tell from the radiograph whether it is on the buccal or lingual surface or whether it is decay, or a radiolucent (dark looking on the radiograph) composite restoration.

restoration than would have been required if it were *clinically* diagnosed at its earliest stages (Fig 12-11). Therefore, the examiner should not depend on radiographs for detection of these lesions. However, when discovering a cervically located radiolucency on a radiograph, the dentist should carefully evaluate the tooth to clinically prove or disprove the presence of Class V caries. Darker (radiolucent) areas of cervical abrasion, as well as older types of radiolucent restorative materials, can appear like Class V or root surface caries on radiographs.

F.   CLASS VI TYPE OF DENTAL CARIES

A Class VI type of dental caries or restoration is not one of Black's original classifications. In Baum's text, it is defined as the cavity or defect found on the tips of cusps or along the biting edges of incisors.[10] In Sturdevant's text, Class VI caries includes lesions on the cusp tips of posterior teeth.[9]

SECTION III. Indications for Restoring a Tooth

A.   CLASS I CARIES: WHEN TO RESTORE

Some Class I lesions are difficult to differentiate from noncarious deep enamel defects. If tug-back occurs with a sharp explorer in a deep pit or fissure, and the surrounding enamel is chalky or less translucent, a restoration is indicated (recall Fig. 12-2). Certainly, by the time caries is obvious on the radiograph, it would be evident clinically and should be restored. However, if tugback is minimal and without the accompanying evidence, the dentist might consider periodically reevaluating the area during recall appointments, especially if the patient is older and has a low caries rate. Beware, however, that tugback can occur when probing in deep fissures even if caries is not present. Generally, multiple signs should be present to make a clinical diagnosis of caries, and then consider the need for a restoration.

B.   CLASS II CARIES: WHEN TO RESTORE

Clinically obvious Class II lesions, when cavitated (with a break or hole in the surface), should be restored (recall Fig. 12-4). The radiographic indication for restoring small lesions is when the lesion has penetrated to the dentinoenamel junction (DEJ) and begins to spread out into dentin (recall Fig. 12-5). If the lesion is small enough to be confined to enamel on the radiograph, the dentist must consider the patient's previous history of carious activity, oral hygiene, and age in order to decide whether to restore now, or to reevaluate at subsequent recall intervals. For example, a young patient with a small carious lesion only two-thirds of the way through enamel, but with many deeper lesions and poor oral hygiene, should probably have this tooth restored, especially since a *lesion extends deeper in the tooth than it appears on the radiograph.*[10]

C. CLASS III CARIES: WHEN TO RESTORE

The indications for restoring a Class III lesion are the same as for a Class II lesion: that is, if the surface is cavitated, or has reached the dentin as seen on the radiograph or through transillumination, a restoration is indicated (recall Figs. 12-6 and 12-7).

D. CLASS IV CARIES: WHEN TO RESTORE

The Class IV restoration is indicated when active caries is detected (recall Fig. 12-8). Many Class IV restorations are indicated, however, not because of caries but because the corner of the tooth has fractured off in an accident. In these instances, the extent of the fracture, the proximity of the exposed tooth structure to the pulp chamber, hypersensitivity to temperature changes, and, most often, the patients' concern for esthetics are important in determining when to restore the tooth. If the fracture is not into the dentin and the patient is not concerned about the appearance of the tooth, smoothing the rough edges of the tooth may suffice. If, however, dentin is involved, or if there is evidence of decay, a restoration is indicated to prevent discomfort from the exposed dentin and to stop the spread of decay.

E. CLASS V CARIES: WHEN TO RESTORE

Not all areas at the cervical of the tooth that are cavitated and white or darkly stained require a Class V restoration, since some of these areas may be either areas of arrested (old, inactive) decay, or noncarious cavitated defects due to abrasion, erosion or **abfraction** (the loss of hard tooth structure which appears similar to abrasion but is caused by flexure or bending of the tooth from heavy occlusal forces). Class V lesions require restorations when tooth structure is *soft* or cavitated (recall Fig. 12-10). Restorations should also be considered for non-carious defects that occur in this part of the tooth if the tooth is severely sensitive and does not respond to desensitizing agents, if the lesion is very deep and cannot be kept clean, or if it appears that it will continue to get worse due to poor oral hygiene.

SECTION IV. Principles of Cavity Preparation

Basic principles of cavity preparation were developed by Dr. Black and were uniquely applied to each class of caries and type of restorative material. Today, the application of his principles has been modified due to the introduction of new dental restorative materials which were not available in his day. Each principle that the dentist must consider when preparing a tooth for a restoration is described here:

A. ESTABLISH AN OUTLINE FORM

The outline form of a preparation is the external shape of the preparation on the tooth. It is developed by *removing the least amount of tooth structure* possible, yet adhering to the following principles:

1. EXTEND THE PREPARATION TO SOUND ENAMEL

The dentist enlarges the preparation outline so it extends to solid enamel that has no signs of cavitation or active caries. Also, the dentist must determine if the integrity of the margins is adequate to support function. In many cases, this involves extending the preparation to enamel that is supported by, or resting on, sound dentin (that is, enamel that is not undermined by the spread of caries within the dentin). Since enamel is brittle, if it is not sufficiently supported by sound dentin and/or bonding techniques, the unsupported enamel rods will fracture off, leaving a gap between tooth and the restorative material.

2. EXTEND THE PREPARATION FOR PREVENTION

The dentist evaluates the need to enlarge the preparation within enamel beyond the specific area of decay in order to include adjacent tooth structure felt to be prone to the development of future decay. This may involve enlarging a preparation for a pit and fissure lesion to include adjacent deep pits and fissures thought to be caries prone, even though they have not yet become carious. Similarly, when developing the cavity preparation for smooth surface carious lesions, the outline of the preparation may be extended to include adjacent smooth surface areas likely to become carious. For example, if one small area of tooth next to the gingiva has decay, the preparation might be enlarged to include more of the tooth adjacent to that caries-prone area (particularly if the adjacent area shows signs of early decay such as white decalcified areas).

Over the past 30 years, there have been a tremendous increase in the use of fluoride (in community water, toothpaste, rinses, and topical applications applied periodically by the dentist), and improved efforts by dental professionals to educate the population in prevention techniques. Therefore, the need for preventive extension on smooth surface lesions must be weighed against the possibility that excellent hygiene and fluoride could stop or even reverse the decay process, especially if it has not progressed too far. The degree of extension should be based on such factors as the age of the patient (younger enamel is more susceptible to caries than mature enamel), his or her rate of caries activity, personal oral hygiene, and dietary habits. For example, extension for prevention for a tooth preparation on a younger patient with multiple areas of active decay, poor oral hygiene, and frequent intake of high sugar snacks and sugar-containing carbonated beverages who is unwilling to change, is more appropriate than it would be on an older patient with a lower caries rate, better eating habits, and good oral hygiene.

3. PROVIDE ADEQUATE ACCESS

A restoration outline must be large enough for the dentist to ensure that all carious tooth structure has been removed, and that instruments required to place the filling material will fit. A small, narrow initial cut through the enamel might not permit the dentist to confirm the removal of all caries that may have spread laterally at the dentinoenamel junction. Further, even when the removal of all caries can be verified visually or by probing, a very small initial preparation might be too small for the instruments required to place the restorative material to be placed into the preparation without voids.

4. PROVIDE RESISTANCE FORM

The dentist must design a preparation to ensure room for an adequate thickness of restorative material for strength, and sufficient remaining solid tooth structure to withstand occlusal forces. If preparation depth is inadequate for the material of choice to withstand occlusal forces, the restoration could break. If the remaining tooth is too thin, it could fracture. One solution to protect thin remaining tooth structure is to cover it with cast metal onlays or crowns, as discussed in Section VI of this chapter. Another solution is to bond on a layer of composite material to increase the strength of the thin remaining enamel.

B. PROVIDE RETENTION FORM

Retention form is the internal design of a preparation that will prevent the restoration from falling out or becoming dislodged. The methods for providing retention differ depending on the restorative material and on the location of the carious lesion. The appropriate methods for establishing retention form with different restorative materials are described later in Section V of this chapter.

C. REMOVE CARIES AND TREAT THE PULP

All principles of the cavity preparation described up to this point assume that caries has spread minimally, not yet beyond the outer 0.5 mm of dentin which is adjacent to the dentinoenamel junction. The dentist usually prepares the outline form and retention for cavity preparations with a high-speed dental handpiece using carbide or diamond burs that cut quickly, minimizing the potentially damaging heat by use of an effective water coolant spray. When removing carious lesions that have progressed deeper than 0.5 mm into dentin, the dentist selects slowly rotating round burs (in slow-speed handpieces) or hand instruments. The slow-speed handpiece permits the dentist to differentiate between the *softer* carious dentin and the harder, sound dentin.

When caries extends close to the pulp, it may be advisable to protect the vital tissues of the tooth (odontoblasts, and blood vessels and nerves within the pulp) with dental liners and cement bases prior to placing the final restoration. Various dental materials have been developed for this purpose. When used in the appropriate combination and in the correct order, they can prevent bacterial penetration, provide thermal insulation, sedate the pulp, and stimulate the production of secondary dentin.

D. FINISH THE PREPARATION WALLS

This step entails using a handpiece with appropriate burs, discs, and hand instruments (chisel type) designed to smoothly plane the walls while removing unsound enamel (i.e., enamel that is crazed or cracked or not supported by sound dentin).

E. CLEAN THE PREPARATION

Prior to the restoration for all cavity preparations, the operator must remove excess cement base that is too close to the preparation margins, along with tooth debris, hemorrhage, and saliva from the walls of the preparation. In this way, the restorative material will contact only sound clean tooth structure.

F. FINAL EVALUATION OF THE PREPARATION

Finally, a most important last step is to evaluate the finished preparation to ensure that all of the principles of cavity preparation have been addressed.

SECTION V. Principles of Cavity Preparation Based on Restorative Material, Class, and Size of Lesion

A. RESTORATIVE (FILLING) MATERIALS

Materials of choice for restoring small conservative defects requiring intracoronal restorations include amalgam, composite, glass ionomer, and porcelain or cast metal inlays that are placed into intracoronal preparations within the tooth. The materials of choice for restoring larger defects that require protection (extracoronal coverage) of thin remaining tooth structure include gold, semi- or non-precious metal, or porcelain, which surround or cover the entire tooth in a relatively thin outer shell.

1. AMALGAM

Amalgam is a widely used restorative material owing to its ease of placement and relatively low cost. It is silver in color and is packed into a preparation in successive small increments which, within several hours, cohere and become hard enough to withstand chewing forces. Therefore, it is used for restorations on the chewing (or occlusal) surfaces of posterior teeth and other restorations when maintenance of proximal and occlusal contacts is important but when esthetics is not a factor (Figs. 12-12 and 12-13). Although amalgam is being used less often than in the past, it is still the restora-

FIGURE 12-12. Class I and II amalgam restorations, mandibular arch. **Left**: Class I OB-A (occlusobuccal amalgam) on tooth number 32. **Left-center**: Class II MOB-A (mesio-occlusobuccal amalgam) with a mesiobuccal cusp build-up or replacement on tooth number 31. **Right-center**: Class II MO-A (mesio-occlusal amalgam) on tooth number 30. **Right**: Class II MO-A on tooth number 29.

FIGURE 12-13. Class I, II, and III amalgam restorations, maxillary arch. **Left**: Class I O-A (occlusal amalgams) on tooth number 3 with two parts separated by a strong intact oblique ridge. **Left-center**: a Class I O-A (occlusal amalgam) on tooth number 4. **Right-center**: Class II DO-A (disto-occlusal amalgam) on tooth number 5. **Right**: Class III D-A (distal amalgam) on tooth number 6. These are all very conservative restorations, extended only as wide as necessary for access and prevention.

tion of choice by dentists for restoring Class II lesions [according to 76.3% of the dentists polled in a 1995 survey].[14]

2. ESTHETIC RESTORATIVE MATERIALS

Esthetic restorative materials, such as composite resin and glass ionomer, are being increasingly used due to patients' demands for esthetic restorations. **Composite resin** is a tooth-colored restorative material which is applied as a plastic-like mass into a preparation. It can be hardened quickly with a light source. Due to initial concerns about the strength and abrasion resistance of composite resins,[15,16] it was historically used primarily for restoring the proximal surfaces of anterior teeth and the facial surfaces of teeth on which esthetics is a chief concern. An example of composite restoration used to close a diastema is shown in Figure 12-14, and to restore Class III lesions in Figure 12-15. Note that

FIGURE 12-14. A. Teeth numbers 8 and 9 with diastema. **B.** Same teeth during final finishing stages after placement of **composite veneers** used to close the diastema. No tooth preparation was necessary. (Courtesy of Dr. Roland Pagniano, D.D.S.)

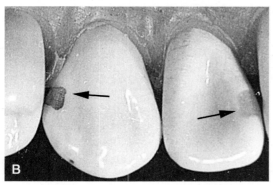

FIGURE 12-15. Class III restorations. A. DF-C: distal composite with labial approach on tooth number 8. **B. Left**: The DL-A: distal amalgam with lingual approach on tooth number 11; metal is used here to maintain the distal contact. **Right**: The ML-C (mesial composite) with lingual approach on tooth number 10. (The dark shade of the composite was used to make the restoration visible in this photograph.)

the shade of the composite restorations in Figure 12-15 are dark in order to visualize the size, outline, and location of these restorations.

As composite resin properties and placement techniques have improved, composite resins are now used more often in posterior surfaces. One longitudinal study rated composite restorations after 10 years (using a United States Public Health system of evaluation) to be over 90% satisfactory for color stability, surface smoothness, anatomical form, lack of recurrent caries, and pulp response.[17] Only marginal adaptation was scored below 90%, with a score of 81%. With recent physical property improvements[18] and a new generation of dentin bonding agents that can etch enamel and dentin simultaneously,[19] and a new generation of packable composite based resins, they will be used even more widely in the future.

When esthetics is a factor, tooth colored materials can be used as inlays or onlays, using either a direct technique (constructed within the mouth) or an indirect technique (constructed outside the mouth and then cemented in place). Also, when there are large cavities, an adhesive (bonded) indirect composite restoration that has adequate wear resistance can be used to strengthen the remaining tooth.[9]

Glass ionomer and related materials such as compomers and resin-modified glass ionomers, are recommended for the treatment of root surface caries and erosion lesions.[20] These materials bond to dentin chemically, are reasonably esthetic and contain fluoride, which reduces the possibility of recurrent caries.

3. CAST METAL RESTORATIONS

Cast gold or semiprecious alloys, when used for inlays and onlays (and full crowns as discussed later), are constructed from an accurate model (or die) of the patient's teeth (Fig. 12-16). These cast metal restorations require considerably more time to construct than composite resin or amalgam restorations because of the laboratory procedures. Consequently, they are more expensive for the patient.

An **inlay** is a cast restoration that fits within the prepared tooth cavity but does not overlay the cusps, in contrast to an **onlay** which overlays or replaces cusps (Fig. 12-16). Onlays and full crowns are recommended when the tooth structure remaining after tooth preparation is frail and needs to be

FIGURE 12-16. Class II cast-metal inlay and onlay restorations. **Left:** An MOD-I (mesio-occlusodistal **inlay**) on tooth number 20. **Center and Right:** MOD-Os (extensive mesio-occlusodistal **onlays**) on teeth numbers 19 and 18.

protected from occlusal forces. The greater strength of the cast metal in thin layers compared to amalgam permits optimum protection and strength with less bulk of metal, resulting in less occlusal reduction of tooth structure. Further, cast metal restorations can be contoured more perfectly on a **die** (which is a precise dental stone reproduction of the individual prepared tooth) than in the mouth. Finally, cast restorations are more inert (less likely to change) in the mouth compared to amalgam (that is, cast restorations have better marginal stability over time). For these reasons, a cast inlay may be selected over amalgam for patients who desire and can afford the cast restoration, even when the restoration will be quite conservative and not require onlaying.

4. **PORCELAIN: INLAYS, ONLAYS, AND VENEERS**

Indirect (i.e., constructed outside of the mouth and cemented) ceramic inlays and onlays are becoming esthetic alternatives to cast inlays and onlays due to advanced processing methods and bonding

FIGURE 12-17. Porcelain veneers. **A.** Teeth numbers 8, 9, and 10 with old composite resin veneers that have chipped and exhibit a loss of translucency. **B.** These same teeth after placement of esthetic porcelain veneers that cover the entire facial surfaces. (Courtesy of Dr. Roland Pagniano, D.D.S.)

techniques which improve fit.[21,22] Advances are also occurring in the generation of these restorations by computer.[23] Conservative techniques for veneering the labial surfaces of anterior teeth to improve esthetics include porcelain (or direct composite) veneers that require minimal or no tooth reduction and fees that are generally less than for a crown with a porcelain veneer. Porcelain veneers used to improve the esthetics of anterior teeth with old, unesthetic composite restorations are shown in Figure 12-17.

B. PRINCIPLES OF CAVITY PREPARATION AND NOMENCLATURE FOR EACH G.V. BLACK CLASS OF CARIES BASED ON MATERIAL USED

The discussion of tooth restoration that follows assumes that the tooth to be prepared is periodontally sound (i.e., has a stable alveolus and healthy gingiva) and that the maintenance of the tooth is an integral part of the overall treatment for that patient. The five classifications of decay devised and published by Dr. G.V. Black in 1908 are still appropriate, although the principles of cavity preparation are now applied uniquely for each class of decay and each new restorative material. Successful cavity preparations for restorative materials such as dental amalgam, composite, resin, or cast metal are designed to allow placement and maintenance of each restorative material and, at the same time, to ensure the preservation of remaining tooth structure.

1. CLASS I CARIES: PRINCIPLES OF CAVITY PREPARATION AND TERMINOLOGY

Pit and fissure sealants can be used as a preventive measure to prevent Class I caries in deep caries prone pits and fissures, especially for the young patient. A sealant is a "flowable" resin that is applied over non-carious but caries prone, unprepared pits and fissures of recently erupted teeth. These sealants have been shown to be an effective means of preventing caries in pits and fissures.[24-26] An initial sealant application for all permanent molars and premolars requires only 15–20 minutes per child.[27] A transitional restoration involving composite resin in a very conservative preparation confined within enamel, plus a sealant over adjacent pits and fissures, is called a **preventive resin** restoration. Conservative preparations can also be formed using an air-abrasion system where abrasive particles are blown forcefully toward the tooth to actually remove tooth structure. This technique permits removal of only the most conservative amounts of tooth structure, but the principles of cavity preparation for this new technology are not necessarily unique. Bonding agents, similar to sealants, can be used for retention when placing composite restorations over the abraded tooth.[28]

Amalgam is frequently chosen for stress-bearing Class I restorations on occlusal surfaces. For small Class I pits or fissures on posterior teeth where esthetics are important, composite resins may be used. Cast gold or porcelain onlays would only be considered for Class I restorations if there were few restorations in the mouth with a low evidence of new decay, or the size of the restoration necessitated onlaying cusps.

Certain of G.V. Black's principles of cavity preparation are uniquely applied when restoring the Class I cavity with amalgam as described here. Differences in preparation requirements will be noted for resin materials.

a. Extension for Prevention (Class I)

Extension for prevention, to include those pits and fissures adjoining the defects with active decay, should be considered when the patient is young, has a high caries rate, and/or exhibits poor oral hygiene. Examples of preparations including all major grooves can be seen in Figures 12-18 and 12-19.

b. Resistance Form (Class I)

When amalgam is used on a stress bearing surface, a minimum depth of 1.5-2 mm is recommended due to the brittleness of amalgam in thinner layers; whereas, if cast metal is used, a thickness of 1 mm may be sufficient to withstand occlusal forces. Ideally, amalgam meets the unprepared tooth surface at right angles to provide resistance form, whereas gold ends in an overlapping bevel (seen later in Fig. 12-24). Resin restorations can be thin in low stress areas (as

FIGURE 12-18. Extending the preparation for access and extending to sound enamel. A. Class I lesion seen as small pits on the occlusal surface. **B.** The same tooth after preparation showing the extension necessary to obtain access (convenience form) to remove decay, which spread out laterally beneath the dentinoenamel junction. This outline form is also necessary to end the preparation on sound enamel walls, which are supported by sound dentin (not softer caries).

when used as a sealant or preventive resin restorations) or as thick as amalgam in areas of high stress. Because the material mechanically bonds to the tooth structure, it can meet the prepared tooth surface at right angles, or be beveled.

c. Retention (Class I)

For amalgam, retention is provided in an occlusal preparation by a slight *convergence* of the buccal and lingual preparation walls towards the occlusal surface, which, due to the slope of the triangular ridges, is coincidentally accomplished by ending the buccal and lingual cavity walls at right angles to the unprepared triangular ridges (seen later in Fig. 12-21C).

For composite preparations, retention is provided by acid etching the enamel to produce *microscopic* irregularities (minute undercuts) on the surface. Then, flowable resin bonding agents can flow into the irregularities to form retentive resin tags that *mechanically* lock into the *microscopic* retentive features of the etched enamel (Fig 12-20). Layers of the stronger composite resin can subsequently be *chemically* bonded to the flowable resin layer.

For inlays or onlays (cast gold or porcelain), retention is provided by preparing the opposing *internal* walls of the preparation with a slight (5–7°) *divergence* toward the occlusal surface (as seen within the Class II inlay preparation in Fig. 12-24), thus allowing the solid casting to be seated snugly within the tooth, somewhat like a glass stopper fitting into the opening of a decanter. The dental cement used between the inlay and tooth provides retention by sealing the margins and by setting to hardness at the interface between the slight irregularities of the enamel walls of the preparation and those of the inlay/onlay. Some dental cements chemically bond to the

FIGURE 12-19. Class I amalgam preparations showing various degrees of extension for prevention. **Left:** Tooth number 3 with an occlusal and an occlusal-lingual preparation. The preparations are separate since in this case, there was no need to cross the oblique ridge. **Center:** An occlusal amalgam preparation of tooth number 31. **Right:** An occlusobuccal amalgam preparation on tooth number 30.

FIGURE 12-20. **The effect of etching enamel. A.** Magnified view of a non-etched enamel surface (x3260). **B.** Magnified view of etched enamel surface (x3600) after application of 50% phosphoric acid. This etched surface allows the resin bonding agent of the composite systems to flow into the irregular microscopic undercuts, thus affording mechanical retention for the material. (Courtesy of Dr. Ruth Paulson, Ohio State University.)

calcium of the tooth, and can be mechanically attached to the etched surface of metal castings (glass ionomer and polycarboxylate cements).

d. Cavity Nomenclature (Class I)

The occlusal preparation can be compared to a room (with no ceiling) that has four vertical walls and a horizontal floor or wall. The four vertical walls are named after the most closely related tooth surfaces, namely, buccal, mesial, lingual, and distal; the horizontal floor is called the **pulpal floor (or wall)** because it is over the pulp (abbreviated as B, M, L, D, and P in Fig. 12-21). A **line angle** in the preparation is the line formed when two walls join. There are eight internal line angles in a conservative Class I preparation (if it is confined to the occlusal surface and is not extended into a buccal or lingual groove). These are named by combining the terms for the two walls that join to make up each line angle, changing the suffix of the first word from "al" to "o." It makes no difference which wall is named first. For example, the junction of the pulpal floor and distal wall is the distopulpal *or* pulpodistal line angle. All possible line angles in a Class I occlusal preparation include four horizontal ones—distopulpal, mesiopulpal, buccopulpal, and linguopulpal—and four vertical ones—mesiobuccal, distobuccal, mesiolingual, and distolingual.

The term that describes the junction of any wall of the preparation with the unprepared tooth structure is called the **cavosurface**. The cavosurface, therefore, is the *outline* that encircles the preparation and restoration. An occlusal restoration where the buccal wall of a preparation meets the uncut surface is the buccal cavosurface; where the lingual wall ends is known as the lingual cavosurface, and so on (Fig. 12-21B).

Finally, there are four **point angles** in a Class I preparation, each formed by the junction of three walls (as in the corner of a room where two walls meet the floor). Point angles are named after the three walls that form them: mesiobuccopulpal (abbreviated MBP in Fig. 12-21), mesiolinguopulpal, distolinguopulpal, and distobuccopulpal. Since the junction of walls in a preparation is often rounded, line angles and point angles may be small, general areas rather than distinct sharp angles or points.

A Class I *restoration* is properly described and identified by naming the surfaces involved and material used. For example, an amalgam on tooth #14 involving the occlusal surface with a lingual extension would be abbreviated OL-A, #14. The letter O represents the occlusal portion of the preparation, the L represents the lingual extension, and the letter A represents the restorative material, amalgam. (Refer to Figs. 12-12 and 12-13) If composite had been used, the representation would have been OL-C #14. A lower right third molar with an occlusal amalgam and buc-

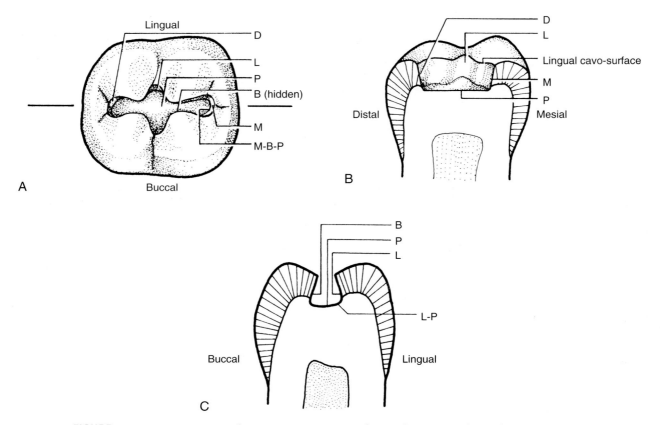

FIGURE 12-21. **A conservative Class I cavity preparation for amalgam** on tooth number 31. **A.** Occlusal surface showing extension for prevention into the major grooves. **B.** Mesiodistal cross-section of the same tooth showing the ideal depth of the pulpal floor, just into dentin (about 0.5 mm). The lingual cavosurface is also identified where the lingual wall of the preparation joins the unprepared surface of the tooth. **C.** Buccolingual cross-section of the same tooth showing the convergence of the vertical buccal and lingual walls toward the occlusal for retention and resistance form. **Key for nomenclature:** **B** = Buccal wall; **L** = Lingual wall; **M** = Mesial wall; **D** = Distal wall; **P** = Pulpal wall or floor. Example of a line angle: **L-P** is the linguopulpal line angle. Example of a point angle: **M-B-P** is the mesiobuccopulpal point angle in A.

cal extension would be an OB-A, **#**32. A buccal or lingual pit restored with composite would be a B-C or L-C, followed or preceded by the tooth number.

2. CLASS II CARIES: PRINCIPLES OF CAVITY PREPARATION AND TERMINOLOGY

The preparation for a Class II carious lesion can be restored with amalgam, direct composite, inlays, or onlays (cast metal or tooth-colored). The larger the preparation (and, therefore, the thinner the remaining tooth structure), the more appropriate a cast metal onlay might be to protect the remaining thin tooth and provide adequate resistance form (recall Fig. 12-16). Recent improvements in composite restorative materials and techniques have resulted in increased use of this tooth colored material for Class II restorations, especially when esthetics is an important factor.

a. Extension for Prevention (Class II)

To reach Class II lesions, the dentist must, in most cases, prepare a **proximal box** that extends apically through the marginal ridge in order to reach the decay which forms just cervical to the proximal contact. The Class II preparation often extends over some of the occlusal surface to include adjacent occlusal pits and fissures as in a Class I preparation, whereas the proximal box might be compared to a stair-step descending gingivally off of the occlusal portion (Fig. 12-22). The Class I portion follows the principles for restoring a Class I lesion already discussed, but the proximal extension (box) adds new features. For example, the buccal and lingual walls of the proximal box of Class II preparations are extended beyond the proximal contact areas just into the buccal and lingual embrasures. In this way, the margins of the restoration can be better evaluated by the dentist and kept clean by the patient.

b. Retention Form (Class II)

For Class II *amalgam* cavity preparations, the buccal and lingual walls of the occlusal portion and the proximal boxes are prepared so that they *converge slightly towards the occlusal* to prevent the restoration from dislodging occlusally as in the Class I preparation. Retentive grooves may be prepared buccally and lingually in a proximal box as extensions of the internal vertical wall of the box that is aligned along the long axis of the tooth, and is therefore called the axial wall. These retentive grooves are designed to prevent the amalgam restoration from dislodging in a proximal direction. They are located at the axiobuccal (A-B), and axiolingual (A-L) line angles seen later in Figure 12-25.

For *cast metal* inlays, opposing buccal and lingual walls must *diverge slightly toward the occlusal*. The two axial walls in a mesio-occlusodistal inlay preparation must *converge slightly towards the occlusal* so that an accurate wax model (pattern) and subsequent casting can be seated within the preparation and then removed while constructing and refining the casting prior to cementation (Figs. 12-23 and 12-24). **Bevels** are angular enamel reductions placed at the cavosurface in order for the margins (or outer edges) of the casting to be thin enough so the dentist can perfect the adaptation and minimize the cavosurface gap between tooth and metal. The goal is to minimize the gap between the casting and tooth since this gap is to be filled with a dental cement, which is not as strong nor as durable as the metal.

c. Cavity Nomenclature (Class II)

Class II lesions can involve just one or both proximal surfaces of a posterior tooth, but since obtaining access into the proximal lesion normally requires breaking through the occlusal marginal ridge, these restorations involve a minimum of two (occlusal and mesial *or* occlusal and distal) or three (mesial, occlusal and distal) surfaces. A proximal box has vertical buccal, lingual, and ax-

FIGURE 12-22. **Models of conservative Class II amalgam preparations. A. Occlusal views: Left:** MO-A (mesio-occlusal amalgam) preparation on tooth number 30. **Left-center**: MO-A, DO-A (mesio-occlusal and disto-occlusal amalgam) preparation on tooth number 3 with the oblique ridge intact. **Right-center**: MOD-A (mesio-occlusodistal amalgam) preparation on tooth number 5. **Right**: DO-A (disto-occlusal amalgam) preparation on tooth number 28. **B. Proximal views** of Class II amalgam preparations. **Left**: MOD-A preparation on tooth number 4. **Right**: MO-A preparation on tooth number 30. Note the convergence of the buccal and lingual walls toward the occlusal for retention and resistance form. When the decay process has progressed deeper and wider, the prepared walls by necessity will be farther apart than these.

FIGURE 12-23. Models of **Class II inlay and onlay preparations. A.** Three inlay preparations. **Left:** An MO-I (mesio-occlusal **inlay**) preparation on tooth number 21. **Center and Right:** MOD-I (mesio-occlusodistal inlay) preparations on tooth numbers 20 and 13 respectively. **B.** Three **onlay** preparations. **Left:** A conventional MOD-O (mesio-occlusodistal onlay) preparation on tooth number 18. **Center:** An MOD-O preparation (for ledge type onlays) on tooth number 19. **Right:** An MODL-O (mesio-occlusodistolingual onlay) with conventional onlayed buccal cusps on tooth number 14. **C.** Proximal views of an onlay preparation (left) and of an inlay preparation (right) showing the continuous **bevel** surrounding the preparation and the divergence of the buccal and lingual walls towards the occlusal. The cavosurface, or outline of the preparation (marked with arrows), is at the outer end of the prepared bevels.

ial walls (the **axial** wall is along the long axis of the tooth), and a horizontal **gingival wall** (or floor) (all labeled with abbreviations in Fig. 12-25).

The line angles that are present in a mesial or distal proximal box are axiopulpal, axiogingival, buccogingival, linguogingival, axiobuccal, and axiolingual. The axiobuccal and axiolingual line angles (labeled A-B and A-L in Fig. 12-25) are where the retentive grooves for an amalgam preparation are placed. In a mesio-occlusodistal preparation, each line angle is differentiated by stating whether it is in the mesial or distal box. For example, there are two axiopulpal line angles in the mesio-occlusodistal amalgam preparation: one is the axiopulpal line angle of the mesial box and the other is the axiopulpal line angle of the distal box. The point angles in each box include axio-

Mesial View

FIGURE 12-24. Diagram of a **conservative Class II MOD inlay preparation** on a maxillary premolar. Note that the buccal and lingual walls of the preparation diverge toward the occlusal, allowing the casting to be seated. Notice also that the preparation ends with a continuous **bevel** that allows a thin overlap of the metal, which can be burnished or adapted more closely to the enamel with a blunt instrument.

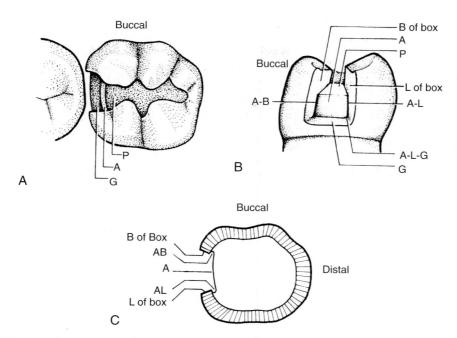

FIGURE 12-25. Conservative Class II preparation for amalgam on tooth number 30. **A.** Occlusal view showing the proximal box extending just through the proximal contact buccally and lingually. **B.** The mesial view showing the slight convergence towards the occlusal of the buccal and lingual walls of the box and axiobuccal (A-B) and axiolingual (A-L) line angles where retentive grooves are placed. An example of a point angle: A-L-G for axiolinguogingival is seen. **C.** A cross-section of this prepared tooth in the middle third of the crown showing the placement of the retentive grooves entirely within dentin at the axiobuccal and axiolingual line angles. Key for nomenclature: Walls, **B** = Buccal; **P** = Pulpal; **L** = Lingual; **A** = Axial; **G** = Gingival. Example of line angles: **A-B** = Axiobuccal; **A-L** = Axiolingual (location of retentive grooves).

linguogingival (A-L-G in Fig. 12-25), axiobuccogingival, axiobuccopulpal, and axiolinguopulpal.

The Class II preparation for amalgam involving only two surfaces, such as mesio-occlusal or disto-occlusal, are traditionally abbreviated MO-A or DO-A (not OM-A or OD-A). A mesio-occlusodistal amalgam preparation is abbreviated MOD-A (not DOM-A). A Class II preparation for composite material involving only two surfaces would be abbreviated similarly, with a suffix of "C" such as MO-C or DO-C. For inlays (I), or onlays (O), the abbreviation would be MO-I, DO-I, MOD-I and MO-O, DO-O and MOD-O, respectively.

3. CLASS III CARIES: PRINCIPLES OF CAVITY PREPARATION AND TERMINOLOGY

Since the Class III lesion occurs in a non-stress bearing area that is often of esthetic concern to the patient, a tooth colored composite resin is usually the restoration of choice. The distal proximal surface of the canine is less visible so it could be restored with a conservative Class III amalgam (Fig. 12-13). However, composite materials are being increasingly used in this Class III area.

a. Extension for Prevention: Class III

Extension for prevention is minimal in the Class III preparation since the dentist wants to preserve as much enamel as possible for esthetic reasons, and because the anterior teeth may be easier to keep clean. For all Class III lesions, the approach to the decay, whenever possible, is from the lingual of the tooth so the facial enamel is preserved for maximum esthetic effect (Fig. 12-26A and C), but when the decay has already destroyed the facial plate of enamel, a facial approach can be used (Fig. 12-26B).

FIGURE 12-26. Class III cavity preparations. A. Model of a DL-A: distal amalgam preparation with lingual approach on tooth number 6. Note the box-like shape and axioincisal retentive groove in the shadow (the axiogingival retentive groove is hidden). **B.** Model of the DF-C: distal composite preparation with facial approach on tooth number 10. Note the generally triangular form. **C.** DL-C: distal composite preparation with lingual approach on tooth number 8. Note the axioincisal retentive feature. (The axiogingival retentive feature is less visible here.)

b. **Retention: Class III**

Retention form may be obtained by simply removing the decay that has spread out at the dentinoenamel junction, resulting in a preparation that is wider internally than externally. Historically, retentive pits or grooves have been used as extensions of the axial wall in order to improve retention for either a composite or amalgam Class III preparation. However, the more conservative method of affording retention and reducing leakage at the cavosurface margin of a composite restoration is by bonding the composite resin to an acid etched enamel surface (recall Fig. 12-20B). The first layer of flowable resin can form resin tags that fill the microscopic etched irregularities and harden, thus locking the restoration in place.

c. **Cavity Nomenclature: Class III**

The preparation for the *lingual approach* for a Class III composite has the same terminology as the lingual approach for a Class III amalgam, and is represented in Figure 12-27 A and B. This lingual approach preparation can be compared to the four-walled proximal box portion of a Class II preparation, which is also cut through the marginal ridge. However, due to the more horizontal alignment of the box of a Class III preparation, the names assigned to the walls differ. Here, the four walls are called gingival, facial, incisal, and axial (as abbreviated in Fig. 12-27 A and B). There are only five internal line angles: gingivofacial, incisofacial, gingivoaxial, facioaxial, and incisoaxial. There are only two internal point angles: gingivofacioaxial and incisofacioaxial.

The preparation for a composite with a *facial approach* may be more triangular in shape with three walls and a floor (Fig. 12-27C). The three walls are the facial, lingual, and gingival walls, and the fourth wall (or floor) is the axial. Subsequently, this preparation has six internal line angles: facioaxial, linguoaxial, gingivoaxial, faciolingual, linguogingival, and gingivofacial. There are only three internal point angles: faciolinguoaxial (abbreviated F-L-A in Fig. 12-27C), linguogingivoaxial, and faciogingivoaxial.

Class III amalgam or composite restorations may be abbreviated by identifying the proximal surface as well as the surface through which access was gained, and the material used. For example, a composite on the mesial surface of tooth #7 with access to the decay through the lingual enamel would be identified as M-C, #7, lingual approach, or more precisely, ML-C, #7. A distal composite restoration on tooth #24 approached from the facial would be identified as D-C #24, facial approach, or DF-C #24. Note that, instead of using "L" to denote the labial (or facial) surface, "F" is used to denote the facial surface in order to avoid confusion with "L" which is used to denote the lingual surface.

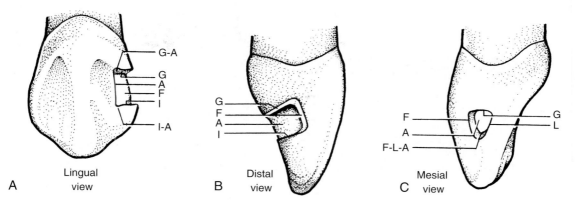

FIGURE 12-27. Class III preparations. A. The lingual view of the Class III amalgam preparation, lingual approach, on the distal of tooth number 6. Retentive grooves are evident at the cavosurface of the gingivoaxial and incisoaxial line angles. B. The distal view of a Class III composite preparation, lingual approach. Note the slight convergence of the incisal and lingual wall toward the lingual for retention. This preparation also has retentive grooves (or pits) at the incisoaxial and gingivoaxial line angles, but they do not extend to the cavosurface. The gingivoaxial groove is in the shadow between G and A. C. The mesial view of a Class III composite preparation, labial approach. Note the triangular shape. Retentive features are found internally at the axiogingival line angle and the faciolinguoaxial point angle. **Key for nomenclature: For lingual approach** (Diagrams A and B): **G** = Gingival; **A** = Axial; **F** = Facial; **I** = Incisal. Example of the angles are the retentive features **G-A** and **I-A** for the gingivoaxial and incisoaxial line angles. **Key for the facial approach** (Diagram C): **F** = Facial; **A** = Axial; **G** = Gingival; **L** = Lingual.

4. CLASS IV CARIES: PRINCIPLES OF CAVITY PREPARATION AND TERMINOLOGY

If a Class IV preparation is conservative, a composite, particularly one that utilizes an acid-etching technique, is the restoration of choice. An alternative treatment is a veneer of porcelain bonded to the facial surface of the tooth, replacing the fractured incisal area (Fig. 12-17). If the preparation is extensive, or if the whole incisal edge of the tooth and both proximal surfaces are involved, but there is sufficient remaining tooth structure, it may be better to recommend a full cast crown with facial porcelain, or a full porcelain crown for the best esthetics and longevity.

Caries removal and smoothing extremely rough or unsupported enamel may be all that is needed to prepare the tooth for a Class IV composite. The occlusion, as always, must be analyzed to be sure that there is room for the restoration when the patient chews and incises, especially in a protrusive direction. Retention is most commonly achieved by acid-etch techniques that permit resin tags to bond the composite to the tooth. A thin sleeve or skirt of excess composite material can cover beveled enamel that has been acid-etched to maximize retention (Fig. 12-28B) and to improve esthetics by blending the color differential between composite and enamel.

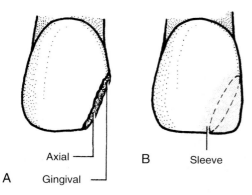

FIGURE 12-28. Class IV carious lesion or fracture on tooth number 8 and the resultant restoration. A. View of the lesion or fracture showing the gingival and axial portions of the defect. B. After smoothing the preparation and acid etching the enamel, the restored tooth with a sleeve or skirt (thin film of bonded resin that extends beyond the original cavosurface margin) of composite overlaps the etched enamel surface, thus establishing maximum retention and enhancing (blending) the color match.

FIGURE 12-29. Class V restorations. A. Two B-As (buccal amalgams) on teeth number 29 and 30. The extent of these amalgams is usually dictated by the extent of the caries. **B.** Class V B-C (buccal composite) on tooth number 27. If the shade of the material is good, these restorations are difficult to detect, and their surface grittiness felt by an explorer or scaler might be confused for incipient calculus formation. (Restorations by Gregory Blackstone, second-year dental student.)

Depending on the degree of involvement, this preparation may have only one flat wall (as in a fracture; similar to the shape seen in Fig. 12-28), or may be made up of two main surfaces: a gingival surface and a more axial surface. These two portions may join at an angle called the axiogingival line angle. There are no point angles.

A composite restoration that restores one incisal angle actually restores parts of four surfaces, so it may be abbreviated as either an MIFL-C or DIFL-C, to denote the involvement of all surfaces of either the mesioincisal or the distoincisal angle of the tooth. If both proximal surfaces are involved, the restoration would be designated as MIDFL-C.

5. CLASS V CARIES: PRINCIPLES OF CAVITY PREPARATION AND TERMINOLOGY

Since a Class V lesion occurs in non-stress bearing areas, when esthetics is a factor a composite may be used, even though it may be less resistant to abrasion than amalgam (Fig. 12-29). In gingival abrasion lesions, the dentist may use a glass ionomer because it bonds to dentin and contains fluoride. Amalgam may be used when the esthetics are *not* of prime concern. In rare cases, primarily at the patient's request, a cast metal inlay (or porcelain inlay) could be used to replace lost tooth contour.

The preparation for a Class V restoration is usually kept as conservative as possible, with little or no extension for prevention (Fig. 12-30). Prevention of future caries occurs through patient education in oral hygiene techniques and from periodic application of topical fluoride. The retention of amalgam restorations is obtained by preparing retentive grooves that are extensions of the axial wall in an occlusal and gingival direction (A-O and A-G in Fig. 12-31B). When using composite, similar retentive grooves could be used, but more often, retention is dependent on beveled enamel surfaces that have been acid etched (recall the discussion under Class III preparations). A glass ionomer restoration in an area of deep cervical abrasion (V-shaped or notched) may require no preparation,

FIGURE 12-30. Class V preparation. Class V labial composite preparation on tooth number 6. [A Class III D-C (distal composite) preparation with labial approach can also be seen in the facial embrasure on tooth number 7.] (Preparations by Gregory Blackstone, second-year dental student.)

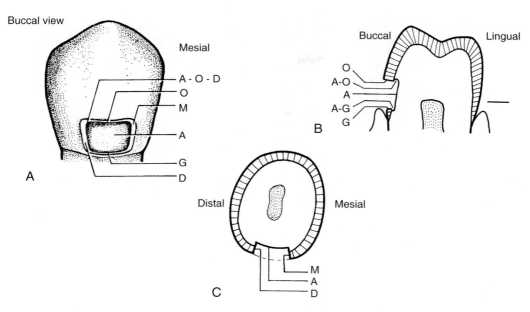

FIGURE 12-31. Conservative Class V preparation for amalgam on tooth number 29. **A.** Buccal view showing the trapezoidal outline form. Example of a point angle is the A-O-D or axio-occlusodistal point angle. **B.** Buccolingual cross-section of the same tooth revealing axio-occlusal (AO) and axiogingival (AG) line angles and retentive grooves. **C.** Cross-section of B showing the axial wall (A) just minimally into dentin (0.5 mm) forming a convex axial wall. **Key for nomenclature: O** = Occlusal; **M** = Mesial; **A** = Axial; **D** = Distal; **G** = Gingival.

only a treatment with a dentin conditioner or primer that aids in the chemical bond between dentin and a glass ionomer restoration. A Class V inlay must have walls *slightly divergent toward the crown surface* to allow the wax model (pattern) removal from the tooth model (die) and, as for all gold castings, there should be short bevels prepared at the cavosurface margins.

The Class V preparation is somewhat box shaped, and consists of five walls: distal, occlusal, mesial, gingival, and axial. There are eight line angles: axiomesial, axiogingival, axiodistal, axio-occlusal, mesiogingival, distogingival, mesio-occlusal, and disto-occlusal. The axio-occlusal and axiogingival line angles are prepared with retentive grooves labeled as A-O and A-G in Figure 12-31B. There are four point angles: axio-occlusodistal (A-O-D in Fig. 12-31A), axio-occlusomesial, axiodistogingival, and axiomesiogingival.

The restoration is identified by surface and material. For example, a buccal amalgam on tooth **#**19 is B-A, **#**19. A facial composite on tooth **#**7 is F-C **#**7, and a glass ionomer on the facial surface of tooth **#**11 would be F-GI **#**11. Typically, the term facial (F) is applied to anterior teeth, whereas buccal (B) is applied to posterior teeth.

6. CLASS VI: TYPE OF DENTAL CARIES OR RESTORATION

The resultant preparation for a Class VI lesion conservatively follows Black's principles of cavity preparation, and the restoration of choice depends on size and location of the lesion and the need for strength and esthetics.

SECTION VI. Restoring Large Tooth Defects and Tooth Replacement

When a tooth is too badly broken down to be restored with an intracoronal restoration because only a thin shell of enamel remains, it may be necessary to remove decay and replace some or all of the lost tooth structure with amalgam or composite to develop a "core" of tooth and filling around and over which an extracoronal crown can be constructed. The core restoration that replaces tooth structure prior to preparing a tooth for a crown may be called a restoration under crown (RUC) or amalgam under crown (AUC). When the remaining tooth

FIGURE 12-32. **A. Crown preparation** on tooth number 20 for a full cast-metal crown that will eventually support the framework of a removable partial denture with clasps. **B.** The resultant solid metal **cast metal crown** in place. The facial surface of a crown like this can be veneered with porcelain if visible when speaking or laughing.

crown is almost completely gone, a cast metal *core* (resembling a tooth prepared to receive a crown) must be designed with a metal *post* which fits snugly into one of the previously endodontically treated and prepared root canals. The post is necessary to provide retention. This restoration is called a cast **post and core**.

On posterior teeth, a crown will often be constructed entirely of cast metal, and can be called a complete crown or a **complete veneer crown** (CVC) (Fig. 12-32B). To prepare a tooth for a complete crown, the previously restored anatomic tooth crown (or prepared core) is externally reduced with diamond burs to make room for the required thickness of the metal cast crown. The preparation usually extends gingivally beyond the core filling material so that the crown margins end on sound tooth structure. Full metal crown preparations end at the gingival cavosurface with a rounded shape called a **chamfer** (Figs. 12-32A and 12-33A).

When esthetics are a factor, especially on anterior teeth and maxillary premolars, further reduction of tooth structure is necessary on the facial surface to not only make room for the thin cast metal, but also an additional thickness of tooth colored porcelain veneer over the metal. This restoration is called a **metal ceramic crown** (MCC) or **porcelain veneer crown** (PVC). The preparation for this type of crown ends at the gingival margins with a ledge that may have a bevel (Fig. 12-33B). Photographs of a crown with a porcelain facing used to improve the esthetics of a severely fractured tooth **#9** is shown in Figure 12-34B. Crowns gain retention from the encompassing shape, nearly parallel walls that slightly converge toward the occlusal, accurate fit, and the cement. Retention of large onlays and crowns may be enhanced through mechanical bonding by etching the tooth or crown, and chemical bonding utilizing a glass ionomer, polycarboxylate, or resin cement.

Even when little or no caries or breakdown are evident, a crown may be recommended if the tooth is cracked, or when needed to support an adjacent false tooth (pontic) which replaces a missing tooth. The crowned teeth and the replaced tooth or teeth together are called a **fixed partial denture** (FPD) (commonly called a fixed bridge) (Fig. 12-35). The false tooth is called a **pontic**, and the teeth that are crowned on either side that are attached to and support the pontic are called the **abutment teeth** which are covered by their crowns called **retainers**. An FPD replacing tooth **#4**, with an abutment metal ceramic crown on tooth **#5** and a complete veneer crown (CVC) on tooth **#3** is shown in Figure 12-35. The metal pontic replacing **#4** is veneered with porcelain.

In the 1980's and 90's, techniques for replacing lost teeth with **dental implants** (titanium alloy roots surgically embedded into the bone) were perfected and widely used (Fig. 12-36). A dental implant involves embedding an artificial root (titanium alloy) into the bone. Three to six months after surgical placement, the em-

FIGURE 12-33. Proximal views: **Crown preparations** with their facial surface toward the right. **A. Full metal crown** (no veneer) preparation on a mandibular premolar with chamfer finish lines. **B.** Preparation on a maxillary canine that will have baked-on **porcelain veneer** covering the facial surface for esthetics. The finish line on the lingual is a **chamfer**, but on the facial, to make room for porcelain, a **ledge with bevel** (arrow) is necessary.

FIGURE 12-34. A. Tooth 9 with a fracture that includes the entire incisal edge. A large Class IV composite could be used to restore this defect but would be more susceptible to fracture and discoloration than a crown with a porcelain facing. **B.** The same patient with an **esthetic cast metal crown and porcelain facing** on tooth 9. (Photographs courtesy of Dr. Steven Rosenstiel, Chair of Restorative Dentistry, Prosthodontics and Endodontics, The Ohio State University.)

bedded implant can be used to provide retention for a crown, or provide support for a removable partial denture. Ten-year success rates of 91% for dental implants in the mandible have been reported.[29]

Groups of lost teeth can also be replaced with multiple implants, fixed partial dentures, or a **removable partial dentures** (RPD). When all teeth have been lost, **complete dentures** (CD, also known as false teeth) can be constructed.

FIGURE 12-35. Fixed Partial Denture or Bridge. A. Buccal view of full-crown preparation on tooth 3 (on left) and a crown-veneer preparation on tooth 5 for the attachment of a bridge to replace tooth 4. **B.** The completed three-tooth fixed partial denture (bridge) for replacing tooth 4. The premolar **retainer** (abutment tooth crown) and **pontic** (replacement tooth) in the photograph are porcelain veneered to metal.

FIGURE 12-36. An Implant. Tooth 29 has been extracted and replaced with a dental implant. It supports a crown veneered with porcelain. **A.** A radiograph of the implant with the screw-retained component and crown. **B.** The screw-retained component (crown support) attached to the implant and extending above the tissue prior to placement of the crown. **C.** The crown cemented on the screw-retained component of the implant. (Photographs courtesy of Ed McGlumphy, D.D.S., M.S., Associate Professor, Ohio State University, College of Dentistry.)

LEARNING EXERCISE

Without looking at the key to each photograph of restorations in this chapter, identify the material used, the surfaces involved, and the abbreviation that could be used to denote the restoration. Do the same with extracted teeth that have existing restorations. Looking in your mouth using a mirror or in a friend's mouth, identify the classification of the existing restorations (according to Dr. G.V. Black). Note that some restorations are extended over more of the tooth than others. Could this be because the dentist extended the preparations or was it due to the spread of caries? Do you suspect any areas of decay? (If so, check with a dentist.)

Answer each of the following test items by selecting the correct answer, or answers, for each item.

1. What is the class of decay found in the buccal pit of tooth #19?
   a. Class I
   b. Class II
   c. Class III
   d. Class IV
   e. Class V

2. Which material is more likely to be used for a conservative class III restoration (mesial and facial surfaces) on tooth #8?
   a. amalgam
   b. cast gold crown
   c. composite resin
   d. cast porcelain inlay
   e. cast gold onlay

3. Caries in the cingulum area of tooth #7 is an example of which class of caries?
   a. Class I
   b. Class II
   c. Class III
   d. Class IV
   e. Class V

4. Throughout the end of the twentieth century, has dental caries occurrence in children increased, decreased, or stayed about the same?
   a. increased
   b. decreased
   c. stayed about the same

5. Which class(es) of caries occur(s) only in posterior teeth but not on anterior teeth?
   a. Class I
   b. Class II
   c. Class III
   d. Class IV
   e. Class V

6. Which class(es) of caries occur(s) *only* in anterior teeth, but not on posterior teeth?
   a. Class I
   b. Class II
   c. Class III
   d. Class IV
   e. Class V

7. A point angle is the junction of how many cavity preparation walls?
   a. one
   b. two
   c. three
   d. four
   e. five

LEARNING QUESTIONS, cont.

8. Which of the following are point angles in a conservative Class I preparation (if it has *not* extended onto the buccal or lingual surfaces to include buccal or lingual grooves)?
   a. gingivobuccoaxial
   b. occlusobuccoaxial
   c. mesiobuccopulpal
   d. distolinguopulpal
   e. buccolinguopulpal

9. Which of the following are line angles within a DO-A preparation?
   a. axiobuccal
   b. axiopulpal
   c. distopulpal
   d. distoaxial
   e. mesiopulpal

ANSWERS: 1–a; 2–c; 3–a; 4–b; 5–b; 6–c, d; 7–c; 8–c; 9–a, b, e.

REFERENCES

1. DiOrio LP. Clinical preventive dentistry. East Norwalk, CT: Appleton-Century-Crofts, 1983.
2. Newbrun E. Problems in caries diagnosis. Int Dent J 1993;43:133–42.
3. Powell LV. Caries risk assessment: relevance to the practitioner. JADA 1998;129:349-353.
4. National Caries Program. The prevalence of caries in U.S. children, 1979–80. NIH Publication No. 82–2245, December 1981.
5. Brown JL, Wall TP, Lazar V. Trends in total caries experience: permanent and primary teeth. JADA 2000;131:223-31.
6. American Dietetic Association: Position of the American Dietetic Association: oral health and nutrition. Available at: www.eatright.org/aoral.html.
7. Hicks MJ, Flaitz CM. Epidemiology of dental caries in the pediatric and adolescent population: a review of past and current trends. J Clin Pediatr Dent 1993;18:43–9.
8. Heinrich R, Heinrich J, Kunzel W. Prevalence of root caries in women. Z Stomatol 1989;86:241–7.
9. Sturdevant, CM. The art and science of operative dentistry, third edition. St. Louis: C.V. Mosby, 1995.
10. Baum L, Phillips RW, Lund MR. Textbook of Operative Dentistry. Philadelphia: Saunders, 1995.
11. Black GV. A work on operative dentistry. Vol. 1. Chicago: Medico-Dental Publishing Company, 1908;203-34.
12. Hannigan, A, et al. Caries susceptibility classification of tooth surfaces by survival time. Caries Research 2000;34:103-8.
13. Radike AW. Criteria for diagnosis of dental caries. In: Proceedings of the Conference on the Clinical Testing of Cariostatic Agents. Chicago; ADA, 1972.
14. Clinical Research Associates Newsletter 1995;19(10):4.
15. Leinfelder KF. Posterior composite resins. JADA 1988;11(Special Issue):21E-26E.
16. Roulet JF. The problems associated with substituting composite resins for amalgam: a status report on posterior composites. J Dent 1988;16:101–13.
17. Ishikawa A. 10-year clinical evaluation of a posterior composite resin [Abstract 2178]. J Dent Res 1996;75:290.
18. Leinfelder KF. Posterior composite resins: the materials and their clinical performance. JADA 1995;126(May): 663–76.
19. Kugel G, Ferrari M. The science of bonding: from first to sixth generation. JADA 2000;131:20S-25S.
20. Shaw K. Root caries in the older patient. Dent. Clin. North Am. 1997;41,4:763-93.
21. Nathanson D, Riis D. Advances and current research on ceramic restorative materials. Curr Opin Cosmetic Dent 1993; 34–40.
22. Leinfelder KF. Porcelain esthetics for the 21st century. JADA 2000;131:47S-51S.
23. Leinfelder KF. Advances in biorestorable materials. JADA 2000;131:35-41.

24. Simonsen RJ. The clinical effectiveness of a colored sealant at 36 months. J Dent Res 1980;59:406.

25. Simonson RJ. Preventive resin restorations: three-year results. JADA 1980;100:535.

26. Craig RG, O'Brien WJ, Powers JM. Dental materials properties and manipulation, Third Edition. St. Louis: C.V. Mosby; 1983;33-44.

27. Harris NO, Cristen G. Primary preventive dentistry. Reston, VA: Reston Publishing, 1982.

28. Guirguis R, Lee J, Conry J. Microleakage evaluation of restorations prepared with air abrasion. Pediatric Dent 1999; 21,6:311-15.

29. Rosenstiel S, Land M, Fujimoto J. Contemporary fixed prosthodontics, Third Edition. St. Louis: Mosby, Inc., 2001.

Guidelines for Drawing, Sketching, and Carving Teeth

I. Drawing Teeth
   A. Materials needed
   B. How to accurately reproduce a tooth outline
   C. Example: accurately reproduce the shape of a mandibular canine (copying an actual tooth or tooth model)
II. Sketch teeth recognizably from memory
III. Carving teeth
   A. Materials needed
   B. How to carve a tooth
   C. Example: how to carve a maxillary central incisor
   D. Notes

OBJECTIVES

This chapter was designed to prepare the learner to perform the following:
- Carefully draw a tooth to reproduce its contours precisely from various views.
- From memory, sketch (quickly) teeth from various views so the sketch is recognizable as that tooth view.
- Reproduce the contours of a tooth in wax.

SECTION I. Drawing Teeth

A. MATERIALS NEEDED

- Graph paper ruled 8 squares to the inch
- Drawing pencil, 3H or 4H, sharpened to a fine point
- Eraser
- Ruler with millimeter scale
- Boley gauge
- Teeth or tooth model
- Chart with dimensions of tooth to be drawn (such as Table 3-2)

B. HOW TO ACCURATELY REPRODUCE A TOOTH OUTLINE

To accurately reproduce the outline of any object, you must not only look at the object; you must also see or visualize it. Rarely is there a person, however lacking in artistic skill, who cannot make a reasonably good drawing of a human tooth. Those who are not skilled in accurate drawing (extensive art training does not necessarily result in accuracy of outline) may find a solution in using graph paper ruled 8 squares to the inch. The tooth specimen is measured in millimeters with a Boley gauge, and the measurements are transferred to the graph paper, allowing 1 square to equal 1 mm. Drawings may be made to scale of each type of tooth: maxillary and mandibular incisors, canines, premolars, and molars. All drawings should depict maxillary teeth with crowns down and mandibular teeth with crowns up, the same orientation they have in the mouth.

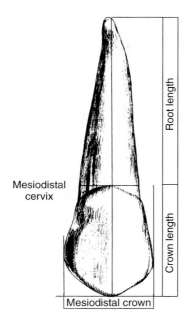

FIGURE 13-1. Facial side of a maxillary right canine tooth model showing how measurements of a tooth may be made to assist in drawing and carving.

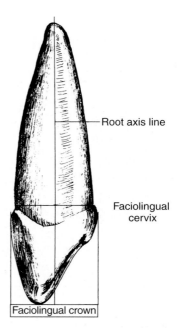

FIGURE 13-2. Mesial side of the maxillary canine depicted in Figure 13-1 showing how tooth measurements can be made and how the incisal portion is compared to the root axis line.

Using an undamaged extracted tooth or tooth model for a specimen, make the following six measurements with the Boley gauge (Figs. 13-1 and 13-2).

- Crown length
- Mesiodistal crown
- Faciolingual crown
- Root length
- Mesiodistal cervix
- Faciolingual cervix

Using a consistent method of measurement avoids confusion. On anterior teeth, measure the crown length on the facial side from the cervical line to the incisal edge. On premolars, measure the crown length on the facial side from the cervical line to the tip of the buccal cusp. On molars, which have more than one buccal cusp, crown length is always to the mesiobuccal cusp tip. Make the other cusps their proper length relative to the measured cusp, that is, either longer or shorter. With more than one root, the overall tooth length will be from the mesial or mesiobuccal root apex to the mesiobuccal cusp (refer to Table 3-2).

Plan how you want to place your drawings on the graph paper. One convenient arrangement is facial aspect, upper left corner; lingual aspect, upper right; mesial aspect, lower left; distal aspect, lower right; and incisal aspect, center (Figs. 13-3 and 13-4). These views will be centered nicely if you allow a four-square border on all sides as shown in the same illustrations.

C. EXAMPLE: ACCURATELY REPRODUCE THE SHAPE OF A MANDIBULAR CANINE (COPYING AN ACTUAL TOOTH OR TOOTH MODEL)

1. FACIAL VIEWS

Use the measurements you have made of the tooth specimen you intend to draw. In the upper left corner of the page, count down from the upper four-square border the number of squares and fraction thereof equal to the crown length in millimeters and draw a horizontal line. From this line, count down the number of squares equal to the root length in millimeters and draw a second horizontal line. From the inside of the left four square border, count to the right the number of squares equal to the mesiodistal crown measurement and draw a vertical line. You will draw the facial aspect of the tooth inside the

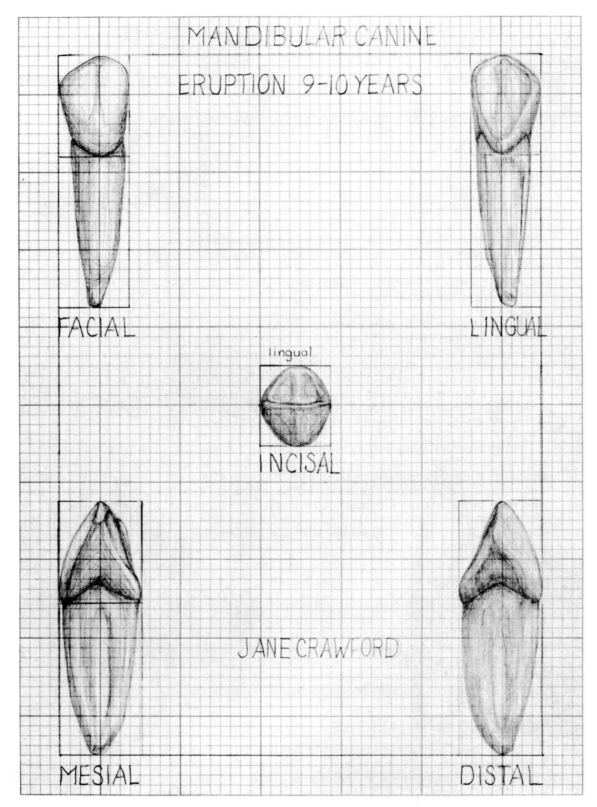

FIGURE 13-3. A precise drawing on graph paper of a model of a mandibular right canine by a first-year hygiene student.

FIGURE 13-4. Professional drawing (by medical artist) of a model of a maxillary canine based on dimensions given in Table 3-2.

box. Make your lines *very light at first*, so that corrections can be made easily. Remember to begin from the four-square margin (top and side) as seen in Figure 13-3.

Before you start to draw, make a light mark at the locations of the mesial and distal contact areas of the crown. (A pencil or straight-edge held against the side of the tooth parallel to the root axis line will help you determine where to put the small marks.) Also, mark the location of the apex of the root. Estimate the location mesiodistally of the cervix of the tooth. When you fit the crown into the box, if you remember to keep the root vertical, the axis will not always be an equal distance from the mesial and distal sides because the crowns of some teeth are tilted distally. Mark off the mesiodistal cervical measurement very lightly.

Now draw in the curvature of the crown at the contact areas (you marked the location), and draw in a portion of the cervical line and the incisal cusp ridges. Draw the root apex and the cervical part of the root. Correct any errors in location or shape, and then connect the lines you have drawn. You have a drawing of a tooth. You may be pleasantly surprised how natural and morphologically correct this first sketch appears. Many professional artists are unable to depict natural teeth accurately because they are unfamiliar with tooth morphology, and they do not have the proportions that were dictated by your measurements.

2. LINGUAL VIEWS

In the upper right corner of the page (Fig. 13-3) use the same set of measurements to make the box in which to draw the lingual aspect of the tooth. Remember that almost all teeth taper toward the narrower lingual surface, but the overall outline from the lingual is the same width as from the facial view. The cingulum is narrower than the cervical portion on the labial sketch, and it should be drawn centered or a little toward the distal.

3. MESIAL AND DISTAL VIEWS

Draw these two boxes in the lower left and right corner of the page (Fig. 13-3) using the same root and crown lengths. However, use the faciolingual crown measurement instead of the mesiodistal measurement. Before you start to draw the tooth, lightly mark the locations of the incisal edge, the labial crest of curvature (that is, where the curve or greatest convexity of the labial surface will touch the line of the box), and the crest of curvature on the cingulum (Fig. 13-2) and the root tip. Mark the faciolingual width of the cervix. Then draw the tooth. Remember to leave the four-square border at each side and below these views.

4. INCISAL VIEW

Near the center of the page draw a box with the distance between the upper and lower horizontal lines the exact number of squares for the faciolingual measurement of the crown in millimeters. The distance between right and left vertical lines of this box should equal the number of the squares of the mesiodistal crown measurement in millimeters. Hold the tooth facial side down and in such a position that you are looking exactly in line with the root axis line. Be sure that the tooth is not tilted up or down. On the sides of the box, mark the places where you are going to put the mesioincisal and distoincisal angles. The incisal edge of the tooth will normally have a slight lingual twist of the distoincisal corner (not evident in Fig. 13-3), and will lie either in the center of the box faciolingually or slightly lingual to the center (in the same position it is shown on your drawings of the mesial and distal aspects). The cingulum is normally centered on, or slightly distal to, the root axis line.

Do you find any straight lines (ruler-straight, that is) on any tooth other than those lines that have been produced by attrition? This would be most unusual.

Using the same approach you will be able to draw other types of teeth. Labeling the grooves, the fossae, and the ridges on the occlusal surfaces of the posterior teeth will help to fix the morphology in your mind.

SECTION II. Sketch Teeth Recognizably from Memory

The extremely precise and accurate drawings described in Section I of this chapter have the value of developing skills to accurately visualize and reproduce the subtle outlines and exact grooves of a specific tooth from various views. However, this time-consuming method of copying teeth may have limited value in helping the student to quickly *sketch* a tooth from memory for a specified view as might be expected during a conversation with an instructor or a patient. Therefore, the authors are adding another set of guidelines to this edition that have been useful at the Ohio State University for dental and dental hygiene students when learning how to *quickly* sketch a specific tooth and view from memory.

In order to sketch a recognizable tooth from memory, the drawer must have knowledge of the following characteristics related to the tooth being drawn: (A) approximate crown to root ratio, (B) approximate crown proportions (width compared to length), (C) location of the crown heights of contour (crests of curvature), (D) crown shape (taper, incisal edge shape or number and size of cusps, and CEJ shape), and, when drawing the entire tooth, (E) root shape (taper and number of roots). If one considers each of these tooth characteristics in the appropriate order, sketching a tooth becomes a relatively easy task, and is an excellent exercise to apply all of the knowledge of dental morphology that has been presented throughout this text.

As an example, consider a sketch of the facial view of *a right maxillary central incisor from the facial view.* Follow along with Figure 13-5 as you read about each step.

Step A: Consider the **root-to-crown ratio**. It is not expected that a student will remember the exact ratio of this tooth (1.16 to 1), but rather the student should recall that all roots are normally longer than the crown. On maxillary central incisors, the root is only *slightly* longer than the crown. Based on this fact, three parallel horizontal lines can be drawn to denote the distance of the *crown length* from incisal edge to the cervical line *relative to* the *root length* (only slightly longer) from cervical line to root apex. Position the smaller *crown length* on top for the mandibular teeth, and on the bottom for maxillary teeth. For this maxillary central incisor, the crown length is on the bottom.

Step B: Consider the **proportions of the crown**, that is, the crown height (incisocervically) compared to its width (mesiodistally). Again, the student does not need to memorize that the average crown width for this tooth is 8.6 mm, and its average length is 11.2 mm, but you should recall that the maxillary central incisor crown is slightly longer than it is wide. Using this knowledge, two parallel *vertical* lines can be placed perpendicular to the horizontal lines to establish the proportion for the tooth crown. Extending these vertical lines along the entire tooth length results in the formation of two boxes: a *crown box* that will surround the crown, and a *root box* that will enclose the root. At this time, label the mesial (M) and distal (D) surfaces of the crown box that is dependent on whether you are viewing a right or left incisor. For this right incisor, the mesial surface is on the right side, and the distal is on the left side, as if you were facing the patient.

Step C: Consider the **heights of contour** (crests of curvature) on the mesial and distal surfaces. Since these two points are the widest parts of the tooth crown where the mesial and distal surfaces bulge out the most, they are therefore the points where the crown outline touches the *crown box* established in the previous step. When the teeth are in ideal alignment, they are the location of the proximal contacts. On all incisors, the proximal heights of contour occur in the incisal 1/3, and are located more incisally on the mesial surface than on the distal surface (EXCEPT on the symmetrical mandibular central incisor). With this knowledge, a dot can be placed on the mesial and distal crown box outline at the appropriate levels. It is not until this step is complete that you actually begin sketching the tooth crown shape (outline).

Step D: Begin sketching the **crown outline**. Use as many of the criteria presented in the Appendix as you can recall to make your sketch recognizable. For example, on a maxillary central incisor, we know that the ar-

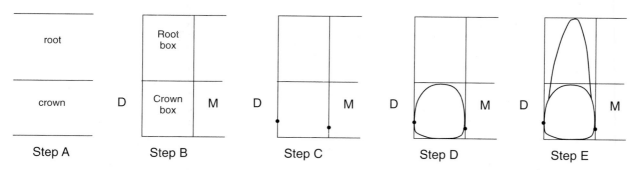

FIGURE 13-5. Five steps involved in sketching the facial view of a tooth (in this case, a right maxillary central incisor).

eas immediately surrounding all contact areas are convex; mesial and distal crown walls taper *slightly* toward the root; and the incisal edge is almost flat or slightly convex and is a little shorter toward the distal. We also know that the cervical line from the facial view is broad and curves toward the apex. Based on this knowledge, begin sketching the crown outline by placing subtle convexities that touch the crown box at the heights of contact points (dots). These convexities blend apically to become the mesial and distal walls, and these walls converge (just slightly) toward the cervical line. The proximal convexities also curve incisally to blend with the relatively straight incisal edge which touches the incisal line of the crown box in the mesial half, and tapers shorter (farther from the box outline) toward the distal. Finally, the cervical line appears as a continuation of the mesial and distal walls, and curves toward the apex, just touching the cervical line of the crown box. If a sketch of the crown is all that you required, you would be finished. If, however, you wish to add the root, proceed to the final step.

Step E: Sketch the **root**. We know that the apex of the root is near or just distal to the center of the tooth root axis (a vertical line in the center of the root). We also know that roots are broadest in the cervical third (but not very much narrower than the width of the crown), may be nearly parallel in the cervical third, and taper toward the rounded apex. Based on this knowledge, you can finish the sketch. Be aware that part of the root outline where it joins the crown is actually visible within the *crown box*, and the rounded apex just touches the apical line of the *root box*.

When sketching other teeth from the **facial views**, use steps A through C as described earlier for developing the "boxes" and crests of curvature, and refer to the Appendix pages for tooth traits when sketching the actual tooth outlines. With practice, teeth can be sketched without the boxes in less than a minute while still maintaining the approximate proportions and heights of contour. See the student sketch of a recognizable molar from the buccal view in Figure 13-6A.

The steps used to sketch the **lingual view** of all teeth are the same as for the facial view EXCEPT the *outline* is a mirror image of the facial view. Also, on this surface of anterior teeth, there is normally evidence of a narrower crown cingulum, marginal ridges, a lingual fossa, and a cervical line that often includes a partial view of

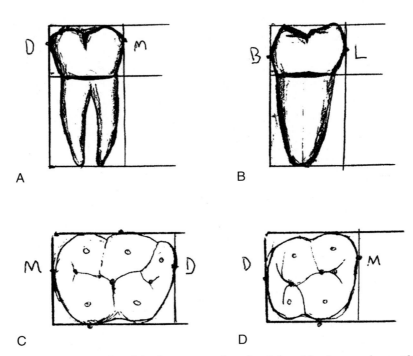

FIGURE 13-6. Four sketches of teeth by first quarter dental and dental hygiene students. Although not perfectly drawn, each sketch is recognizable as the tooth being drawn. **A.** Right mandibular second molar, facial (buccal) view. **B.** Right mandibular first molar, mesial view. **C.** A right mandibular first molar, occlusal view. **D.** A Right maxillary first molar, occlusal view. Sketches A and B would look nicer if the lines were not so wide and dark.

the proximal CEJ due to the taper of teeth toward the lingual. On maxillary molars, the lingual root is now in the foreground.

When sketching the **proximal view** of teeth, the first two steps are similar to steps A and B above except the crown outline box is developed for this view by using the faciolingual and mesiodistal *crown proportions*. The *facial crest of curvature* is similar for **all teeth**: in the cervical third. *Lingually*, the crest of curvature is in the cervical third on the cingulum for anterior teeth, but in the middle third for posterior teeth. Develop a *crown and root shape* according to guidelines in the Appendix. See the student sketch of a mandibular molar from the mesial view in Figure 13-6B.

Posterior teeth from the **occlusal view** are viewed looking directly down along the axis of the root. Crown to root ratios do not apply from this view. The crown outline box is developed for this view by using the mesiodistal and faciolingual *crown proportions*. On **mandibular premolars**, the crown proportions are slightly longer buccolingually than mesiodistally, but close to square. **Maxillary premolars** from the occlusal view are similar to mandibular premolars except crown proportions are less square, more rectangular: proportionally wider bucco-lingually than mesiodistally. **Mandibular molars** from the occlusal view are wider mesiodistally than buccolingually, whereas **maxillary molars** are slightly wider bucco-lingually than mesio-distally.

The *crests of curvatures* on molars and premolars on the mesial and distal surfaces are located in the center or slightly to the buccal of the bucco-lingual midline. The buccal and lingual crests of curvature for molars are located mesial to the middle, except on the buccal of the mandibular first molar where it is close to the middle. After the outline "box" is sketched and crests of curvature have been noted, sketch the crown outlines using descriptions from the Appendix pages. An additional challenge on these views involves reproducing the location of the *cusp tips, grooves, pits* (as must be accomplished by dental personnel every time a restoration is placed on an occlusal surface, finished and polished, or constructed or carved in wax in the laboratory).

Cusp tips can be identified by placing small dots or circles on the sketches at these locations. It may be helpful to remember these basic guidelines regarding *pits and grooves*. Most premolars have a mesial and distal pit connected by a groove running mesiodistally between buccal and lingual cusps. Molars (and three-cusped mandibular second premolars) have three pits (mesial, central and distal) that are also connected by a groove passing mesiodistally between buccal and lingual cusps. Molars also have one or two buccal grooves that separate the two or three buccal cusps, respectively. On mandibular molars, the lingual groove comes off near the central pit, but on maxillary molars, a lingual (distolingual) groove comes off of the distal pit and parallels the oblique ridge. Developmental or supplemental grooves may angle off from the mesial and distal pits of most posterior teeth, directed toward the "corners" of the tooth. See the student sketches of two recognizable molars in Figure 13-6C and D.

SECTION III. Carving Teeth

A. MATERIALS NEEDED

- Blocks of carving wax (34 x 17 x 17 mm for molars or 32 x 12 x 12 for other teeth)
- Boley gauge (Vernier caliper)
- Millimeter ruler
- Office knife and sharpening stone
- Roach carver, No. 7 wax spatula, and PKT-1 (for melting and adding wax)
- No. 3, No. 5-6, 6C, and PKT-4 carvers
- Sharpened 3H or 4H drawing pencil
- Large or small tooth model and its measurements

B. HOW TO CARVE A TOOTH

Carving a tooth helps you to see the tooth in three dimensions and also to develop considerable manual skill and dexterity. While eventually you may be able to carve a tooth from a block of wax without preliminary measurement, the beginner can only do well by approaching the carving systematically in the same way you approached the drawings: first, by outlining a box on the wax block; second, by sketching an outline of the tooth in the box; and third, by carving around the sketch or outline, one view or aspect at a time (sequence is shown in Fig. 13-8).

When approaching the task of carving a tooth, consider Michelangelo, who conceived of his task of producing a marble statue by "liberating the figure from the marble that imprisons it." And remember that he, too, sometimes made mistakes and had to discard a half-finished statue of St. Matthew, which appears to the casual observer to be all right from the front, but from the side, the leg, bent at the knee, is seen to be hopelessly out of position. The same can happen to your tooth carving. To minimize this, as you cut away wax, repeatedly examine your carving from all sides; turn it round and round and compare it with your specimen from each view. Where it is too bulbous, the fault is easily correctable by further reductions. Where too much wax has been removed, you have one of three choices: add molten wax to the deficient region, make the entire carving proportionally smaller, or start with a new block of wax.

C. EXAMPLE: HOW TO CARVE A MAXILLARY CENTRAL INCISOR

Refer to Figures 13-7 and 13-8 as you follow the following guidelines.

1. Use the measurements you used for drawing. (Again, use the measurement of the buccal cusp on premolars and of the mesiobuccal cusp and mesiobuccal or mesial root on molars.) This consistency of method prevents confusion. Allowance is made for the greater length of some lingual cusps, which are longer than the measured buccal cusp.
2. Shave the sides of the block flat, and make all angles right angles.
3. Measure 2 mm from one end of the block and draw a line at this level, encircling the block (on all four sides). (This end of the block will be the incisal or occlusal end of the tooth and the 2-mm allowance here is to provide for the extra length of the lingual cups on molars that are longer than the mesiobuccal cusp which established crown length. Although it is convenient to allow the 2 mm on all carvings, it is essential only for molars.)
4. From the 2-mm line, measure the crown length and draw a second line around the block at this level. This line is the location of the cervical line on the facial, mesial, distal, and lingual sides of the tooth (Fig. 13-8A).
5. From this cervical line, measure one-half of the length of the root and draw a third line around the block. (The end of the block beyond this line will be referred to now as the base.)
6. On the base of the block, carve, on appropriate sides, F (facial), L (lingual), M (mesial), and D (distal). Be sure to put M and D in the proper relation to F and L so that you will carve a right or a left tooth, whichever you intend.

FIGURE 13-7. Maxillary central incisor wax carvings by first year dental hygiene students as seen from the mesial (M), lingual (L), incisal (I), facial (F), and mesial-facial (M, F) aspects. The crown and half of the root were carved to specific dimensions that were proportional to the tooth model they viewed during the carving. These excellent carvings were each done in less than 3 hours as a required skill test.

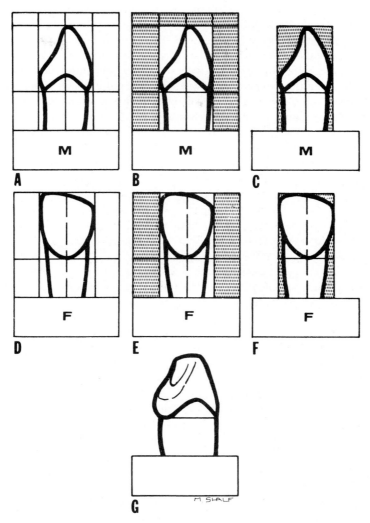

FIGURE 13-8. The sequential method described in this chapter for carving a tooth from a block of wax. The final product should look like those shown in Figure 13-7. The large letter M denotes the mesial aspect of the carving. Likewise, F indicates the facial side of the block.

7. Using a very sharp pencil, draw a shallow line lengthwise on the block in the center of the mesial surface. Do the same on the distal surface, and **be sure that these lines are exactly opposite.**

8. Add 0.5 mm to the faciolingual measurement of the crown. Divide this number by 2. Using this measurement, draw a line this distance on either side of the center line on the mesial and distal sides of the block (Fig. 13-8A). These two outer lines should be parallel to the center line and extend from the top of the block to the base. These two lines form a box whose dimension faciolingually is equal to the crown dimension plus 0.5 mm. The extra 0.5 mm is an allowance for safety in carving. Do not make trouble for yourself by allowing more than this extra 0.5 mm.

9. On the *mesial* side of the block marked M, draw, within the box, an outline of the mesial side of the tooth as you drew it on the graph paper. Be careful to place the incisal edge and the labial and lingual crests of curvature accurately. Your carving will probably be no better than this drawing.

10. Draw a similar outline on the *distal* side of the block. Be sure that on both sides, the drawings are oriented so the facial surface of the tooth is toward the side of the block you have marked F. (It is easy to make a

mistake here.) These drawings of the crown may appear slightly fat due to the extra 0.5 mm width allowance confining the crown size faciolingually.

11. Carve away the shaded portions of wax in Figure 13-8B from the facial, lingual, and incisal sides of the block so it is now shaped like Figure 13-8C. At this time, do not carve around the outline of the tooth, but rather carve into the straight vertical lines that form the box in which the tooth picture is drawn.

12. Check the distance between the two parallel carved surfaces carefully with your Boley gauge. Be sure they are perfectly flat and smooth. Be sure the thickness of the column of wax between these parallel surfaces exactly equals the given faciolingual crown dimension plus 0.5 mm.

13. Now carve away the shaded regions seen in Figure 13-8C around and down to the facial and lingual outlines of the tooth. Follow the drawing carefully, making the tooth shape the same all the way through the block. Keep the carving surface smooth; if it becomes chopped up, it will be impossible to smooth it without losing both the shape and the size of the carving.

14. With a sharp pencil, very lightly draw center lines on the curved facial and lingual sides of the carving as in Figure 13-8D. Be sure they are exactly opposite.

15. Add 0.5 mm to the mesiodistal crown measurement and draw two lines one-half this distance on either side of the center line. This makes a box on the curved surface as wide as the greatest mesiodistal crown measurement plus 0.5 mm (Fig. 13-8D).

16. Redraw a horizontal line the exact crown length distance from the incisal edge on the facial and lingual sides (since the original line was carved away). Then draw the facial outline of the crown and half of the root on the curved facial side of the block (Fig. 13-8D).

17. On the lingual surface of the block, draw an outline the same shape as the one on the facial surface except, of course, that it is a mirror image; the distal side of the tooth must be toward the same side of the block in each case. Check the crown length on the lingual surface too, so the crown won't be too long.

18. Carve away all the wax outside the drawing box, removing all the shaded portions as shown in Figure 13-8E. On some first molars their spreading roots may extend beyond the box lines, and these roots should be carved accordingly. Check your measurements again.

19. Shape the tooth by carefully carving the mesial and distal contours by removing the shaded portions of Figure 13-8F so that it resembles your tooth specimen outline from the facial and lingual sides.

20. Now it is time to round off the corners, narrow the lingual surface, shape the cingulum (it is distal to the center line, and the mesial marginal ridge is longer than the distal), and carve out the lingual fossa. Be sure to look at all aspects of the tooth as you are finishing the carving. Include, of course, the incisal (occlusal) aspect (Fig. 13-7). Four nice carvings of maxillary canines, made by dental hygiene students at Ohio State University, are shown in Figure 13-9. Five aspects of another very fine carving by a dental student are seen in Figure 13-10.

21. Carve your initials on the bottom of the base of the block. Be an honest critic of your work, constantly looking for regions where the carving could be improved.

You can work toward becoming proficient in drawing teeth by sketching in outlines (lightly at first) in the blank boxes which are proportionally the correct size for the view and tooth listed in Figures 13-11,

FIGURE 13-9. Maxillary canine wax carvings viewed from the distal (D), lingual (L), incisal (I), and facial (F) aspects. These were done by first-year dental hygiene students during a skill test (2 hours, 50 minutes time limit).

FIGURE 13-10. Maxillary right canine carving done by senior dental student Keith Schmidt. Observe the nearly perfect contours from all aspects and that the root is not becoming narrower as it joins the crown (a very common carving error in attempting to refine the cervical line).

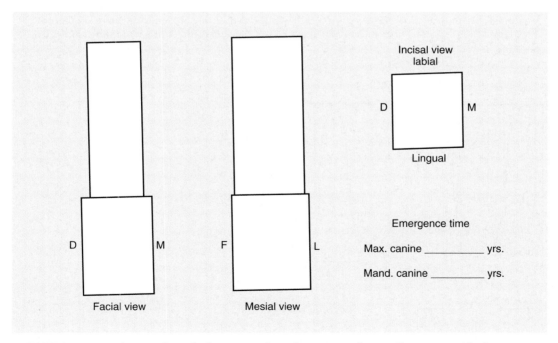

FIGURE 13-11. Outlines within which you may draw three views of a maxillary canine. The boxes are proportional to the natural teeth measured in Table 3-2. The widest portions of the crown (mesial and distal contacts) should touch the sides of the wider lower box. Only the widest part of the root should touch the sides of the narrower box above with the root apex touching the top of this box. On the incisal view, be sure to position the incisal ridge just labial to the faciolingual middle of this box. Drawing these three views will be helpful to you when you outline similar contours on a block of wax for carving a maxillary canine.

FIGURE 13-12. Outlined proportional boxes for drawing several views of the maxillary first and second premolars in their usual relationship to each other. Use the same guidelines given in the legend for Figure 13-11. A dental hygiene student's drawing of these two teeth within the outlined boxes is seen in Figure 13-13.

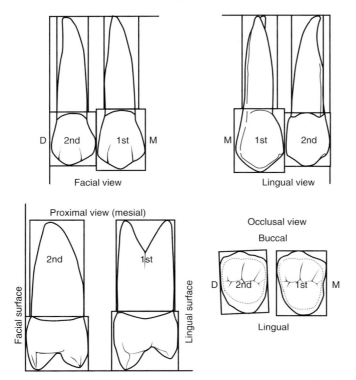

FIGURE 13-13. A dental hygiene student's drawings within the outlined boxes is an example for your own drawings in the blank boxes in Figure 13-12. Study these and perhaps you can make even better drawings. For example, in the lingual view, the maxillary first premolar's lingual cusp is too long. It is the correct length in the drawing of the mesial aspect.

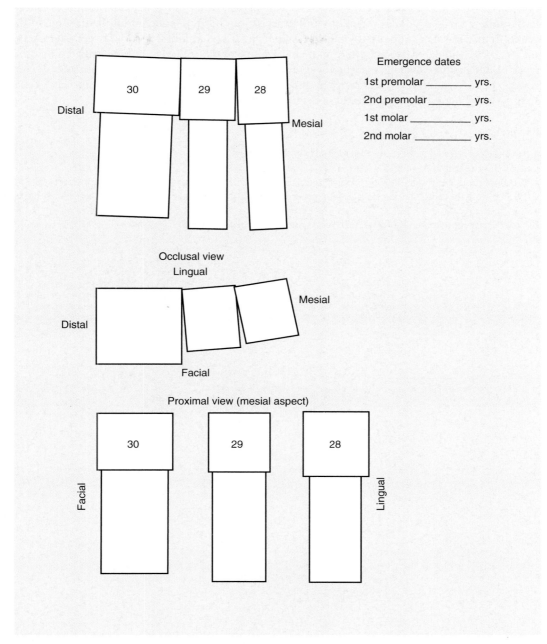

Emergence dates

1st premolar _____ yrs.

2nd premolar _____ yrs.

1st molar _____ yrs.

2nd molar _____ yrs.

FIGURE 13-14. Proportionally outlined boxes for drawing the lower right first and second premolars and first molar in their usual relationship to one another. Select three nice tooth specimens or tooth models and go to work.

13-12, and 13-14. You should have a tooth model or extracted tooth specimen to view as you make these sketches. One example of how to sketch teeth into the blank boxes of Figure 13-12 is shown in Figure 13-13.

D. NOTES

Practice makes perfect, or at least you will see pronounced improvement in your later carvings. Therefore, do not discard your first ones, but keep them for future comparisons. The most difficult task is to begin for the very first time. We have found from many years of experience, however, that the inexperienced people who follow these or similar directions and proceed step-by-step, often end up with some of the best carvings in the class. Do not be afraid to begin. When you become skillful at carving teeth, it may surprise you that it is possible to carve a tooth from memory alone of the contours, possibly aided only be several important dimensions. Average measurements from 4,572 extracted teeth are given in Table 3-2. Should you draw or carve a tooth to these average dimensions, it might surprise you how normal it looks. You may find the following books helpful in perfecting your carving techniques.

General References

Ash MM Jr. Wheeler's atlas of tooth form. Philadelphia: W.B. Saunders, 1984.

Beaudreau DE. Tooth form and contour. JASPD 1973;3:36–37.

Burch JG. Coronal tooth contours: didactic, clinical and laboratory. 3rd ed. Worthington: James G. Burch, 1980.

Grundler H. The study of tooth shapes: a systematic procedure. Berlin: Buch-und Zeitschriften-Verlag "Die Quintessenz," 1976.

Linek HA. Tooth carving manual. Pasadena, CA: Wood and Jones, Printers, 1948.

Forensic Dentistry

This chapter was contributed by Theodore Berg, Jr., D.D.S.

   I. Dentistry and human identification
  II. Civil litigation (including abuse)
 III. Bite marks
  IV. Mass disasters
   V. Conclusion

OBJECTIVES

This chapter is designed to prepare the reader to perform the following:

- **Cite examples of the importance of dentistry in human identification and crime investigation.**
- **Recognize the role of the dentist in identifying and reporting cases of abuse.**

Forensic dentistry is an investigative aspect of dentistry that analyzes dental evidence for human identification. The forensic dentist plays an important role in our justice system. This field of dentistry is divided into forensic odontology and jurisprudence (the science of law). *Forensic odontologists* study and identify teeth, jaws, prostheses, dental appliances, bite marks, dental injuries, and dental records in the interest of justice.

This chapter provides an overview and introduction to forensic dentistry, while illustrating its elemental dependence on dental anatomy. This textbook is cited as the prime dental anatomy reference in the American Society of Forensic Odontology Manual on this subject.

Forensic dentistry is one of a number of forensic sciences. Other forensic sciences are listed below:

1. **FORENSIC ANTHROPOLOGY** examines and interprets skeletal evidence with methods used by archaeologists and with knowledge of human biological variation. This evidence includes bones, teeth, hair, clothing, artifacts, and scene analysis. The examination considers time of death, aging, sexing, race, body size and weight, individualization, and the cause and manner of death.
2. **FORENSIC PATHOLOGY AND BIOLOGY** utilizes autopsy, tissue study, and review of medical records in the investigation of injury or death as a result of accident, homicide, or suicide. Legal responsibility usually resides with a medical examiner or coroner. The criteria for death is irreversible cerebral function. The forensic pathologist attempts to determine and report on the (a) cause, (b) manner (homicide, suicide, accident, or unknown), and (c) mechanism of death.
3. **CRIMINALISTICS** includes fingerprints, ballistics, tool marks (chisel, hammer, etc.), and scene investigation to identify and analyze physical evidence in order to reconstruct the crime and to connect or eliminate suspects and victims.
4. **TOXICOLOGY** utilizes chemistry, photography, and biology to identify harmful substances within a body. These include medications, poisons, and illegal drugs.
5. **FORENSIC PSYCHIATRY** examines and testifies about the aspects of legal sanity, human motivation, and possible personality profile.
6. **FORENSIC ENGINEERING** uses engineers to investigate incidents such as airplane crashes, auto accidents, and structural collapse.
7. **QUESTIONED DOCUMENTS TECHNICIANS** study and report about printing, typewriting, handwriting, ink, paper, and other features of documents.
8. **GENERAL FORENSICS** involves other specialists who are qualified to analyze specific evidence such as designers, photographers, and technical experts. They might report, for example, in a case of product liability associated with death or injury.

9. **FORENSIC JURISPRUDENCE** involves criminal and civil lawyers using the earlier described specialists, reports, and testimony to pursue their case in our system of justice.

Forensic dentistry as a science is represented in the United States of America by numerous forensic dentistry teams on local levels, including the Odontology Section of the American Academy of Forensic Sciences, the American Board of Forensic Odontology, and the American Society of Forensic Odontology. Each year more dentists become involved as law enforcement becomes increasingly aware of dentistry's potential and reliable contribution.

SECTION I. Dentistry and Human Identification

Dentistry often has much to offer in identification because teeth are the most durable parts of the body and dentitions are as individual as fingerprints. Situations involving decomposition and skeletal remains will yield no recognizable facial features or fingerprints. Postmortem (after death) teeth, jaws, prostheses, and appliances can yield a positive identification, given antemortem (before death) records (Figs. 14-1 and 14-2).

Erroneous suspected identifications are often eliminated. The benefits of this are such that even with the lack of antemortem records, the effort is worthwhile to aid investigators with information from dental aging, sexing, and estimated socioeconomic grouping derived from restorative materials, attrition patterns, periodontal status, eruption patterns, skeletal features, and serology (Figs. 14-3 and 14-4).

Forensic dental techniques most commonly include collection and preservation of dental and jaw remains, dental radiology, photography, impressions and casts, antemortem and postmortem charting, and the comparison of these records. Features are referred to as Points of Comparison and include (a) the number and identity of teeth, (b) tooth rotation, spacing, and malposition, (c) anomalies, (d) restorations and prostheses or appliances, (e) caries, (f) endodontic treatment, (g) implants and surgical repairs, (h) pathology, (i) bone patterns, and (j) occlusion, erosion, and attrition (Figs. 14-3 and 14-4).

FIGURE 14-1. Deciduous tooth J and permanent tooth 14 were recovered in an air crash involving many adults and several children. The fully erupted position and root completion of tooth 14, the resorbed roots of J (deciduous second molar), and the crypt for tooth 13 (arrow) suggest that this specimen is from a person in the 10–14-year-old age group. The victim was identified by dental records and the radiographs in Figure 14-2. Modeling clay is often useful to position postmortem specimens for radiographic survey.

FIGURE 14-2. The postmortem radiograph of the specimen in Figure 14-1 (at right) shows consistent points of comparison to one of the antemortem radiographs (at left) gathered in the investigation of an air crash and subsequently led to the victim's identification.

FIGURE 14-3. The maxillae and teeth offer many clues to age, origin, and identity, including a missing premolar on each side, erupting third molars, type of restorations, arch form, morphology of incisors, and the occlusal and incisal attrition in an otherwise young-appearing specimen.

FIGURE 14-4. A mandible, teeth, restorations, and orthodontic arch wire offered a high probability for the eventual identification of a victim. Positive identification depends on adequate antemortem records. Postmortem radiographs will define the unique internal configurations of restorations and the status of the third permanent molars.

FIGURE 14-5. Separate, standardized dental charts are carefully completed during examination of both antemortem records and radiographs and postmortem specimens and radiographs.

DNA can be recovered from periodontal and pulpal tissues, and although DNA analysis has become an important tool in the forensic science armamentaria, it too has limitations including, but not limited to, time and cost. Forensic Dentistry techniques retain a valuable place in the scope of forensic sciences.

A well-organized approach results in accurate comparisons and minimizes the chance of error. The examiner should record each feature of the postmortem teeth and jaws and the radiographs on a standardized dental chart (Fig. 14-5). The same is done for antemortem records, radiographs, casts, and pictures on a separate, but identical, chart. Great caution must be exercised with antemortem record interpretation. Records vary widely in quality and completeness. Some dentists mount radiographs as viewed from the front (film bump out) and others prefer mounting them as viewed from the lingual (film bump inward)! Charting tooth identification is not always done in the Universal System (see Chapter 3 for other tooth identification systems such as Palmer and International). The forensic dentist must carefully organize all evidence so that it is analyzed in a systematic manner using consistent and standardized methods.

FIGURE 14-6. Preincident and postincident dental radiographs can be crucial evidence in the investigation and adjudication of fraud and malpractice cases. A radiograph shows marginal overhangs, marginal insufficiency or caries, inadequate endodontic therapy, and apical pathology. In identification cases, these features or even the unique contours of teeth and restorations, as in the second molar, are a "fingerprint" to that individual.

SECTION II. Civil Litigation (Including Abuse)

A person might claim that improper dental care was rendered or that damage was sustained at the hands of another person (Fig. 14-6) or by food contaminated with a foreign body (glass, shell, etc.). Investigators of claimed malpractice and fraud often require examinations, comparisons, and testimony by expert witnesses. This may involve examining a person and studying records and radiographs from prior dentists. All of the techniques and careful comparisons described previously are useful.

Dentists and other health caregivers have a responsibility to report suspected *abuse* of their patients by others. This includes recognition and differentiation of the signs, symptoms, and body areas involved in accidents compared to injuries sustained in child, spousal, assault, and elder abuse. As an example, the author had a young adult male bring his girlfriend in to the dental office for emergency treatment of several broken front teeth and lacerated lips. The woman was silent while the man related an accident as the cause of the injuries. The man insisted on being present during the treatment and was evasive about answering questions. Toward the end of treatment the police were called and the man was arrested. Radiographs, the dental record, and the dentist's testimony were critical since the victim was fearful of future revenge from her abuser. Injuries the dentist might observe include fractured bones and teeth, bruises, lacerations, and bite marks.

SECTION III. Bite Marks

Numerous homicides and attack cases have been solved by bite mark identification, analysis, and comparison (Figs. 14-7 through 14-10). Many bites are severe and leave telltale marks long after an assault. One of several techniques of comparison and analysis is shown here, comparing bite mark tracings to the suspect's or defendant's tooth imprint pattern tracings (Figs. 14-8 and 14-9). Dental casts (Fig. 14-10) and photographs from the suspect are made after obtaining a court-ordered search warrant. These techniques can be useful in solving some child abuse cases in addition to many assaults and homicides.

New technologies are coming to use in bite mark analysis to recover saliva DNA, digitalize photographic images, and preserve the unalterable original image on computers. Details may be highlighted to better see patterns but without physical change to the image. This method has withstood "chain of evidence" requirements. In the past, bite mark analysis had the vulnerability of some subjectivity and the inability to numerically quantify certainties. Today, when DNA can be collected, amplified, and analyzed with the standard accepted mod-

FIGURE 14-7. A bite mark was found on the abdomen of a crime victim. Color and black and white photographs were taken with a reference rule along side the mark. Other investigative techniques include saline swab washing for residual saliva blood-typing and a free-flowing, high-detail silicone impression of both the bite mark and the surrounding area.

FIGURE 14-8. Wax test imprints from casts of a suspect's teeth can be made at various penetration levels (A). A composite overlay tracing of the suspect's 1 mm and 2 mm wax penetrations (B) can be compared to the tracing from another cast of "very similar" teeth and then both compared to a tracing of the bitemark as in Figure 14-9.

FIGURE 14-9. A bite mark tracing of a black and white photograph, taken in direct frontal position to the victim's bite mark and printed in 1:1 scale referenced to a ruler included in the photograph, can be compared to 1:1 scale tracings from test bites and wax penetrations as in Figure 14-8. The mandibular teeth marks are highly consistent with the defendant's tooth marks (Fig. 14-8B) but do not match with the other "suspect" (Fig. 14-8C). (Tracings in these illustrations are not reproduced here in 1:1 scale.)

FIGURE 14-10. Potential occlusal positions with articulated casts of the suspect/defendant might suggest bite pattern potentials and possible orientation of the defendant when a bite was made. Casts can be compared to 1:1 scale photographs and compared to replicas of the bitemark in stone and silicone.

ern methods, it is possible to quantify the numerical probability of the association between the biter and the bite mark injury.

The forensic dentist must first establish the mark as a human bite mark, then identify, if possible, the teeth involved in the mark. Possibilities may involve missing, extruded, hypoerupted, rotated, tilted, chipped, and anomalous teeth. The chapter in this text on anomalies should be reason enough to remain open-minded and diligent when considering bite marks! The dental forensic examiner must also consider the possibility of animal bites, victim self-bites, and marks from foreign objects that might be mistaken for a bite mark. Separate analysis of those markings may be useful to law enforcement agencies by connecting the victim's injuries to a tool or instrument owned by a suspect.

Law enforcement agencies are becoming increasingly aware of potential identifications from the dental profession. In a landmark bite mark case in California, *State vs. Marx*, Dr. G. Vale, a forensic dentist, recognized bite marks on the autopsy photograph of a nose. After alerting investigators, the body was exhumed and studied with the resultant identification and conviction of the murderer based on the victim's nose bite mark and the suspect's dentition! An appeal was made to the Supreme Court on the grounds that the dental techniques were unique, untested, and not scientific. The appeal was denied, making this the first United States bite mark case to withstand the appellate process. Thus, the reliability of this method of identification was legally verified [People (of California) versus Marx, 54 Cal. App. 3rd 100, 126 Cal. Reptr. 350, Dec. 29, 1975.] Since the outcome of the decision in this landmark case, it has been cited 52 times in 19 states, 10 times in State Supreme Courts (Arkansas, Connecticut, Florida, Iowa, Kansas, Mississippi, West Virginia, New York, North Carolina, and South Carolina) and 9 times in State Court of Appeals (Alabama, California, Ohio, Oklahoma, Oregon, Pennsylvania, Texas, Washington, and Wisconsin). It has also been cited before the military justice system and in Federal Court of Appeals (3rd Circuit Court). In addition to these numerous citings, there have been 22 law review articles mentioning this landmark case.

The notorious mass murderer Ted Bundy (executed January 1989) was positively identified as the responsible person by his bite marks found on the buttocks of one of his young female victims. John Wayne Gacy of Chicago, convicted of 33 counts of murder, became a real test of the vital role forensic dentistry plays in the identification of the involved victims. Only five of the human remains found still had soft tissue, making the identification process a challenge. However, 20 of the 33 known victims were identified through their dental records.

SECTION IV. Mass Disasters

Forensic dentists have made many contributions in the identification of bodies involved in air crashes, mass homicides, structural collapses, floods, and similar disasters. The large volume of specimens and records demands a team approach with excellent organization. The coroner's or medical examiner's office commonly develops a mass disaster medical/dental team, with a Center Team Chief. The *dental team* has a chief who both organizes and schedules the team members and provides a consistent communication link with the Center Team Chief and the other teams, including those working in radiology, autopsy, and fingerprints.

The ground search teams are organized with a *site grid chart.* These teams collect bodies and body parts while carefully charting locations. Remains are sent to storage and examination sites with adequate security, lighting, and support equipment for preservation and study.

The *dental team* is best organized into antemortem and postmortem teams of two examiners per team. One person handles the specimen and examines the radiographs while the other person charts findings (Fig. 14-5). The examining pair then reverses roles and checks each other's efforts. Ideally, a third person, usually the Dental Team Chief, reviews the work of the team. Antemortem charting will usually come later as records arrive. Antemortem charting and records must be done separately and stored separately from postmortem evidence during the investigation. An air crash investigation, for example, can result in dozens to hundreds of records and take days to weeks to complete. Long hours of work are involved, as authorities and families seek answers and identifications quickly. There must be organization to avoid errors and oversights from fatigue and to provide the numbers of team members required to complete a project.

In mass disasters and in single human identifications, success at the task goes to the undaunted and determined examiner. Knowledge of dental anatomy as represented in this text is a basic. The examiner refers to texts such as this book for calcification and eruption tables, charting systems, and suggestions for rare or anomalous tooth identifications or relationships. Dental forensic examiners also use close-up photography systems and commonly used equipment, as suggested in the forensic dentistry books referenced at the end of this chapter.

What may seem of no value, or what may actually be overlooked by site searchers who are not dentists or anthropologists, may be the key to an identification (Figs. 14-11 through 14-14). Even a removable partial denture (Fig. 14-11) or a piece of a denture (Fig. 14-12) may be useful and critical. A lay person might not imagine that one or two teeth could be useful, but nothing should be overlooked if possible (Fig. 14-13). An edentulous jaw, which might seem useless at casual glance, may be correlated with a prosthesis or with dental casts and radiographs, and offers unique trabecular bone patterns and, perhaps, impactions, old fracture sites, implanted metals, foreign bodies, and pathologic disorder (Fig. 14-14). Often identifications are established by comparing unique features of restorations that show up on both antemortem and postmortem radiographs.

One particular disaster highlights vividly the unique skills and tremendous value of a forensic dental team in the accurate identification of bodies. Few can ever forget the horror that occurred at 8:30 p.m., 17th July

FIGURE 14-11. A mandible broken in three pieces with several teeth and a removable partial denture was recovered from a crash and burn accident. The survivors directed investigators to the suspected victim's dentist. The dentist provided antemortem records and a working cast for the partial denture that permitted identification.

FIGURE 14-12. The dental stone cast of an upper denture (**A**) was obtained in evidence collection for investigation of an airliner crash. A denture fragment (**B**) recovered from the crash site, with teeth numbers 2, 3, and 4 present, matches the antemortem cast. The impact broke off a distal piece of tooth 2. Unique horizontal grooves in the buccal resin of the denture precisely match those seen in the antemortem cast.

FIGURE 14-13. Although one or two teeth might seem scant evidence for identification, they should be thoroughly examined and radiographed. The labial laminate bonded veneer (arrow) made this specimen especially unique since this was in the early period of such technique. Also useful can be crown, root and pulp shape, tooth positions, other restorations, pin and base buildups, endodontic therapy, posts, and bone trabecular patterns.

FIGURE 14-14. Even an endentulous jaw might provide a big clue to identification with some unique feature such as the dentigerous cyst shown in the maxillary canine region. Each case challenges the investigator to carefully consider all possibilities and to make no premature assumptions.

1996 off East Moriches, New York: the explosion of a 747 airplane, TWA flight 800 bound for Paris, France, with 230 passengers aboard. Within the first 12 hours, a team of 30 dentists, headed by Dr. B. K. Friedman, D.D.S., American Board of Forensic Dentistry, began the painstaking work of identifying the recovered bodies, which were devoid of clothing. Two and a half weeks later, 208 of the 210 recovered bodies and body parts had been positively identified. Identification of 95 was by dental records alone, another 60 by dental records along with medical records (radiographs, MRI's, etc.), medical anomalies, fingerprints, etc.

For the first time ever, all relatives were screened for DNA samples to compare with the more than 400 recovered body parts, enabling the return of each to the families for an appropriate resting place. Nuclear DNA samples were extracted from both bone and dental pulps, which was all that remained after the first week. Mitrocondrial DNA was also extracted from ground tooth structure, but it is only effective in matching females.

One victim was identified by examining DNA on toothbrushes in his home (Columbus Dispatch, Columbus, Ohio, Tuesday April 1, 1997). During toothbrushing, microscopic bits of tissue from the gums and mucosa are scrubbed off. In all, seven people were identified by DNA alone because no other method was available.

Altogether, 61 dentists and 22 auxiliary dental personnel participated in this important forensic project. Thirty-five to 40 of these dentists had worked with Dr. B. K. Friedman as part of his forensic dentistry team for $5^{1}/_{2}$ years. Such dedication and professionalism by these dentists was a great service to the community and the families of the victims.

One month later, Norwegian researchers were able to identify 139 of 141 people who died in a plane crash in Spitsbergen, Norway August 1996 (*Journal of Nature Genetics*, April 1997). They proved that 257 recovered body parts belonged to 141 people. They collected DNA samples from close relatives. When relatives were not available, investigators collected DNA from hairbrushes, dirty laundry, and toothbrushes in the victims homes.

SECTION V. Conclusion

Even if the average dentist does not intend to be involved in forensic dentistry, the probability is that eventually he or she may be contacted regarding questions about quality of care, observed injuries (such as suspected child or spousal abuse), or from law enforcement agencies requesting help. A valuable contribution can be made by understanding the role of dentistry in forensic science, by recognizing dental evidence or a bite mark, and by helping to properly preserve crucial evidence for later analysis.

You will find dental anatomy the foundation or basis for any forensic dentistry investigation. The references offered with this chapter were selected to give the novice a practical and representative introduction to the field and techniques of forensic dentistry.

Acknowledgments

This chapter was contributed by Theodore Berg, Jr., D.D.S., who is Clinical Professor Emeritus, Department of Advanced Prosthodontics, Biomaterials, and Hospital Dentistry at the School of Dentistry, University of California, Los Angeles; Diplomate, American Board of Prosthodontics; member of the American Society of Forensic Odontology and the Forensic Odontology Team of the Los Angeles Coroner's Department, Los Angeles, California.

For the most part, photographs and tracings were made by the author while serving with the Los Angeles County Coroner's Forensic Odontology Team under Dr. G. Vale. The author thanks the staff of the UCLA School of Dentistry's Photography and Illustration Departments for help in preparing the materials for publication.

General References

American Board of Forensic Odontology. Guidelines for bite mark analysis. JADA 1986;(Mar).

American Society of Forensic Odontology's information source via the Internet World Wide Web: http://www.asfo.org.

Bowers CM, Bell GL, eds. Manual of forensic odontology. American Society of Forensic Odontology, 3rd Ed. 1995. This manual can be obtained from: Forensic Science Foundation, PO Box 1669, Colorado Springs, CO 80901–0669.

Harvey W. Dental identification and forensic odontology. London: Henry Kimpton Publishing, 1976.

Lampe H, Roetzcher K. Age determination from adult human teeth. Med Law 1994;13(7–8):623–628.

Luntz L, Luntz P. Handbook for dental identification. Philadelphia: J.B. Lippincott, 1973.

Nuckles DB, Herschaft EE, Whatmough LN. Forensic odontology in solving crimes: dental techniques and bite mark evidence. Gen. Dent. 1994;42(3):210–214.

Rothwell BR. Bitemarks in forensic dentistry: a review of legal, scientific issues. 1995;126(2):223–232.

Sopher M. Forensic dentistry. Springfield, IL: Charles C. Thomas, 1976.

Standish SM, Stimson PG. Symposium on forensic dentistry: legal obligations and methods of identification for the practitioner. Dent Clin North Am 1977;21.

Krogman W. The human skeleton in forensic medicine. Springfield, IL: Charles C. Thomas Publ., 1973.

Cottone, JA, Standish SM. Outline of Forensic Dentistry. Chicago; Year Book Medical Publishers, Inc., 1982.

Journal of California Dental Association: Dec. 1974 (Sognnaes: M. Borman mystery); May 1975 (Vale: SLA shootout); March 1986 (Vale and others: several areas covered, a good short overview); and May 1996: Vol.2(5): 28-66) (seven concise articles with overview introduction on subjects of bite marks, crime investigation, child abuse, photography, computers, and mass disasters).

Guidelines for bite mark analysis by the Am. Board of Forensic Odontology. Journal of Am. Dent. Assoc.: March 1986.

Gill GW, Rhine S., Symposium Ed: Skeletal attribution of race—Methods for forensic anthropology; Manual available from Maxwell Museum of Anthropology at Univ. of New Mexico, Albuquerque, NM, 1990.

Clark DH, Ed. Practical forensic odontology. Wright (Butterworth-Heinman Ltd.), 1992.

Manual of Forensic Odontology. Am. Soc. of Forensic Odontology, Forensic Science Foundation, Colorado Springs, CO, 1975.

Stimson and Mertz, Ed. Forensic Dentistry: a formidable tool for identification. Boca Raton, FL: CRC Press, 1997.

deVilliers CJ et al. Person identification by means of a single unique dental feature. J. Forensic Odontostomatol. 16(1): 17-19; Jun 1998.

Wright FD. Integrating new technologies in bitemark analysis. Am. Soc. Forensic Odontology News. Saratoga Springs, NY: Winter 1999.

Index

Page numbers in *italics* denote figures; those followed by a "t" denote tables.

Appendix

This Appendix includes numerous drawings of permanent and primary teeth which are labeled (with letters) to highlight features of each tooth. Traits represented by each letter are described on the back of each page following the same letter used on the drawings.

The pages in this Appendix are designed to be torn out to facilitate study for Chapters 4 through 9 thus minimizing page turns.

General Class Traits of All Incisors
(Using the maxillary right lateral incisor #7 as an example)

Class Traits

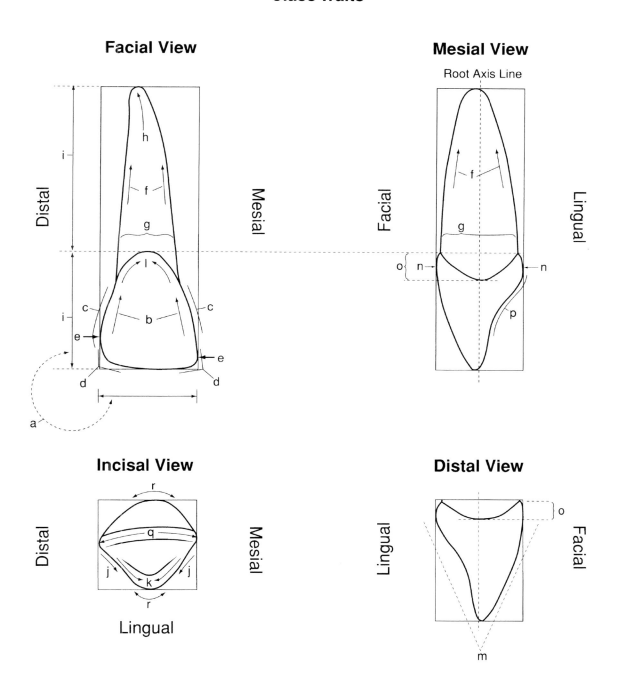

Facial View

Mesial View

Root Axis Line

Incisal View

Distal View

Refer to letters a–r on back which describe these features.

GENERAL CLASS TRAITS OF ALL INCISORS

a. Crown shapes are rectangular; longer incisogingivally than mesiodistally (facial views).

b. Crowns taper from the contact areas to cervical lines (facial views).

c. Crown outlines on the distal are more convex than on the mesial (facial views) EXCEPT on mandibular central incisors, which are known for their symmetry.

d. The mesioincisal angles are more square (or acute) than the distoincisal angles which are more obtuse (facial views) EXCEPT on mandibular central incisors.

e. Mesial contact areas are in the incisal third; distal contact areas are more cervical than the mesial (facial view) EXCEPT on mandibular central incisors where mesial and distal contacts are at same height (facial views).

f. Roots taper from the cervical line toward the apex (facial and proximal views) and from the facial toward the lingual (best seen on an actual tooth or model).

g. Roots are wider faciolingually than mesiodistally (comparing proximal to facial view) EXCEPT maxillary central incisors where dimensions are about equal.

h. When bent, roots often bend to the distal in the apical third (facial views).

i. Roots are slightly-to-considerably longer than crowns (facial and proximal views).

j. Crowns taper from proximal contact areas toward the lingual (incisal views).

k. The mesial and distal marginal ridges converge toward the lingual cingulum (incisal and lingual views).

l. Cervical lines on the facial (and lingual) surfaces are convex (curve) toward the apex (facial and lingual views).

m. Proximal outlines are wedge shaped (proximal views).

n. Facial and lingual crests of curvature are in the cervical third (proximal views).

o. Proximal cervical lines are convex (curve) toward the incisal AND more so on the mesial than on the distal surfaces (compare mesial to distal views).

p. Lingual outlines are "S" shaped with a concave lingual fossa and convex cingulum, and the lingual outlines of the marginal ridges are more vertical than horizontal (proximal views).

q. Incisal edges terminate mesially and distally at the widest portion of the tooth crown (incisal views).

r. Facial outlines are more broadly rounded than lingual outlines due to lingual convergence (incisal views).

Incisors

Refer to letters a–r on back which describe these features.

TYPE TRAITS THAT DISTINGUISH THE MAXILLARY CENTRAL INCISOR FROM THE MAXILLARY LATERAL INCISOR

a. Although the crowns of both types of maxillary incisors have a larger cervicoincisal dimension than mesiodistal, maxillary central incisors are closer to square. Lateral incisors are more oblong cervicoincisally (facial views).

b. On both maxillary incisors, the mesioincisal angles are close to 90°; the distoincisal angles are more rounded (facial views), but both angles are more rounded on the lateral versus central incisor (facial views).

c. Incisal edges slope cervically toward the distal (facial views); more so on lateral incisors (facial views).

d. Maxillary central incisors have crowns and roots closer to the same length. Lateral incisors have proportionately longer roots relative to crowns (facial views).

e. When the incisal edges are aligned horizontally, cingula of maxillary central incisors are off-center to the distal versus cingula of lateral incisors which are centered (incisal views).

f. Mesial marginal ridges are longer than the distal marginal ridges (in central incisors due to the distally displaced cingulum, and in lateral incisors, due to the cervical slope of the incisal edge to the distal) (lingual views).

g. From the incisal view, when the crest of curvature of the cingulum is positioned directly downward, the incisal edge of maxillary central incisors has a slight distolingual twist with the distoincisal corner more lingual than the mesioincisal corner. Lateral incisor ridges run mesiodistally with no twist (incisal and mesial views).

h. Mesiodistal dimensions on central incisors are considerably wider than faciolingual dimensions (rectangular shaped). On lateral incisors these dimensions are more nearly equal (closer to square) (incisal views).

TYPE TRAITS THAT DISTINGUISH THE MANDIBULAR CENTRAL INCISOR FROM THE MANDIBULAR LATERAL INCISOR

Mandibular central incisors are very symmetrical versus lateral incisors which are not. Examples of asymmetry in lateral incisors include the following:

i. Lateral incisors have the distal proximal contacts more apical than the mesial contacts. Central incisor contacts are at the same level (facial views).

j. Lateral incisors have the distoincisal angles more rounded than the mesioincisal angles. On central incisors the mesio- and distoincisal angles are quite similar (facial views).

k. Incisal edges of lateral incisors have a slight distolingual twist (relative to a line bisecting the cingulum). Central incisors have their incisal edges at right angles (with no twist) to this bisecting line (incisal views).

l. The crown of the mandibular lateral incisor tips slightly to the distal relative to the root (facial views).

ARCH TRAITS THAT DISTINGUISH MAXILLARY FROM MANDIBULAR INCISORS

m. Lingual fossae are more pronounced on maxillary incisors (often with a lingual pit, especially on the maxillary lateral incisor). Mandibular incisors have smoother lingual anatomy without grooves and pits (lingual views).

n. Maxillary incisors have roots that are more round in cross-section. Mandibular incisors have roots that are more ribbon like (i.e., are thin mesiodistally and much wider faciolingually). Compare proximal views to facial views.

o. Incisal edges of maxillary incisors are often labial to the root axis line. Mandibular incisal edges are often lingual to the root axis line (proximal views).

p. Mandibular crowns are smaller and narrower mesiodistally relative to the length compared to maxillary incisors which are wider (facial views).

q. Mandibular crowns have outlines mesially and distally that are flatter than on maxillary incisors (facial views).

r (compared to i). Proximal contact points (crests of curvature or heights of contact) are closer to the incisal edge on mandibular incisors (i) than on maxillary incisors (r) (although all incisor proximal contacts are in the incisal third of the crowns) (facial views).

General Class Traits of All Canines
(Using the maxillary right canine #6 as an example)

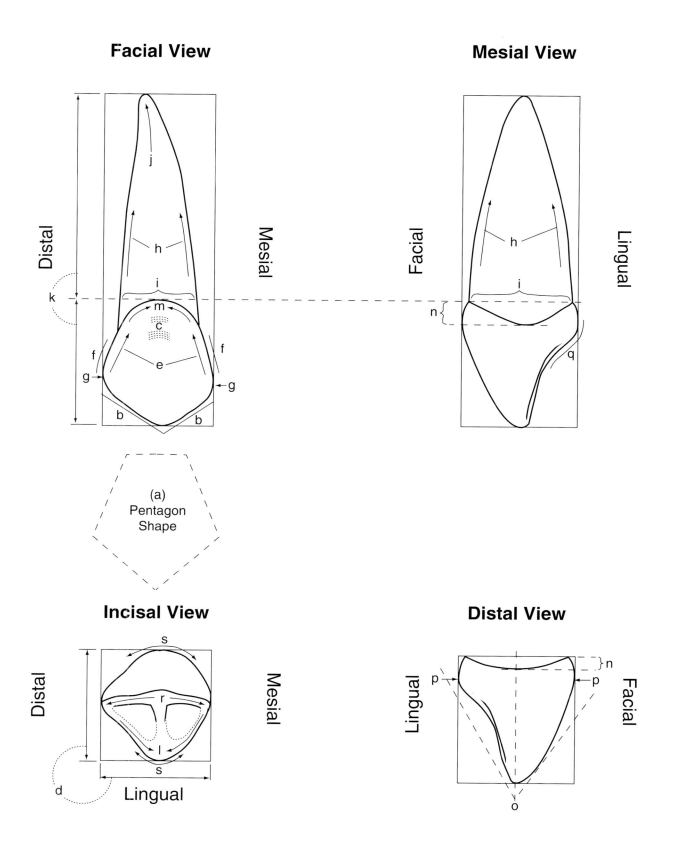

Facial View

Mesial View

Incisal View

Distal View

(a)
Pentagon
Shape

Refer to letters a–s on back which describe these features.

GENERAL CLASS TRAITS OF ALL CANINES

a. Crowns are pentagon shaped (facial views).
b. Cusps have mesial cusp ridges shorter than distal cusp ridges (facial views).
c. Vertical labial ridges are prominent (more so on maxillary canines) (facial views).
d. Crowns are wider faciolingually than mesiodistally (similar to mandibular incisors) (incisal views).

General Canine Characteristics Similar to Incisors

e. Crowns taper from contact areas toward the cervical line ((facial views).
f. Crown outlines are more convex on the distal and less convex (flatter) on the mesial (facial views).
g. Mesial contact areas are located in the incisal third of the crown; distal contact areas are more cervically positioned (facial views).
h. Roots taper from the cervical line toward the apex (facial and proximal views), and from facial toward lingual (which is best viewed on an actual tooth or model).
i. Roots are wider faciolingually than mesiodistally (compare proximal to facial views).
j. If roots are bent, they more often bend toward the distal in the apical third (facial views).
k. Roots are considerably longer than crowns (facial views).
l. Crowns taper from the proximal contacts toward the lingual (incisal views), so the mesial and distal marginal ridges converge toward the cingulum (incisal views).
m. Cervical lines on the facial (and lingual) surfaces curve toward the apex (facial and lingual views).
n. Proximal cervical lines curve toward the incisal, more so on the mesial than on the distal surface (compare proximal views).
o. Canines (like incisors) are wedge-shaped when viewed from the proximal.
p. Facial and lingual crests of curvature are in the cervical third (proximal views).
q. Lingual outlines are "S" shaped with a concave lingual fossa and convex cingulum; the marginal ridges are oriented more vertically than horizontally (proximal views).
r. Incisal edges run toward the mesial to the distal contact areas (incisal views).
s. Facial outlines are more broadly rounded than lingual outlines due to lingual convergence (incisal views).

Canines

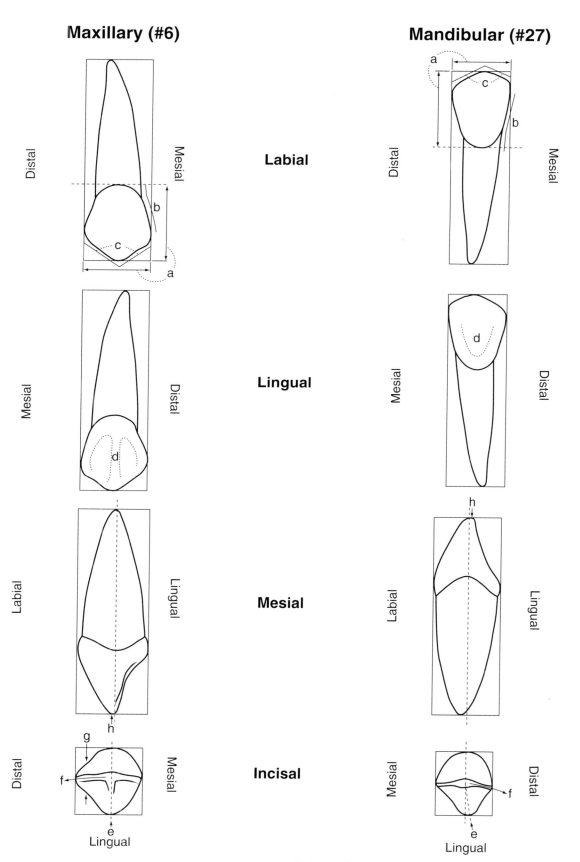

Maxillary (#6)

Mandibular (#27)

Labial

Lingual

Mesial

Incisal

Refer to letters a–h on back which describe these features.

TYPE (AND ARCH) TRAITS THAT DISTINGUISH THE MAXILLARY CANINE FROM THE MANDIBULAR CANINE

a. Both maxillary and mandibular canine crowns are oblong (rectangular) with the mesiodistal dimension less than the incisocervical dimension, but the mesiodistal dimension is narrower on mandibular canines than on maxillary canines (facial views).

b. Maxillary canines have mesial crown contours convex to flat cervically versus mandibular canines which have mesial crown contours more in line with the contour of the root (facial views).

c. The angle formed by the cusp slopes of maxillary canines is more acute (averaging about 105°) resulting in a sharper cusp, compared to the broader (less sharp) angle on the mandibular canine which averages 120° (facial views).

d. Lingual ridges with mesial and distal fossae are more prominent on maxillary canines than on mandibular canines (lingual views).

e. Cingula on maxillary canines are large and centered mesiodistally. On mandibular canines they are often slightly to the distal (incisal views).

f. Incisal ridges on maxillary canines are straighter mesiodistally. On mandibular canines the distal cusp ridge bends distolingually (incisal views).

g. The distal half of the crown of maxillary canines is compressed (squeezed) faciolingually more than on mandibular canines (incisal views).

h. The cusp tip of the maxillary canine is on or labial to the root axis line whereas the mandibular cusp tip is lingual to this line (proximal and incisal views).

General Class Traits of All Premolars
(Using the maxillary right second premolar #4 as an example)

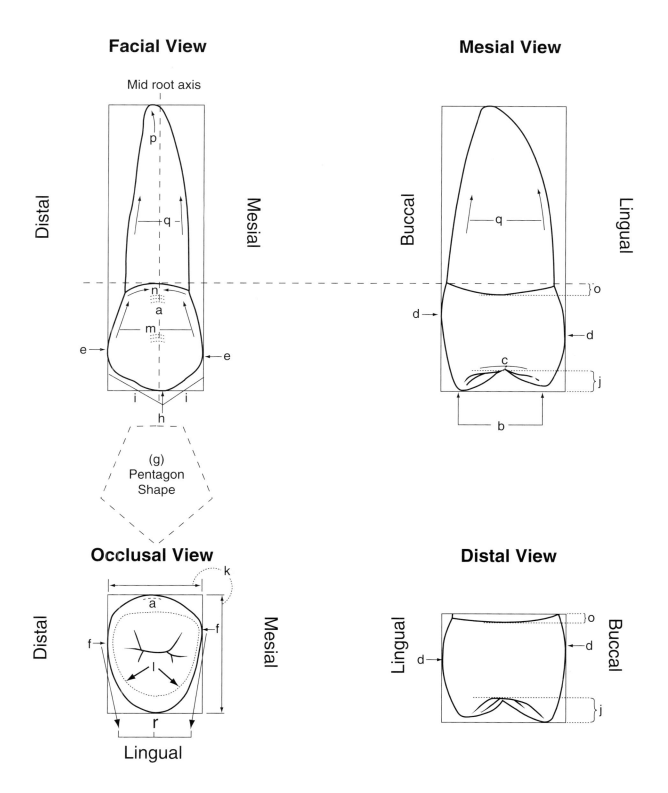

Facial View

Mid root axis

p

q

Distal

Mesial

n

a

m

e → ← e

i   i

h

(g)
Pentagon
Shape

Mesial View

Buccal

q

Lingual

} o

d →

← d

c

} j

b

Occlusal View

k

a

Distal

Mesial

f →

← f

l

r

Lingual

Distal View

Lingual

Buccal

} o

← d

d →

} j

Refer to letters a–r on back which describe these features.

GENERAL CLASS TRAITS OF ALL PREMOLARS

a. Buccal ridges are present (similar to canine labial ridges) (facial and occlusal views).

b. Usually premolars have two cusps: one buccal and one lingual cusp (EXCEPTION is the mandibular second premolar which often has three cusps: one buccal and two lingual) (proximal views).

c. Marginal ridges are aligned relatively horizontally (EXCEPT on mandibular first premolars where the mesial marginal ridge is closer to a 45° angle from horizontal) (proximal views).

d. Buccal and lingual crests of curvature are more occlusal than on anterior teeth (still in cervical third on the facial, but in the middle third on the lingual) (proximal views).

e. Mesial proximal contacts (heights of contour) are near the junction of the occlusal and middle thirds, and the distal contacts are often slightly more cervical in the middle third (EXCEPT on mandibular first premolars where mesial contacts are more cervical than the distal contacts) (facial views).

f. Proximal contacts (crests of curvature) from the occlusal view are buccal to the center faciolingually (occlusal views).

g. From the facial, premolars are roughly pentagon shaped (similar to canines) (facial view).

h. The buccal cusp tip is mesial to the mid-root axis (EXCEPT on the maxillary first premolar where the cusp tip is distal to the mid-root axis) (facial views).

i. The mesial cusp ridge of the buccal cusp is shorter than the distal cusp ridge (EXCEPT on the maxillary first premolar where the mesial cusp ridge is longer) (facial views).

j. Mesial marginal ridges are generally more occlusal than distal marginal ridges which are more cervical (EXCEPT on mandibular first premolars where distal marginal ridges are in a more occlusal position) (compare the proximal views).

k. Crowns are oblong from the occlusal view, wider faciolingually than mesiodistally relative to anterior teeth (maxillary premolars are decidedly oblong or rectangular, whereas mandibular premolars are closer to round or square in shape) (occlusal views).

l. Cusp slopes and marginal ridges form the boundary of the occlusal surface or occlusal table (occlusal views).

m. Crowns taper from proximal contact areas toward the cervical (facial views).

n. Cervical lines curve apically on the facial and lingual surfaces (facial and lingual views).

o. Cervical lines curve occlusally on the proximal surfaces, with the mesial cervical line more convex than the distal (proximal views).

p. The apical third of roots bend distally more than mesially (facial views).

q. Roots taper toward the apex (both proximal and facial views).

r. The crowns taper narrower from the contact areas toward the lingual (occlusal views).

Premolars

Maxillary

Second (#4)   First (#5)

Mandibular

Second (#29)   First (#28)

Buccal

Lingual

Mesial

Occlusal

Lingual
(three cusps)

Lingual

Lingual
(two cusp)

**Refer to letters a–u on back which describes these features
(t is not shown).**

ARCH TRAITS OF PREMOLARS THAT DISTINGUISH MAXILLARY FROM MANDIBULAR PREMOLARS

a. Mandibular premolar crowns tilt to the lingual so mandibular lingual cusp tips may be lingual to the root (proximal views). Maxillary crowns do not tip noticeably.

b. The outline of the mandibular premolars are rhomboid in shape, and the maxillary premolars are trapezoidal (proximal views).

c. (Compared to p). Although lingual cusps are shorter than buccal cusps for all premolars, the mandibular lingual cusps are relatively much shorter than buccal cusps (p) compared to maxillary lingual cusps which are closer to the same length (c) (maxillary second premolar cusps are almost equal in length) (proximal views).

d. Mandibular premolars are more square or round from the occlusal view; maxillary premolars are more rectangular or oblong (relatively wider buccolingually) (occlusal views).

TYPE TRAITS DISTINGUISHING MAXILLARY FIRST FROM MAXILLARY SECOND PREMOLARS

e. Buccal cusps of maxillary first premolars are tipped more to the distal with mesial cusp ridges are longer than distal cusp ridges. (THESE ARE THE ONLY PREMOLARS WITH THIS TRAIT.) (Facial and occlusal views.)

f. Buccal cusps of maxillary first premolars are more pointed (average: 105°) than on second premolars where they are more obtuse (120°) (facial views).

g. Buccal ridges are more prominent on maxillary first premolars (occlusal and facial views).

h. Maxillary first premolars usually have a divided root versus second premolars which usually have one root (proximal views).

i. Maxillary premolars have their lingual cusps tipped (bent) toward the mesial (lingual and occlusal views).

j. Both maxillary premolars have mesial and distal *root* depressions but only the maxillary first premolars exhibit a mesial *crown* concavity (mesial views).

k. Mesial marginal ridge grooves are almost always present on maxillary first premolars and are less common on second premolars (occlusal views).

l. The central developmental grooves on maxillary first premolars are longer (from mesial to distal pit) than those of second premolars where they are only one-third or less of the mesiodistal dimension (occlusal views).

m. Occlusal outlines of maxillary first premolars are more *a*symmetrical with the lingual cusp tip positioned more to the mesial and the buccal cusp tip more to the distal, versus second premolars which are more symmetrical overall (occlusal views).

TYPE TRAITS DISTINGUISHING MANDIBULAR FIRST FROM SECOND PREMOLARS

n. Mandibular first premolar buccal cusps are more pointed (110°) versus on second premolar where they are more obtuse or blunt (130°) (facial views).

o. Mesial proximal contacts (and marginal ridges) of mandibular second premolars are more occlusal than distal contacts (following the general rule), whereas the reverse is true on mandibular first premolars (EXCEPTION) where *mesial* contacts and marginal ridges are more cervical (facial views).

p. Lingual cusps of mandibular first premolars are very small and nonfunctional. On second premolars the lingual cusps function and are relatively longer (proximal views).

q. Lingual cusps of mandibular second premolars are positioned to the mesial (or, if there are two lingual cusps, the mesiolingual is the more prominent) (lingual views).

r. Mandibular first premolars have a mesiolingual groove separating the mesial marginal ridge from the lingual cusp. Second premolars do not (lingual and mesial views).

s. Mesial marginal ridges of first premolars slope cervically toward the lingual at about 45° from horizontal. On second premolars they are more horizontal (mesial views).

t. The mesial root surfaces of mandibular second premolars are the only premolar root surface (maxillary and mandibular, mesial and distal) not likely to have a mid-root depression (best seen on models or actual teeth, not labeled in drawings).

u. Mandibular first premolars are the only premolars that have the mesiolingual corner, with its mesiolingual groove and low marginal ridge, pinched or squeezed in, forming about a 45° angle with the lingual surface. This makes the occlusal outline somewhat diamond shaped (occlusal views).

General Class Traits of All Molars
(Using the second mandibular molar #31 as an example)

Facial View

Mesial View

Occlusal View

Distal View

Refer to letters a – g on back which describe these features.

GENERAL CLASS TRAITS FOR ALL MOLARS

a. Molar crowns are wider mesiodistally than cervico-occlusally (facial views).

b. Crowns taper (get narrower) from the buccal to the lingual, that is, the mesiodistal width on the buccal half is wider than on the lingual half (EXCEPT some maxillary first molars with large distolingual cusps where crowns taper to the buccal and the mesiodistal dimension on the lingual is greater than on the buccal) (occlusal view).

c. Crowns taper (get narrower) from the mesial to the distal (that is, the buccolingual width is less on the distal half than on the mesial half (occlusal view).

d. Crowns taper (get shorter) from mesial to distal (that is, the crown height on the distal half is less than on the mesial half) (facial view).

e. As with premolars, the buccal crests of curvature (heights of contour) of crowns are in the cervical one-third, and the lingual crests of curvature are in the middle third (proximal views).

f. Proximal contacts (heights of contour) on the mesial are at or near the junction of the occlusal and middle thirds; and distal proximal contacts are more cervical: in the middle third near the middle of the tooth (facial views).

g. Lingual cusps on mandibular molars (and mesiolingual cusps on maxillary molars) are longer than buccal cusps when molars are oriented on a vertical axis (facial, mesial and distal views).

Molars

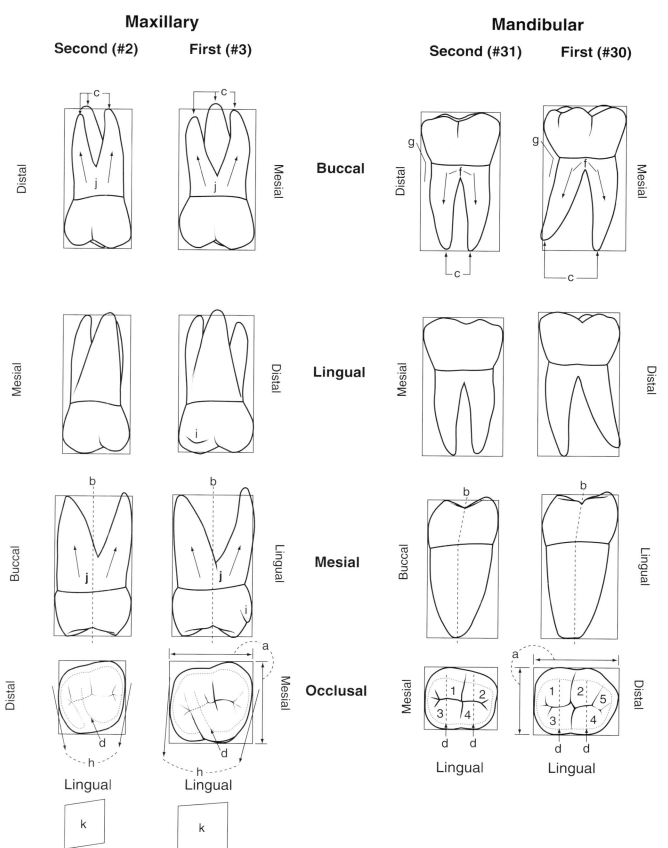

Maxillary

Second (#2)   First (#3)

Mandibular

Second (#31)   First (#30)

Buccal

Lingual

Mesial

Occlusal

Refer to letters a–k on back which describe these features.

ARCH TRAITS THAT DISTINGUISH MAXILLARY FROM MANDIBULAR MOLARS

a. Mandibular crowns are wider mesiodistally than faciolingually resulting in a more rectangular or pentagon outline. Maxillary molar crowns have the faciolingual dimension slightly greater than the mesiodistal dimension, and are more square or rhomboid in outline (k) (occlusal views).

b. Mandibular molar crowns tilt lingually at the cervix (like mandibular premolars), whereas maxillary crowns are aligned directly over the roots (proximal views).

c. Mandibular molars usually have two roots (a larger mesial and a smaller distal root) versus maxillary molars which have three roots (the longest lingual root, the shorter mesiobuccal, and the shortest distobuccal root) (facial or lingual views).

d. Maxillary molars have oblique ridges that run diagonally across the tooth from the mesiolingual to the distobuccal cusp compared to mandibular molars which primarily have two transverse ridges that run directly buccolingually (occlusal views).

TYPE TRAITS THAT DISTINGUISH MANDIBULAR FIRST FROM MANDIBULAR SECOND MOLARS

e. Mandibular second molars have four cusps (mesiobuccal = 1, distobuccal = 2, mesiolingual = 3, and distolingual = 4) with a "cross" pattern of occlusal grooves compared to first molars which have five cusps, the same four cusps as the second molar plus a smaller distal cusp (distal = 5) with a zigzag occlusal groove pattern. (facial or occlusal views; see corresponding numbered cusps, not labeled as "e")

f. First molar roots are more divergent and widely separated compared to second molars roots which are more parallel and closer together (facial and lingual views).

g. There is more taper (narrowing) from the distal proximal contact to the cervical line on first molars than on second molars due to the presence of the distal cusp on first molars (facial views).

TYPE TRAITS THAT DISTINGUISH MAXILLARY FIRST FROM MAXILLARY SECOND MOLARS

h. There is more taper (narrowing) from the buccal to lingual on second molars due to their smaller distolingual cusp, compared to less taper on maxillary first molars with their wider, prominent distolingual cusps (occlusal views).

i. First molars are more likely to have a fifth cusp, the cusp of Carabelli (located on the mesiolingual cusp) compared to second molars which rarely have the cusp of Carabelli (occlusal, lingual, and mesial views).

j. Roots of first molars are more spread apart than on second molars (similar to mandibular molars) (facial and proximal views).

k. The parallelogram outline shape of maxillary molars (with more acute or sharper mesiobuccal and distolingual angles and more obtuse or less sharp distobuccal and mesiolingual angles) is more twisted on second molars than on first molars (that is, acute angles are more acute and obtuse angles are more obtuse on maxillary second molars) (occlusal views).

Primary Anterior Teeth

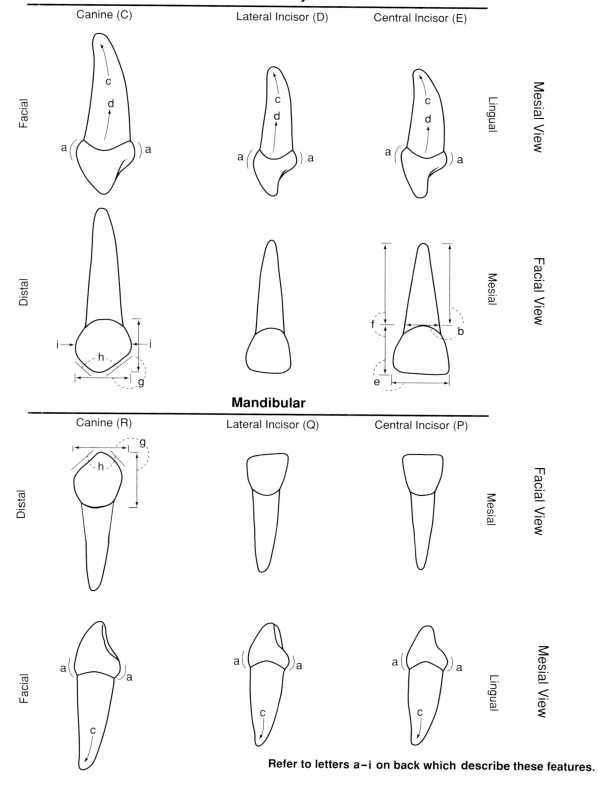

Refer to letters a–i on back which describe these features.

UNIQUE PROPERTIES OF ANTERIOR PRIMARY TEETH

a. Primary anterior tooth crowns have bulges in the cervical third of the labial and lingual surfaces. The lingual bulge is seen as a relatively large cingulum which occupies up to one-third of the cervicoincisal crown length, and the labial bulge is seen as a prominent convex cervical ridge (proximal views).

b. Roots are long in proportion to crown length, and narrower (thinner) mesiodistally than secondary anterior teeth (facial view).

c. Roots of maxillary and mandibular primary anterior teeth bend as much as 10° labially in their apical third, less so in mandibular canines (proximal views).

d. Roots of maxillary incisors bend (bow) lingually in the cervical third to half, whereas the mandibular incisors are straight in their cervical third (proximal views).

e. Primary central incisors are the only incisors, primary or permanent, where the crown is wider mesiodistally than incisocervically (facial views).

f. Primary central incisor crowns are shorter relative to the root length compared to permanent teeth (facial views).

g. Primary maxillary canines are about as wide mesiodistally as they are long incisogingivally. Mandibular canines are longer incisocervically and narrower mesiodistally (facial views).

h. Primary mandibular canines have their distal cusp slopes longer than on the mesial (as do all secondary canines and premolars EXCEPT secondary maxillary first premolars) (facial views). Primary maxillary canines have their mesial cusp slopes longer than the distal cusp slopes (which is UNIQUE to only this tooth and maxillary first premolars).

i. Primary maxillary canines have mesial proximal contacts more cervical than the distal (which is UNIQUE to this tooth and the permanent mandibular first premolar) (facial views). All other primary and permanent teeth have the distal contact area more cervically located than on the mesial.

Primary Molars

Maxillary

First (B)   Second (A)

Mesial View

Buccal   Lingual

e   e

c

Buccal View

Distal   Mesial

g   e
f   e

l   d   a

Occlusal View

First (B)   Second (A)

m
Distal
o
3   1
4   2
n   i
i
Lingual   Lingual   h
Mesial

Mandibular

First (S)   Second (T)   a

Buccal View

Distal   Mesial

d
q
e   f
g   e

c

Mesial View

Buccal   Lingual

e   e

Occlusal View

First (S)   Second (T)

r   j
Mesial   Distal
q   t
s   v
u
Lingual   Lingual

Refer to letters a−v on back which describe these features.

GENERAL CHARACTERISTICS OF ALL PRIMARY MOLARS

a. Primary molars crowns are wider mesiodistally and shorter cervico-occlusally, as on secondary molars (buccal views).
b. Primary first molars are decidedly smaller than primary second molars (compared to permanent or secondary molars where the first molars are larger) (compare all views, not labeled as "b").
c. Primary molar crowns have a narrow chewing surface, or occlusal table, buccolingually compared to the entire tooth width buccolingually (proximal views).
d. Buccal cusps are not sharp; cusp ridges meet at a wide (obtuse) angle (buccal views).
e. Mesial cervical ridges are prominent (proximal views) with cervical lines curved more apically on the mesial half of the buccal surface (buccal views).
f. Root furcations are nearer to the crown with little or no root trunk compared to secondary molars (buccal views).
g. Roots are thin, slender, and widely spread (buccal views).

Additional Characteristics Unique to Primary Maxillary Second Molars (which most closely resemble the permanent [secondary] maxillary first molars)

h. Mesiolingual corner of the occlusal surface is compressed toward the distal (occlusal views).
i. Primary mesiobuccal cusp is about equal in size to the mesiolingual cusp (compared to permanent or secondary teeth where the mesiolingual cusp is larger than the mesiobuccal cusp) (occlusal views).

Additional Characteristics Unique to Primary Mandibular Second Molars (which most closely resemble the permanent [secondary] mandibular first molar)

j. The three buccal cusps are of nearly equal size, versus permanent first molars where the distal cusp is usually considerably smaller. (buccal views).

Additional Characteristics Unique to Primary Maxillary First Molars (which, from the occlusal view, somewhat resemble permanent maxillary premolars)

k. There are often four cusps: two larger cusps (like a maxillary premolar), the mesiobuccal cusp (1) is widest and longest, the mesiolingual cusp (2) is smaller but sharpest; and two smaller cusps, the distobuccal (3) and the inconspicuous, sometimes absent, distolingual (4) (occlusal views; see corresponding numbered cusps).
l. A notch (distal to center) divides the large mesiobuccal cusp from the indistinct distobuccal cusp (buccal views).
m. The crown is wider faciolingually than mesiodistally like a maxillary premolar (occlusal views).
n. The mesial marginal ridge is directed distolingually (occlusal views).
o. There are three fossae: a large mesial triangular fossa, a medium central fossa, and a minute distal fossa (occlusal views).
p. The grooves form an "H" pattern (somewhat similar to a maxillary premolar) (not labeled with a letter; seen on occlusal views).

Additional Unique Characteristics of Primary Mandibular First Molars (resembling no other tooth)

q. The mesial marginal ridge is overdeveloped, almost resembling a cusp (buccal and occlusal views).
r. The occlusal table is wider mesiodistally than buccolingually like secondary (permanent) mandibular molars (occlusal views).
s. The mesial surface converges to the lingual with an acute and prominent mesiobuccal angle of the occlusal table (occlusal views).
t. The mesiobuccal cusp is the largest and longest cusp covering nearly two-thirds of the buccal surface (occlusal views), but is not wide buccolingually (occlusal views).
u. A pronounced transverse ridge runs between the mesiobuccal and mesiolingual cusp (occlusal views).
v. The occlusal table is larger distal to the transverse ridge with a larger distal fossa and a smaller mesial triangular fossa (no central fossa) (occlusal views).